# Abortion
## Understanding Differences

# THE HASTINGS CENTER SERIES IN ETHICS

A Continuation Order Plan is available for this series. A continuation order will bring delivery of each new volume immediately upon publication. Volumes are billed only upon actual shipment. For further information please contact the publisher.

# Abortion
## Understanding Differences

Edited by

## Sidney Callahan

*Mercy College*
*Dobbs Ferry, New York*

and

## Daniel Callahan

*The Hastings Center*
*Institute of Society, Ethics and the Life Sciences*
*Hastings-on-Hudson, New York*

**Plenum Press • New York and London**

Library of Congress Cataloging in Publication Data

Main entry under title:

Abortion: understanding differences.

(The Hastings Center series in ethics)
Includes bibliographical references and index.
1. Abortion—United States—Addresses, essays, lectures. 2. Pro-life movement—
United States—Addresses, essays, lectures.3. Pro-choice movement—United States
—Addresses, essays, lectures. 4. Social values—Addresses, essays, lectures. I. Callahan,
Sidney Cornelia. II. Callahan, Daniel, 1930–      . III. Series.
HQ767.5.U5A28   1984                    363.4'6                         84-9965
ISBN 0-306-41640-9

© 1984 The Hastings Center
Institute of Society, Ethics and the Life Sciences
360 Broadway
Hastings-on-Hudson, New York 10706

Plenum Press is a division of
Plenum Publishing Corporation
233 Spring Street, New York, N.Y. 10013

Printed in the United States of America

# Contributors

**Virginia Abernethy** is Professor of Psychiatry (Anthropology) and Director, Program on Human Behavior, at Vanderbilt Medical School. She received a B.A. from Wellesley and her M.A. and Ph.D. from Harvard. She is the author of *Population Pressure and Cultural Adjustment*, and collected and edited the original papers published as *Frontiers in Medical Ethics: Application in a Medical Setting*. Patient autonomy and allocation of scarce health-care resources are continuing interests.

**Lisa Sowle Cahill** is Professor of Theology at Boston College. She received a Ph.D. from the University of Chicago Divinity School and is Associate Editor of *Religious Studies Review, Journal of Religious Ethics,* and *Horizons*. She is the author of many articles on medical and sexual ethics and is currently working on a book on Christian sexual ethics.

**Daniel Callahan** is Director of The Hastings Center. A philosopher by training, he received his Ph.D. from Harvard and a B.A. from Yale. He is the author of *Abortion: Law, Choice and Morality* and of *The Tyranny of Survival*. He is an elected member of the Institute of Medicine, National Academy of Sciences.

**Sidney Callahan** is Associate Professor of Psychology at Mercy College in Dobbs Ferry, New York. She received a B.A. from Bryn Mawr, an M.A. from Sarah Lawrence, and a Ph.D. from the City University of New York. She is the author of books and articles dealing with women and with the family and values, and she is currently at work on a book on the self.

**Jean Bethke Elshtain** is Professor of Political Science at the University of Massachusetts at Amherst and received a Ph.D. at Brandeis University. She is the author of *Public Man, Private Woman: Women in Social and Political Thought;* and of many articles in scholarly and popular journals. She is the editor of *The Family in Political Thought.*

v

**Sandra Harding** is Associate Professor of Philosophy and Sociology at the University of Delaware. She received a Ph.D. in philosophy from New York University. She has written on issues in the philosophy of science and social science and on feminist theory. *Discovering Reality: Feminist Perspectives on Epistemology, Metaphysics, Methodology and Philosophy of Science* was coedited with Merrill Hintikka and published in March 1983.

**Mary Ann Lamanna** is Associate Professor of Sociology at the University of Nebraska at Omaha. She received a B.A. from Washington University (St. Louis) in political science; an M.A. at the University of North Carolina, Chapel Hill (sociology); and a Ph.D. from the University of Notre Dame (sociology). She is the coauthor of a textbook on the sociology of the family, *Marriages and Families*; and of a monograph on Vietnamese refugees, *Transition to Nowhere: Vietnam Refugees in America.*

**Kristin Luker** is Associate Professor of Sociology at the University of California, San Diego. She is the author of *Taking Chances: Abortion and the Decision Not to Contracept.* The research reported here is part of a larger study funded by the Ford Foundation, the Commonwealth Fund, and Hope Aldrich, and it will be published in 1984 under the title *Abortion and the Politics of Motherhood.*

**Mary B. Mahowald,** who received her Ph.D. in philosophy from Marquette University, is Associate Professor of Medical Ethics at Case Western Reserve University School of Medicine. Her publications include *An Idealistic Pragmatism, Philosophy of Woman,* and articles in American philosophy, ethics and social philosophy.

**Mary Meehan** is a free-lance writer who graduated from Trinity College, Washington, D.C., with a B.A. in history. Her articles have appeared in *America, Commonweal, Human Life Review, Inquiry, Los Angeles Times, New York Times, The Progressive, Washington Post,* and other publications.

**Theodora Ooms,** M.S.W., is Director of the Family Impact Seminar, which moved in 1982 to the Catholic University of America to become the policy unit of the National Center for Family Studies. Prior to her interest in policy, she worked for many years as a social worker and family therapist with children, youth, and their families.

**Mary C. Segers,** Ph.D., Columbia University, is Associate Professor of Political Science and Director of Women's Studies at Rutgers University in Newark, New Jersey. She is coauthor of *Elusive Equality: Liberalism, Affirmative Action, and Social Change in America* and has contributed to *Political Theory, Polity, The Review of Politics,* and the *Hastings Center Report.*

# Acknowledgments

A book of this kind (irenic in purpose) on a topic of this kind (divisive in impact) requires the help of many people. We should first thank the Ford Foundation for support of the project and for the spirit that animated that support: their desire to make a helpful contribution to the national debate. Oscar Harkavy and his colleagues at the foundation were helpful observers along the way. We must next thank some colleagues at the Hastings Center. Joyce Bermel, Managing Editor of the *Hastings Center Report,* worked hard to edit the manuscript and contributed a number of useful ideas along the way. Ellen McAvoy and Eva Mannheimer skillfully turned untidy copy into an orderly manuscript. Finally, we must thank the contributors. They took part in two meetings and wrote at least three draft versions of their papers. We asked them to give a lot and to do a lot—and they cheerfully and enthusiastically complied. As a group, they were a pleasure to work with. We were sorry to see the project end, if only because we found our mutual discussion most fruitful.

SIDNEY CALLAHAN

DANIEL CALLAHAN

# Contents

# Introduction

SIDNEY CALLAHAN AND DANIEL CALLAHAN

This book, like many other things to do with abortion, is a product of long controversy. Though carried out with cooperation, it was conceived in conflict. The conflict between the coeditors has persisted for years—in fact, for at least half of their thirty-year marriage. One, Sidney, is prolife; the other, Daniel, is prochoice. Ever since the topic of abortion became of professional interest to us, in the 1960s, we have disagreed. At one time, while Daniel was writing a book on the subject, *Abortion: Law, Choice and Morality* (1970), we talked about the subject every day for the four years of the book's gestation. On many occasions during the 1970s, prolife articles written by Sidney were passed out at Daniel's lectures in order to refute his prochoice views. Over the years, every argument, every statistic, every historical example cited in the literature has been discussed by the two of us. As Eliza Doolittle says about "words" in *My Fair Lady*, "There's not a one I haven't heard."

And yet we still disagree. How can it be, we ask ourselves, that intelligent people of goodwill who know all the same facts and all the same arguments still come down on different sides of the controversy? As we well know, it is possible to agree about many things and have great love and respect for an opponent, and still differ. Our curiosity, not only about why we differ, but about why others differ as well, was the impulse behind this book. As a psychologist, Sidney had earlier investigated the differing characteristics and views people have about promises and promise keeping. She saw that moral positions on that issue reflect very deep, pervasive premises about the self and the world. In his own work in biomedical ethics in recent years, Daniel has similarly observed that people bring to specific moral issues their broad outlooks toward themselves and the world, and that these can have a profound influence on the way they deal with particular moral questions. Why not, then, look at the problem of abortion from this perspective, considering the differences in people's backgrounds that produce either prolife or prochoice positions?

Since the abortion debate seems to have reached a stalemate, why not back up, shifting the focus of attention to those prior assumptions and deeper values that inform abortion? The Ford Foundation was generous enough to encourage this approach and to support the project.

The purpose of the project out of which these essays developed was to illuminate, enrich, and deepen the dialogue on abortion. We did not aim for any specific practical outcome: We sought no compromises, new solutions, consensus statements, or political recommendations. Instead, our hope was to reach some deeper understanding of why people differ on this issue, and so to pave the way for different, richer discussions in the future. We also hoped to provide some insights into how and why individuals weigh and order their values when dealing with abortion.

The working assumption behind the project was that abortion is particularly troubling because it is so closely linked to broader, more encompassing world views and life commitments. Conflicts over abortion reflect various views about how to live a good life in a good society. We hoped to understand better not only why we differ, but also whether greater understanding could be promoted by examining our differing background values. We asked those writing papers to make explicit their implicit linkages between abortion and the values and views they hold on other fundamental issues. We were looking for a shift in focus from the tip of the iceberg—the public debate on abortion morality and policy—to the submerged underlying mass. Assuming that abortion convictions are part of a broader system of values, how do people situate their abortion positions in relation to their other values and commitments?

Those familiar with the growth of cognitive psychology can recognize here the influence of gestalt psychology. Each perception is organized into a figure emerging from its background. The figure–ground organization can change so that the background becomes the focus of attention and the new figure. In essence, this is what we asked of the participants: to make the background of their views the focus of attention. Another important principle of gestalt psychology is that the whole is greater than the sum of its parts and that the organization of the whole can determine how the parts or the individual elements are used. As we, the editors, could testify, the same elements can be incorporated into very different pictures of abortion. Asking how persons see the larger whole can illuminate how they weigh certain facts and arguments.

Another guiding idea of the project is the concept of "personal knowledge," initially proposed by Michael Polanyi. Personal knowledge is the informal, contextual knowledge that determines how facts and other arguments are evaluated and used. It provides a framework into which other information is fitted and arrayed. We asked the authors to make an attempt to tap their personal knowledge of abortion.

In sum, the project participants were asked to relate their personal understanding to the specific issue of abortion. That was to be the spirit of the project. At the same time, in order to give greater specificity to the discussion, we decided to ask a prolife and a prochoice participant each to focus on a particular aspect of the abortion debate and to engage in dialogue with the critic from the other side. Thus, we selected the four background topics that seem most closely linked to the abortion issue: women and feminism, the role of the family, the child and child rearing, and social and cultural life. Naturally, these areas interrelate in many ways, and the resulting papers inevitably reveal considerable overlap. But we felt from the start that those four topics touch precisely the kind of deep background values that are likely to shape the way people think about abortion; and in this respect, the discussions bore out our initial beliefs.

How was the project organized, and how did we go about picking the participants? Although a good set of papers was the final objective of the project, we also felt it was important to see if those with differing views on abortion could find a profitable and mutually fruitful way of carrying out discussions together. We sought out participants who were willing to talk with those who hold different positions; willing to make the effort to empathize with those who hold opposing views; and willing to take account of the views of others in developing their own more formal positions. We were not looking for still another abortion debate; hence, it was important to find participants who would try hard to engage in a process of mutual exploration rather than adversarial confrontation.

With those general criteria in mind, we first looked for two social scientists who could provide us with the available social-science knowledge about the way people relate their broader values to the abortion issue. Mary Ann Lamanna was asked to examine and analyze the research data from public opinion surveys, and Kristin Luker to make available to us the results of her recent work analyzing the world views of prolife and prochoice activists.

For the remainder of the participants, we sought a group equally divided between prolife and prochoice. Because we wanted a relatively small group for our discussions, we realized that it would not be possible to have all possible religious, cultural, or intellectual backgrounds represented, and we simply hoped to get a fair sprinkling of people from different backgrounds. We also sought participants whose professional work has some bearing on the subject matter. Eventually, we also decided to select an all-female group, with the exception of Daniel Callahan (who was not easily unselected). That was not our original intention, but as we began talking about the project with others and with many of the potential participants, it struck us that a discussion among a predominantly female group might be both fruitful and possibly unique. It is still the case that a good many writings and books on abortion are dominated by male voices. We hope that our own project may correct that balance a bit.

In order to explore the background values that people bring to the abortion issue, we felt it important that all of the project participants give us a fairly good sense of themselves as persons. Hence, at our meetings, we asked them to speak about themselves and the development of their ideas; and we have included an autobiographical statement from each participant. As their backgrounds make clear, most of the group are academics, a disproportionate number come from a Roman Catholic background, and there is some variation in the degree with which they take a prolife or a prochoice position. Indeed, some of the participants felt uncomfortable with these labels. When they are used in this book, they mean more-or-less what is commonly understood: *prolife* is meant to represent the view that abortion ought to be outlawed or severely restricted; *prochoice*, by contrast, represents the position that women ought to be free to make their own decisions on abortion, and that abortion ought to be legally available.

The papers in this book emerged from two lengthy meetings. During the first meeting, early drafts were presented by the authors, and a number of comments and criticisms were provided. The authors were then asked to take into account those comments and to prepare a more polished version for a later meeting. At that later meeting, a further lengthy discussion was held, and in the aftermath, the authors were provided with an opportunity to rewrite yet again. Each author was also assigned a formal commentator from the opposite perspective and was asked to worry about the particular problems raised by that commentator.

The plan of the book follows the general logic of the project. It opens with the two social-science papers, by Mary Ann Lamanna and by Kristin Luker. Dr. Lamanna discerns that, although a plurality of Americans have taken a prochoice position on abortion, most Americans prefer to steer a middle course, and many different factors enter into the way in which they understand the issue. Her paper is very nicely complemented by Kristin Luker's research on the world views of prolife and prochoice activists. Through personal interviews and a comparison of the socioeconomic backgrounds of the two groups, she provides insight into the very different visions that animate the actual workers in the two movements. She avoids any crude theory of determinism, but she does point to the large number of interrelated factors that influence the abortion positions that people take. Whereas Mary Ann Lamanna's paper takes a broad view of the situation, emphasizing the large number of people in the middle, Kristin Luker provides a closeup of those most intensely committed to the abortion cause. With those two social-science papers as background, the remainder of the book is given over to papers on the four major themes mentioned earlier, and to papers by the editors.

The first section is devoted to abortion and the family, with papers by Jean Elshtain and Theodora Ooms. Elshtain begins the section with a statement of the positive values that inspire many prolife advocates, as well as a critique of values that are destructive and dangerous to society. After a discussion of the uses and abuses of language in the abortion debate, Elshtain describes a model of the social compact that is not based on what she takes to be the reigning utilitarian ethic. She describes and advocates what she calls the "modern traditional family," a family that is dedicated to the nurture of others. The paper by Theodora Ooms also emphasizes the importance of the family. Although she holds a prochoice position, she no less strongly argues that the family ought to be factored into the abortion debate and an abortion decision. Although they may differ on many points, both Elshtain and Ooms are trying to conserve values that lead to the familial support of individuals in a stressful world.

The two papers devoted to childbearing and child rearing are much more divergent in the values and the ideology that they represent. A strong prochoice position is taken by Virginia Abernethy, and a very dedicated prolife position is articulated by Mary Meehan. Abernethy analyzes the value of children cross-culturally and throughout the span of history. She believes that the fluctuating value of children is related to many factors in a society or culture, and that it is society that defines the personhood of the child and has the right to do so. She defends the centrality of the concept of personhood in the abortion debate and stresses the need to keep religious values separate from secular policy decisions.

For Mary Meehan, the right to life is fundamental and does not rest on social or cultural definitions. She emphasizes the potentiality of the fetus to become a child and sees the child as a sign of hope for the future. She criticizes the "unwanted-child" concept as one more manifestation of a consumer culture that does not have clear values regarding peace and war or help for the needy. Although Mary Meehan advocates social changes that would help to give each life its dignity, she also believes that some common prolife and pro-choice efforts can be made to better the situation of men, women, and children in our society.

The question of women and abortion is taken up in the next section, with papers by Mary B. Mahowald and Sandra Harding, both philosophers by training. Mahowald gives a deep and penetrating analysis of the various possible positions on abortion, explicating the various implications of each stance. She works toward a model of equality that can give proper weight to the interrelated social realities in which we live. How can one be just to all and properly weigh all the values at stake? She also defends a Marxist-feminist view as a helpful framework for analysis.

Sandra Harding, by contrast, criticizes Marxist and liberal ide-ologies, citing both as being inadequate to effect the kind of change that women need. She advocates a new epistemology founded more on personal experience. Both prochoice and prolife women share many experiences and basic needs that have been ignored in the existing social and political order. Harding holds that, with the rise of feminine consciousness, new insights can be called on to clarify the abortion debate and the full meaning of reproductive freedom. Women can become full members of the species only when they can choose freely.

In the next section, on abortion and the culture, Mary C. Segers continues the quest for a feminist prochoice perspective. She is in-terested in the larger question of what the relation is of law to morality and how, in particular, the women's situation in contem-porary society should be evaluated. She is also interested in whether a specifically feminine moral consciousness comes into play in abor-tion decisions. Once the right of women to make the choice has been granted, she sees the need to explore ways in which the best moral choice can be made. Mary Segers reaffirms her commitment to liberal individualism, but she sees the need for guidance in the individual's free and responsible moral choice.

Lisa Sowle Cahill's prolife paper emphasizes the concept of the common good as a better governing ideal for the society than liberal individualism. As a moral theologian, she thinks abortion is not a religious issue but nonetheless has connections to overall views of the world. An important prior assumption is whether we are going to take the body–mind unity seriously or continue in an age-old dualism that dismisses the body. Cahill sees that taking the body seriously will have implications for the status of pregnancy and for the development of the fetus. She is also interested in what she takes to be the harmful side effects of the prochoice position: Does it make us less capable of dealing with suffering and our common human condition?

Finally, we, the coeditors, have included our own papers in the book. Daniel asks whether progress is possible in the abortion debate and, at the same time, proposes what progress might consist of. He also analyzes the values displayed on both sides of the debate and provides some prescriptions for a more fruitful future discussion. Sidney takes up certain critical issues that she thinks generate differences in abortion positions. Like Daniel, she both analyzes the debate and advocates her particular position. She is interested in discerning those deeper differences that ultimately tip the scale in one direction or another. She examines the issues of sexuality, meaning, suffering, and emotion as they impinge on the debate.

Although we hope that the papers provide provocative reading independently, papers alone never manage to fully capture the flavor of personal discussion and conversation that a project conveys. In this case, the conversations and exchanges were exceedingly rich, and we do hope that the papers catch some of that flavor. Moreover, although it will not be readily obvious to the reader, many of the papers changed significantly between the first and second drafts in response to discussion. All of the authors made a strong effort to be sensitive to the criticisms that they had received, and to try to better understand those who held different positions. Although it is difficult to claim, in a debate as long-standing as that on abortion, that anything absolutely fresh and original had been said, we believe that some new perspectives are aired here more strongly than usual. And what might be called the liberal, feminist prolife position gets more of a hearing.

It is often assumed that those who take a prolife position are automatically political or moral conservatives on most other issues. A number of the papers in this collection should dispel that notion and should perhaps also provide an interesting contrast with the views of prolife activists reported by Kristin Luker. Significantly, many overlapping concerns and commitments are voiced by those on both sides of the abortion argument, and the family as an institution is seen as positive or problematic by those with opposing points of view. Almost all of the papers reject extremely individualistic attitudes and refuse to take an atomistic view of society. Yet, there are also important differences in how decisive the social group should be as arbiter or decision maker. Very different attitudes toward the law and political process are expressed on both sides of the question.

Indeed, some of the papers suggest that people can agree very closely on some of the moral issues and yet disagree fundamentally on how abortion ought to be handled politically and legally.

The participants brought to the project a fine group spirit of mutual sympathy and inquiry. If some of that feeling—dare we call it a feminine nurturing spirit?—is conveyed in the papers, then all our efforts have been well spent.

## CHAPTER 1

# Social Science and Ethical Issues
## The Policy Implications of Poll Data on Abortion

MARY ANN LAMANNA

## AUTOBIOGRAPHICAL STATEMENT

*I have had more of a struggle with abortion than with any other moral or social issue. In fact, I began to write on the abortion issue as a way of clarifying my thoughts after a long period of trying very hard not to think about it at all.*

*My views on abortion are probably affected by my Catholicism. That this is problematic may surprise some people. But the Catholic influence here cannot be taken for granted, as my views on contraception, nonmarital sexuality, homosexuality, divorce and remarriage, women in the priesthood, and even authority are all in disagreement with the orthodox Catholic position, with little trauma on my part. Furthermore, when I was growing up Catholic, the abortion issue was not all that important. One learned that abortion was wrong, but it was an abstract wrong with little emotionality attached.*

*The Catholic influence on my views in this area was more general and more positive. It was not that abortion was wrong, but that babies were right. From Catholic sense of family, I drew a sense of the joy of children and the value of fetal life. The value I ascribed to conception intensified with my fertility problems, my threatened miscarriages, and eventually my pregnancy; my first child was often "at play" prenatally and very responsive to music.*

---

MARY ANN LAMANNA ● Sociology Department, University of Nebraska at Omaha, Nebraska 68182.

*I was, then, opposed to abortion in principle. I was very uneasy when abortion was supported by population experts or planned-parenthood representatives, whom I generally supported, and by colleagues in sociology. As the abortion rights movement developed in the 1960s and the early 1970s, I tried to ignore it, because I found accounts of women seeking abortion threatening to my position. I could put myself in the place of these women and think that I, too, might find no other solution, even though in the abstract I opposed abortion.*

*After a long period of tension, I concluded that the claims of fetal life are limited. The claims of others—the woman, sometimes the family—are strong ones. I came to believe that abortion should be permitted in some cases and that it would be difficult to limit the cases.*

*This change of views was an intellectual rather than a personal development. Having avoided the abortion issue for so long, I decided to plunge into the sociological literature on the subject, in the hope that I might learn something that would help me deal with the issue. In fact, I found myself disagreeing with the prochoice position on many points, including the efficacy of abortion as a solution to various personal and social problems. Nevertheless, I came to believe that there are situations, perhaps many situations, in which the well-being of the already-formed human being takes priority over fetal life, especially early embryonic life. The situation of the pregnant teenager was especially convincing here, because it had the potential of damaging so many young lives. I am sure a personal intensification again, that my daughter's arrival at puberty made this point important in my thinking. Thus, though I think fetal life has value, partly from personal experience, I hold other claims paramount, partly out of concern about the risk that any teenager, such as my daughter, might encounter today.*

Abortion is by all accounts the most difficult public-policy issue in contemporary America. "No end to the dispute over abortion policy can be foreseen"[1] by policy analyst Gilbert Steiner, who sees no "philosophical resolution" to the question of when life begins.

The abortion debate is polarized. It is polarized in argumentation (the familiar "right to life" versus "a woman's right to her own body"). It is polarized in the political process, as prolife and prochoice forces struggle in Congress and on the campaign trail. Public figures are asked to commit themselves to one side or the other, with no middle ground for refuge.

---

[1]Gilbert Y. Steiner, *The Futility of Family Policy* (Washington, D.C.: The Brookings Institution, 1981), p. 53.

Yet, the data on American attitudes toward abortion look very different. In the strict statistics of attitude surveys, I see a *consensus* on abortion on the part of the American public. Numerous polls[2] indicate that a substantial majority, perhaps even three quarters, of Americans favor the legal availability of abortion in at least some circumstances. Does the fact that certain people are asked questions and that their answers are summed and percentaged have anything to do with a moral and ethical issue such as abortion?

As a sociologist carefully brought up in the value-free tradition, I tend to resist the "research shows . . ." ploy often encountered in the abortion debate—as in "the research shows . . . that a conceptus is human life"; "the research shows . . . that unwanted children [whatever that means] have lives not worth living." *Human life* and *worth living* are socially created concepts, judgments of quality and value, not scientific facts. The research never shows us the way. The ethical decision and the just policy are derived from social norms that may take the form of religious principles or humanistic ethical systems.

But what "the research shows" in the realm of community attitudes toward abortion ultimately does provide some direction in policy-making and in moral decisions. Our moral judgments are dependent on the possibilities of our society and the level of moral sensitivity and responsibility present in the culture. Societies have varying capabilities in this regard. The moral sensitivity of individuals is dependent on the cognitive, affective, and evaluative tools provided by their societies. These are reflected in surveys of public opinion on moral issues.

---

[2]ABC News/Washington Post Poll, June 1981; the Roper Center, *Analysis of the ABC News/Washington Post Poll, June 1981* (Storrs, Conn.: University of Connecticut, 1981); Yankelovich, Skelley, and White Poll, 1981 (see editors of *Life*, "Abortion: Women Speak Out, An Exclusive Poll," November 1981, pp. 45–54); G. Gallup, "Seventy-Five Percent Back Abortions but Most Say Only in Certain Circumstances," *The Gallup Poll* news release (Princeton, N.J., 22 January 1978); The Gallup Organization, *U.S. Catholics and the Catholic Press: Summary and Analysis* (Princeton, N.J.: January 1978); Judith Blake and Jorge H. del Pinal, "Predicting Polar Attitudes toward Abortion in the United States," pp. 29–56, in James T. Burtchaell, C.S.C., ed., *Abortion Parley* (Kansas City, Mo.: Andrews and McMeel, 1979), (NORC, Gallup, and National Fertility Survey); Editors of *Better Homes and Gardens, What's Happening to the American Family?* (Des Moines, Iowa: Meredith Corporation, 1978); Stanley K. Henshaw and Greg Martire, "Abortion and the Public Opinion Polls," *Family Planning Perspectives* (March–April 1982), pp. 53–60; Frederick S. Jaffe, Barbara L. Lindheim, and Philip R. Lee, *Abortion Politics: Private Morality and Public Policy* (New York: McGraw-Hill, 1981); William Roy Arney and William H. Trescher, "Trends in Attitudes toward Abortion, 1972–1975," *Family Planning Perspectives* (August 1976), pp. 117–124.

## "THE RESEARCH SHOWS"

Pollsters and social researchers have done a good job on the abortion issue. An enormous amount of attitudinal data is available on the topic of abortion. The data have a basic tripartite pattern that is consistent across researchers and time periods. Almost 20% support the prolife position, defined as forbidding abortion under any circumstances except to save the mother's life. About 25% support prochoice as defined in *Roe* v. *Wade*. About 55% are in between, approving of abortion in some circumstances, but not in others.

Acceptance of abortion varies considerably with the circumstances. For example, in the Yankelovich, Skelley, and White survey, circumstances that compel approval are:

> 92% woman's health at risk;
> 88% woman has been raped;
> 87% woman is carrying a fetus with a severe genetic defect;
> 86% woman is the victim of incest;
> 79% woman is physically handicapped; and
> 72% if the woman is a pregnant unmarried teenager.[3]

Many observers distinguish between "hard," or convincing reasons for abortion and "soft," less compelling reasons. The hard reasons are considered to be a risk to the mother's life, to her physical health, or to her mental health (narrowly defined), the risk of a genetically defective child, and pregnancy due to rape or incest. The soft reasons include being unmarried and/or being a teenager, not being able to support a child, and simply not wanting a child. In general, the public supports abortion for hard reasons and opposes it for soft reasons with the proportions varying with the reasons.[4]

[3]Yankelovich, Skelley, and White Poll, 1981.
[4]The Yankelovich poll surveyed women only. However other surveys of both sexes obtained similar results. For example, the *Redbook* 1979 Gallup Poll (cited in James Tunstead Burtchaell, C.S.C., *Rachel Weeping: And Other Essays on Abortion* [Kansas City, Mo.: Andrews and McMeel, 1982], and adapted to reflect percentages of the total sample) reported approval for legal abortion as follows:

> *Under no circumstances*          18%
> *Under certain circumstances**      54%
>     when woman's life is endangered 46%
>     when woman's physical health is endangered 27%
>     when woman's mental health is endangered 24%
>     chance of deformed baby 28%
>     rape or incest 41%
>     family cannot afford child 8%
>     don't want child 8%
> *Under any circumstances*         25%

*To obtain the total percentage approving each circumstance, of course,

Acceptance of abortion also varies with the trimester of the abortion. Approval for second trimester abortion is approximately 10% less than for first trimester abortion in all three categories of reasons.[5] At present, 91% of abortions do take place in the first trimester.[6]

---

one must add to the percentages in this section of the table the 25% who approved in all circumstances. Of the total sample, 79% approved in at least one circumstance.

With regard to approval or disapproval of the four justifications for legalizing abortion, Blake and del Pinal (1981) reported a 1980 NORC poll in which only 8% disapproved of all justifications, and 7% approved mother's health, 24% approved mother's health and child defect, 6% approved those two plus financial stress, and 40% approved in all circumstances; an additional 37% approved in the circumstances detailed above, for a total percentage of 77% approving in at least one circumstance. The items seem to form a rough scale, with the so-called hard issues followed by unwed status and financial need, then the unspecific desire to terminate pregnancy. Fifteen percent gave inconsistent answers (Blake and del Pinal, 1981).

A bit more detail is offered in answer to a different question in the Yankelovich 1981 poll on whether abortion is morally wrong. The sample viewed abortion as not morally wrong in cases when:

| | |
|---|---|
| Woman has been raped | 80% |
| Woman's health at risk | 80% |
| Woman is incest victim | 78% |
| Genetic defect of child | 75% |
| Physical handicap of mother | 64% |
| Unwed teenager | 48% |
| Welfare mother who can't work | 48% |
| Married woman with large family | 48% |
| Single woman using contraceptives that didn't work | 44% |
| Married woman using contraceptives that didn't work | 44% |

[5] Gallup Poll, 1979, cited in James Tunstead Burtchaell, C.S.C., *Rachel Weeping: And Other Essays on Abortion* (Kansas City, Mo.: Andrews and McMeel, 1982), p. 102:

Approval of Abortion (percentage)

| | First trimester | Second trimester | Third trimester |
|---|---|---|---|
| Woman's life is endangered | 78 | 66 | 59 |
| Woman's physical health is endangered | 52 | 46 | 33 |
| Woman's mental health is endangered | 42 | 31 | 22 |
| Chance baby will be deformed | 45 | 37 | 28 |
| Rape or incest | 59 | 32 | 19 |
| Family cannot afford to have the child | 15 | 6 | 4 |
| No opinion | 9 | 9 | 21 |

[6] U.S. Center for Disease Control, *Abortion Surveillance, Annual Summary*, 1978 (Washington: Government Printing Office, 1980).

Although some variation in wording produces different outcomes (as Judith Blake[7] noted some time ago), most polls have now gone beyond a simplistic single question referring to the magic "a woman and her doctor" and present results in the detailed form summarized above. The pattern of results reported above does not appear to be an artifact of the way the question is worded.

So the poll data are rather clear. Their interpretation is less so.

## CONSENSUS ON ABORTION

I read the abortion poll data as indicating a consensus on abortion. Approximately three quarters of Americans favor access to abortion in at least some circumstances. The consensus extends to most subsections of American society. For example, the Yankelovich *et al.* poll of women over 18 commissioned by *Life* magazine showed that 67% of the total sample believed that abortion should be legal.[8] In no subgroup—the categories were age, religion, race, family income, education, type of place, current marital status, number of children, employment status, political party, political outlook, religiosity, or whether or not the woman had ever had an abortion—was the approval percentage less than 50%, and the only categories with less than 60% approval were women with family incomes less than $10,000 (58%); women from small-town or rural areas (54%); widowed women (59%); and women who attended church more than once a week. (There is undoubtedly some overlap among these categories.) These levels of approval were given in response to a general question, which did not detail the circumstances. (Note also that here we are talking about approval of another's choice or about legal permission for abortion, and not about the morality of one's own behavior.)

Percentages in polls surveying both men and women are slightly lower, but they follow the same general pattern and level of response. Consistently, about 20%–25% of Americans accept abortion under any circumstances, and about 20% reject it under all circumstances. The other 55% accept it under certain circumstances. If we contrast those who condone abortion in at least one circumstance beyond saving the mother's life—that is, those who are not in principle opposed to all abortions—with those who are unequivocally opposed

[7]Judith Blake, "The Abortion Decision: Judicial Review and Public Opinion," in William T. Liu, Edward Manier, and David Solomon, eds., *Abortion: New Directions for Policy Studies* (Notre Dame, Ind.: University of Notre Dame Press, 1977).
[8]Yankelvich, Skelley, and White Poll, 1981.

to abortion, then three fourths or more of the public support legal access to abortion. These percentages have been quite correctly reported as, for example, 83%[9]; 78%[10]; and 77%.[11]

There is a consensus of sorts here. It is not a consensus in support of *Roe* v. *Wade*, that is, of elective abortion (with limited governmental regulation for health reasons in the second trimester and for fetal protection or other policy purposes in the third trimester). Only about 25% support abortion as defined in *Roe* v. *Wade*. When the *Roe* v. *Wade* decision was delivered in 1973, observers correctly noted that this decision did not have public support,[12] and others have pointed this out since.[13]

However, today, the issue is framed differently, as proposed legislation would forbid abortion under *any* circumstances or would allow it only to save the life of the mother. When the issue is put in these terms, there *is* a consensus: Approximately 75% oppose complete delegalization of abortion such as the Human Life Amendment would impose. This consensus extends to virtually all segments of American society; Catholics have percentages only slightly lower than those of the general public.[14]

These data have policy implications and potential political importance. Until recently, however, when the defeat of restrictive abortion legislation in the 1982 Congress undoubtedly reflected lack of support for the prolife position,[15] the consensus I describe had little political impact.

[9]ABC News/Washington Post Poll, June 1981.
[10]1980 Gallup Poll; NORC 1980.
[11]NORC 1980; Blake and del Pinal, 1981.
[12]Judith Blake, "The Supreme Court's Abortion Decisions and Public Opinion in the United States," *Population and Development Review* (March 1977), pp. 45–62.
[13]Burtchaell, *Rachel Weeping*.
[14]Francis X. Murphy, C.S.S.R., *Catholic Perspectives on Population Issues, II.* Population Bulletin 35, no. 6 (Washington: Population Reference Bureau, 1981); Blake and del Pinal ("Predicting Polar Attitudes") did point out that there was more differentiation (less consensus) among subgroups in the population in 1978 than in 1975; "Beginning with 1973, the variance started to decline, and it reached a low in 1975; after that it started to rise, and it has risen steadily ever since. In effect, the country was divided on the extremes of the abortion issue in 1972, it reached more consensus during the mid-1970s (a period of more positive views on abortion), and since 1975 differences among people according to their background characteristics have risen sharply" (p. 15).
   Blake and del Pinal's analysis of relative variance does not refute the claim of extensive support for this position.
[15]Joan Beck, "Abortion Battle Defies Compromise," *Omaha World Herald* (24 August 1982, *Chicago Tribune*); Steven v. Roberts, "Abortion Rights Camp Has Clout," *Omaha World Herald* (22 September 1982, *New York Times* service).

# THE POLITICS OF ABORTION

In particular, the central position, that of conditional access to abortion, has had little political representation. As Blake and del Pinal commented:

> Supreme Court decisions on abortion have been, by and large, victories for those favoring the legalization of voluntary pregnancy termination. Yet these decisions have precipitated the rise of highly organized antiabortion action groups. These groups are ideologically committed to outlawing abortion altogether or to allowing only when the mother's life would be threatened by a continuation of the pregnancy. Their success in impending the implementation of the Court's decision is well known.[16]

Changes in abortion attitudes over time seem related to these events. Approval for abortion increased immediately following the 1973 U.S. Supreme Court decision by about 6%–7% per category.[17] Arney and Trescher commented that, while more than three fourths of respondents approved of abortion for "hard reasons" even before 1973,

> before the Supreme Court decisions, none of the soft reasons obtained approval from as many as half of all respondents; afterward, about one-half of those surveyed approved of abortion for reasons of poverty, and nearly half approved for the other two soft reasons.[18]

Abortion was legitimated by this respected institution, and no strong opposition had been organized. Arney and Trescher also noted that increased approval was especially likely to occur among the less educated. They attributed this fact to toughening economic conditions, as well as to consciousness raising by the women's movement.

But "following the substantial increase in approval for all reasons in 1973, two months after the decisions, approval did not continue to increase between 1973 and 1975."[19] Later studies by Blake and del Pinal,[20] for example, note increasing disapproval of abortion in the late 1970s (1975–1978) Blake and del Pinal also reported that, during the peak of favorable attitudes toward abortion in the mid-1970s, subgroups identified according to religion, education, size of community, race, sex, and age were closer together in their attitudes. The polarization on this issue that had characterized the earlier period, before the U.S. Supreme Court decision, began to reappear in

---

[16]Blake and del Pinal, "Predicting Polar Attitudes."
[17]Arney and Trescher, pp. 117–124.
[18]Ibid., p. 118.
[19]Ibid.
[20]Blake and del Pinal, "Predicting Polar Attitudes."

the late 1970s. In particular, fundamentalist Protestant and Baptist groups, which had become more favorable toward abortion, became less so again, distancing themselves from the highly approving main-stream Protestants. This was the period of increasing right-to-life activity, which brought the issue into sharp focus. At this point, the prochoice movement had not responded to the right-to-life move-ment very effectively. In 1980, the right-to-life movement was rel-atively successful politically.[21] Despite this political impact and the drop in attitudinal support, approval for abortion remains at rather high levels.[22]

One observer has attributed the apparent political support for right-to-life legislation "more to the rising conservative tide than to increased opposition to legal abortion among the American people" and has speculated that "the majority of people who voted for Ronald Reagan do not support such an amendment."[23] The lack of real support for the prolife position became clear in the 1982 elections, and in the failure of the Human Life Amendment in Congress in the fall of 1982.

We are left with the question: What policy might be supported by those who are not dedicated to the prolife position? Here, we need to take a closer look at the center, which did not make itself felt politically during the 1970s.

## Policy in the Center

The center consists of perhaps 50%–55% of those Americans surveyed who support abortion under some circumstances, but not under others. The circumstances vary; particularly, there are sub-stantial differences in support of abortion for hard reasons and for soft reasons. We have been thinking about this group as part of a consensus.

But is this a consensus in support of some policy? It is not, as Burtchaell[24] and others have noted, a consensus in support of *Roe* v.

---

[21]Donald Granberg, "The Abortion Activists," *Family Planning Perspectives 13* (July and August 1981), pp. 157–163. On its earlier impact, see also J. I. Rosoff, "Is Support of Abortion Political Suicide?" *Family Planning Perspectives* (July 1975), pp. 13–22.
[22]Yankelovich, Skelley, and White Polls, 1981; Henshaw and Martire.
[23]Granberg.
[24]Burtchaell, *Rachel Weeping*.

*Wade*. Only 25%, not 75%, support abortion under all circumstances, the way the issue was originally posed in response to *Roe* v. *Wade*.

But the issue has been reframed by the introduction of legislation in Congress to completely outlaw abortion. Now logic sets up a dichotomy of people who favor such laws—the 20% or so in polls who oppose abortion under any circumstances—and those who oppose such laws, the remaining three quarters.

Logic aside, is this how the middle group will really act? As Burtchaell[25] noted, many in the middle are supporters of abortion only for hard reasons—and those are not the reasons that most people are having abortions. Blake and del Pinal[26] noted the demographic and attitudinal similarity of the center conditionals to the negatives; they anticipated that, if those in the center act, it will be to assimilate to a prolife position. Blake and del Pinal anticipated that this "wobbly assent" would wobble off to the right.

That is a possibility and may partially account for the fact that the rather large center has not been the basis for a distinctive policy.

Let us consider the policy implications of the middle, of conditional assent to abortion. A logical extrapolation of the poll data is a policy of regulated access to abortion in which each abortion must be justified by a reason, or "indication." Some reasons would be acceptable, others would not. Theoretically, such a policy should satisfy the center, which would neither support open abortion nor deny all abortions. This was the policy of many states when only "therapeutic" abortions were permitted. The states specified what conditions permitted therapeutic abortion, usually mental health, narrowly or broadly defined. In many European countries, formal approval was or is required for an abortion.[27] The decision model was the presentation of a sufficiently compelling reason; some abortions were refused, particularly repeat abortions. But in the post-Supreme Court–decision era, such a solution to the abortion dilemma—that is, a policy of regulated abortion with indications comprised of various hard or soft reasons—has not been seriously considered. Among other things, it would not be acceptable to the politically powerful polar movements.

[25] Ibid.
[26] Blake and del Pinal, 1981.
[27] Henry P. David, "Eastern Europe: Protonatalist Policies and Private Behavior," *Population Bulletin*, vol. 36, no. 6 (Washington: Population Reference Bureau, 1982); Bogdan Mieczkowski, *Social Services for Women in Eastern Europe* (Charleston, Ill.: Association for the Study of Nationalities, 1982); Murray Gendell, "Sweden Faces Zero Population Growth," *Population Bulletin*, vol. 35, no. 2 (Washington: Population Reference Bureau, 1980).

Regulated access to abortion would not fulfill the goals of either the prolife or the prochoice movements: Saving all fetal life or giving the woman the right to choose. Although the prolife movement would save some fetuses and the prochoice movement would gain some abortions (not over the status quo, but over the situation should the Human Life Amendment pass), neither side would win a substantive or symbolic victory.

Some policy analysts[28] assume that resolution of the abortion issue will come through compromise, not victory for either side. Steiner sees this compromise as not substantive, but political. That is, he envisions no philosophical resolution on the issue of when human life begins, but he believes that the Hyde Amendment restricting funding (a prolife victory) and the failure to pass a Human Life Amendment (a prochoice victory) give us a stable political balance between the two groups. This is not, though, a policy that follows from the values of the center, but a tug-of-war between the two ends.

Aside from political opposition from the small, but strong, polar movements, could a feasible policy be built on the center, which is, after all, a numerical majority? Immediate political problems emerge *within* the majority, for the indicators for abortion are differentially supported. But there are even more serious problems of principle and practice.

## Costs of Allocation

Whatever its political and moral claims, regulated access to abortion poses almost impossible problems of implementation. These include (1) the setting up of a judicial apparatus (Who should decide? What are the criteria?) that will not be contaminated by "vocabularies of motive"[29]; (2) problems of evasion and a sideline industry; (3) considerations of timing,[30] the worry that administrative or judicial process might push many abortions beyond their safe limits[31]; and (4) bureaucratic intrusion of the state.[32]

---

[28]Steiner; Jaffe et al. Luker (this volume) thinks compromise is unlikely because of the extremely different world views of prolife and prochoice activists.

[29]C. Wright Mills, "Situated Actions and Vocabularies of Motive," *American Sociological Review* (May 1940), pp. 904–913.

[30]Gendell.

[31]Marilyn French, "Review of Linda Bird Francke, *The Ambivalence of Abortion,* and James C. Mohr, "Abortion in American" *Conscience* (1982).

[32]Mieczkowski.

A less obvious, but more compelling, objection was raised by
Guido Calabresi and G. Philip Bobbitt in their book *Tragic Choices*.[33]
It is a problem of value conflicts—conflicts, that is, between such a
policy and other important social values. Calabresi and Bobbitt talk
about the allocation of scarce goods in a society. The question of
why goods are scarce and whether this scarcity can be altered is part
of the discussion. But let us assume that society for whatever reasons—here moral—will allocate only so many abortions. A democratic society then has to face the imperfections of allocation systems:

> There are (of course) symbolic and rhetorical purposes prompting the
> demand for laws allowing abortion-on-demand. But few people would
> be willing to support the absolute rule were it not that such a rule
> minimizes the cost of equal access to abortions. Any rule which dis-
> criminates between some situations in which abortion will be allowed
> and some in which it may not gives greater access to the articulate and
> the well-represented; in this way new inequities are introduced by a
> rule intended to avoid (other) unjust results. If inequalities of access
> based on differences in wealth and articulateness are perceived as se-
> rious enough, some, even many, become willing to endorse an absolute
> rule which eliminates those costs, even though it means in some specific
> cases they must live with results which they regard as objectionable in
> terms of other values.[34]

Calabresi and Bobbitt offered a reason for assimilating the middle group to the committed prochoice supporters to produce a consensus in favor of continued permissiveness on abortion. They argued
that if abortion is deemed a legitimate good in some cases, then (as
they analyze the allocation system issues) open access will be the
ultimate result. Too few support the complete elimination of abortion
to make that the solution; this is a key point apparent from the poll
data. And defects in allocation rules will render partial access in-
operable. Given that values other than the sanctity of life are crucial
to our society (equality, for one), and given that various sorts of
market and political allocation systems contravene such values, the
majoritarian preference for regulated access to abortion is unacceptable. We are left with a bipolar choice, and, according to Calabresi and Bobbitt, when faced with a bipolar choice, the majority of
Americans will continue, as they did in the fall of 1982, to favor
retaining open access to abortion.

   If a policy of regulated access to abortion would be unacceptable

---

[33]Guido Calabresi and G. Philip Bobbitt, *Tragic Choices* (New York: Norton, 1978).
[34]Ibid., p. 207, fn. 7.

given certain societal values, the remaining possibility is a coalition between the center and one of the polar positions.

Though some[35] do not agree with me, I, and others,[36] believe that the middle group and the prochoice forces compose a consensus opposed to the delegalization of abortion and that this consensus will dominate the resolution of this issue in the foreseeable future. The percentages will ultimately carry some weight politically, and in fact, they began to do so in 1982.[37]

I speak of the impact of public opinion on this issue, but my analysis is not a simple extrapolation of poll data; it depends on the American value system. Given this distribution of public opinion in combination with certain values, what are the possibilities? The American value system is a far less precise cognition than the percentages of respondents holding a certain view on abortion. Nevertheless, sociologists are ready to deal with values; a classic statement on values in American society is that of Robert Williams.[38]

## EQUALITY AND EFFICIENCY

Calabresi and Bobbitt based their argument on the value of "equality." Persons who might prefer a system of regulated access to abortion will see that one of the costs of an allocation system would be its threat to equality, an important American value.[39]

Williams also talks about the American value of "efficiency." Again, one of the costs of a system of regulated access to abortion would be the likelihood that any administrative or judicial process would not produce a decision in time for an abortion to take place during the first trimester when it is safest. Williams's discussion of efficiency expands into the statement that Americans do not give any single value priority over others; rather, they rationally weigh a variety of values and try to give each its due.[40] Consequently, it seems

---

[35]Blake and del Pinal, 1981; Burtchaell, *Rachel Weeping*.
[36]Jaffe et al.; Calabresi and Bobbitt.
[37]Beck; Roberts.
[38]Robin M. Williams, *American Society* (New York: Knopf, 1951). Readers interested in human values *per se* might want to consult the work of Rokeatch (Milton Rokeatch, *The Nature of Human Values*, New York: Free Press, 1973), who presents research on the values of some American samples. His focus is more on personal values than on societal values and is less applicable to my point.
[39]Williams.
[40]Ibid.

unlikely that any large segment of the population will commit itself to "single-issue politics."[41]

## INDIVIDUAL RIGHTS

Individualism and pluralism are other American values that seem more compatible with the prochoice than with the prolife position. Williams discussed the value that Americans place on "individual personality." The value of "democracy" includes a concern with formal civil rights. The "right-to-privacy" rubric for the *Roe* v. *Wade* decision combines the reluctance to "invade individual integrity," which Williams associates with the value of individual personality, and the notion of inalienable rights that arises from "democracy."[42] That strong individualistic ethic in American society not only provided the basis for the *Roe* v. *Wade* (1973) and *Doe* v. *Bolton* (1973) decisions, and the decision in *Danforth* v. *Planned Parenthood* of *Central Missouri* (1976), but also shapes the abortion problem as one of rights in conflict. Many papers in this volume attack both prolife and prochoice positions as being similar in their dependence on an individualistic perspective. These papers view an advocacy of the individual rights of the woman or the fetus as neglectful of the valid interests of the entire community, of other family members, and of other individuals who might legitimately be included in the abortion decision.[43] Such individualism also discounts community responsibility toward the woman, women in general, and born and unborn children. Instead, values of equity or equality in resource distribution are asserted.[44] The implication is that, if adverse conditions are removed and scarce resources are allocated, the woman can bear the child and abortion will not be a forced choice.

This consideration of community and the social fabric is inherently appealing to me as a sociologist. Sociology emerged in the nineteenth century as a critique of social contract theory and laissez-

---

[41]A typical statement illustrating this point is that of Father Theodore Hesburgh, President of the University of Notre Dame: "Our stand is clear; we are against abortion [but] we have witnessed the fact that political candidates who agree 95 percent with Catholic principles of social justice in most issues of public policy have been defeated by their opposition on this one issue and have been replaced by candidates who, agreeing superficially on this issue of abortion, disagree with us on almost every other issue bearing on justice and equality." (Hesburg, 1979, pp. vii–viii.)

[42]Williams.

[43]Elshtain, Chapter 3; Ooms, Chapter 4; Mahowald, Chapter 7; Cahill, Chapter 10 (this volume).

[44]Elshtain, Mahowald, and Cahill (this volume).

faire individualism.[45] Such early sociologists as Émile Durkheim (1893) had as their central concern the maintenance of social bonds in the new industrial order. Despite the revolutionary rhetoric of individualism and individual rights, Durkheim saw that new institutions and individual rights could flourish only in a setting in which social bonds and community norms supported the new individual freedom. Durkheim and other nineteenth-century social scientists, philosophers, and political theorists "discovered" this social level of analysis. The conference papers are very appealing in their extension of the abortion issue beyond individual rights to the social level of analysis— considering, for example, the involvement of other persons besides the potential mother and child in the abortion decision, and considering the community's responsibility to provide for its members.

Another challenge to an individualistic ethic comes from Carol Gilligan's recent work on the psychology of women and moral perspectives on abortion.[46] Gilligan asserted the sexual ethnocentricism of an individual rights perspective. She pointed out that women have been roundly criticized by therapists,[47] feminists,[48] and psychological researchers[49,50] for their propensity to sacrifice themselves to others' needs and expectations; to be dependent on others; and to give priority to attachment rather than to individual development and self-assertion. Gilligan asserted the validity of a typically feminine "morality of attachment" as against a not-quite-so-evolved "morality of rights."

Although the prolife and prochoice positions can both be seen as individualistic, I divide things a little differently.[51] Calabresi and Bobbitt entitled their book *Tragic Choices*, and in this realm, prolife and prochoice part company. Prolife opts for the sacrifical choice,

[45]Robert Nisbet, *The Sociological Tradition* (New York: Basic Books, 1966); Émile Durkheim, *De la Division du Trávail Social*. Paris: Alcan, 1893.

[46]Carol Gilligan, *In a Different Voice: Psychological Theory and Women's Development* (Cambridge: Harvard University Press, 1982).

[47]Inge K. Broverman, D. M. Broverman, F. E. Clarkson, P. S. Rosencrantz, and S. R. Vogel, "Sex-Role Stereotypes and Clinical Judgments of Mental Health," *Journal of Consulting Psychology* 34 (1970), pp. 1–7.

[48]Colette Dowling, *The Cinderella Complex: Women's Hidden Fear of Independence* (New York: Pocket Books, 1981).

[49]Matina S. Horner, "Femininity and Successful Achievement: A Basic Inconsistency," in Judith M. Bardwick et al., eds., *Feminine Personality and Conflict* (Monterey, Calif.: Brooks/Cole, 1970).

[50]My examples.

[51]It is true that the prolife position is construed in this framework, by bringing in the fetus under the rights umbrella. However, in a confrontation, the rights of the visible adult woman seem likely to prevail; hence, the prochoice position seems more identified with individual rights.

in which the individual woman accepts her pregnancy for the sake of the other: The baby-to-be, the family, the community. Sacrifice is virtuous and has social value; tragedy can be redeemed. This theme, which illuminates several of our papers,[52] reflects a value system which, I think, favors the community over the individual.

I view this approach as utopian—in other words, unworkable—because the real world, our American social world, is constructed on an individual rights basis. Although certainly our society requires and constitutional law recognizes "compelling state interest," the ethos of our political-legal system, reflecting the philosophical bent of the age in which our country was founded, is strongly individualistic. So is our economic allocation system, and Williams noted the strong value we place on "achievement," which makes our society highly competitive and not very nurturing. In the absence of profound social change, the woman who sacrifices will very likely not be able to claim dependence despite the best efforts of some helpful individuals or voluntaristic groups. A shift to the societal perspective advocated by other papers in this volume implies to me not that the woman's right to choose ought to be constrained by a sense of social responsibility and the inclusion of others in her decision, but that a change in the social system is called for when we see the paucity of choices offered. Because we do have an individualistic system, we need to take this framework into account in making policy. Otherwise we exploit individual women by treating their cases "as if," while not actualizing the "as if."

I also refuse to lose sight of the positive side of individualism, the concern for individual integrity and individual rights. *Roe v. Wade* and related decisions were certainly individual rights decisions. They considered the rights of two categories of persons or entities and the rights of others and came down in favor of one of the primary parties. But the essays in this volume move beyond the confrontation of fetal rights and maternal rights. They posit community responsibility and community rights in decision making about abortion. This stand represents a contribution to our thinking on abortion and a possible direction for policy.

However, to resolve the abortion issue in a communitarian rather than an individual rights framework would seem impossible, however appealing the "morality of attachment." It would require a restructuring of our entire society in a socialistic direction; although I might find that desirable, I view it as utopian. I am also uneasy about the corporatism and the coercion that seems inevitable if our application

[52]Cahill and Elshtain, chapters; commentary by Abernethy (this volume).

of community goes beyond providing resources and support to a community determination of the pregnant woman's decision. As one socialized into our culture, I find the value of individual rights powerfully appealing.

## PLURALISM

Pluralism is another distinct feature of the American sociopolitical system. I believe that the resolution of the abortion question will take us in the direction of open access, partly because of our pluralistic values.

Williams referred to our values of "democracy," "freedom," and again "efficiency." Although our democratic system has a strong "moral orientation," he said, it is morality as defined by the individual. Our emphasis on freedom means that Americans tend to think of rights rather than duties and that we prefer control by diffuse cultural structures (ethical systems embodied in individuals or churches) rather than a definite social organization (laws and police enforcement of abortion mores).

Thus, Americans may personally object to abortion and find it morally reprehensible without necessarily endorsing laws against it. Data suggest, in fact, that a posture of moral disapproval and legal permissiveness is not uncommon. In Yankelovich, Skelly, and White's poll of women for *Life* magazine,[53] 56% stated their personal belief that "abortion is morally wrong," and only 35% agreed that "it is not a moral issue." Nevertheless, 67% of the sample agreed that "any women who want an abortion should be able to obtain it legally."[54] More precisely,

> 49 percent of the women who believe abortion is morally wrong nevertheless believe that any woman who wants an abortion should be able to obtain it legally. Thus the belief that abortion is morally wrong does not necessarily lead to the conclusion that women should be prevented by law from obtaining abortions.[55]

When considering the circumstances,

> only 13 percent believe that abortion is morally wrong under all circumstances. . . . Support for legal abortion in these circumstances is widespread, even among those who believe abortion generally should be illegal.[56]

---

[53]Yankelovich, Skelley, and White Poll, 1981.
[54]Editors of *Life*, 1981, p. 47.
[55]Henshaw and Martire, p. 55.
[56]Ibid. (See article for more details on what the circumstances are.)

These views are in keeping with our pluralistic society. We do not have a consensus on abortion as a moral issue. Because pluralistic moral views derive from our cultural pluralism, especially religious pluralism, our society has to

> develop a public policy that will allow us to disagree—even on the bitterly contested question of ending unwanted pregnancy. . . . It is a policy which neither encourages nor discourages abortion. It would protect the right of those morally opposed to abortion by offering adequate maternal and child-welfare services. It would protect the right of physicians, nurses, and ancillary workers with moral or religious objections to refuse to participate in abortion procedures and would exempt Catholic hospitals and those operated by other religious denominations opposed to abortion from participation. It would also ensure the right to obtain abortions of women who, in consultation with their physicians, believe that termination of a pregnancy is necessary for preservation of their health and well-being; and it would protect the right of health-care providers, individual practitioners, and institutions to perform abortions.
>
> . . . Such a public policy . . . is the only kind of policy acceptable in a democratic, pluralistic society that contains many persons and institutions who hold and will continue to hold sharp divergent beliefs on the morality of abortion.[57]

Such reasoning as this—about pluralism, individualism, and equality—leads me to believe that, when forced to make a bipolar choice, the wobbly center will shift toward the prochoice position. We will thus have a consensus supporting the retention of legalized abortion.

## COMMUNITY STANDARDS

A number of my policy conclusions are drawn from the tripartite structure of abortion attitudes presented in the poll data. But who is more worthy of attention in a moral issue, a prophet or a pollster? Why not simply assert and argue the moral rightness of a view on abortion? Is the percentage of public support for a position relevant?

Interestingly, both prolife and prochoice spokespersons point to survey and other social-science data. Prochoice activists claim the support of a substantial majority of Americans for their position. Prolife activists attempt to refute this claim by attacking the data (biased questions) or the interpretation that indicates support for *Roe v. Wade*. Having public opinion on one's side is apparently important enough to argue about.

[57]Jaffe et al., p. 5, p. 196.

Considering the relevance of attitudinal data requires a distinction between moral problems and legal rules. This distinction is readily realized by the Catholic Church, for example, with regard to divorce. Civil divorce is permitted, but the sacramental marriage continues to be recognized.

Poll data as evidence of community standards clearly have *legal* relevance. There is a precedent for tying legal decisions, legislative and judicial, to public opinion. Referenda represent the direct enactment into law of public opinion (that is, the opinion of the voters). Legislation is generally taken to be the will of the people enacted into law by their elected representatives.

As legal scholar Lawrence Friedman noted, however, "what makes the law is not 'public opinion' in the abstract, but public opinion in the sense of *exerted social force* [which] depends on power and intensity."[58] Because of this possible disjuncture between public opinion and "exerted social force," we have a system of checks and balances in which the courts, particularly the U.S. Supreme Court, can overrule legislation. Since legislative bodies can be

> influenced by momentary impulses or overriding emotions . . . an independent body, the Court, should independently scrutinize empirical evidence relating to the operation of a severe penalty so as to insure that the penalty in fact reflects community attitudes of decency and is not merely a reflection of what the public will allow to be placed on the statute books, to be enforced on a non-regular basis.[59]

The implication is that it is important to base laws on community standards of decency and that these cannot always be ascertained from legislation *per se*.

In the *Furman* case, in which the U.S. Supreme Court ruled against the death penalty as then applied, some justices permitted the introduction of attitude surveys as representative of "evolving community standards of decency."[60] In fact, new legislation in this area is required to be tested against "evolving standards of decency."[61]

It seems reasonable, then, and consistent with legal precedent, to use attitude surveys as important sources of information on community standards relating to moral issues.

[58]Lawrence M. Friedman, *Law and Society: An Introduction* (Englewood Cliffs, N.J.: Prentice-Hall, 1977), p. 99.
[59]Welsh S. White, "The Role of Social Sciences in Determining the Constitutionality of Capital Punishment," in Hugo Adam Bedau and Chester M. Pierce, *Capital Punishment in the United States* (New York: AMS Press, 1975), p. 11.
[60]Ibid.
[61]Ibid, p. 4 and fn. citing *Trop* v. *Dulles*, 356 U.S. 86, 101, 1958, Warren, c.j., plurality opinion.

## EMPIRICAL DATA AND MORAL ISSUES

Is there anything wrong with having an ethical choice turn on a social survey? What is the proper role of empirical data in the abortion controversy?[62] Empirical data can help us in ethical decision making in several ways. It can tell us about the effects of a practice such as abortion: What is its social impact? Does it solve problems? Does it cause suffering?[63] Social science data have demonstrated the effects of an existing or proposed policy, for example, the effect of segregation on black children's self-concept[64]; the impact of the death penalty[65]; and the stress caused by fear of nuclear accidents.[66]

---

[62]Though I do not reflect on the role of the sociologist *per se* in the body of the paper, there are a variety of models for the role of the sociologist vis-à-vis "value questions" of ethics, morality and public policy. I shall briefly sketch some:

1. Value-free model—total separation of the sociologist's role (knowledge) from the private citizen-advocate's role (values). The sociologist has no interest in what happens to his or her knowledge, which is generated apart from his or her values.
2. Applied model—sociologist uses his or her technical expertise at the service of a client, who may have certain values or goals.
3. Sociology of knowledge perspective—tells us that knowledge is not value-free, as problems are framed and data are collected in a value framework. Intellectuals strive to be "detached," however, and to attain successively close approximations to an objective truth.
4. Critical theory model—in which the sociologist develops a model of ideal human society and a critique of contemporary society, generated by comparison. This does not tell us precisely how a sociologist should integrate science, law, and ethics around a particular policy issue, but it does provide a basis for the advocacy of particular public policies.

Although none of these models adequately addresses the problem at hand, the critical theory model comes closest. Applied social scientists can also inform legislative or judicial bodies, as clients, of the effects of a policy and community standards.

[63]Mary Ann Lamanna, "Science and Its Uses: The Abortion Debate and Social Science Research," in James T. Burtchaell, C.S.C., *Abortion Parley* (Kansas City, Mo.: Andrews and McMeel, 1979).

[64]Kenneth Clark and Mamie Clark, "Racial Identification and Racial Preference in Negro Children," in T. M. Newcomb and E. L. Hartley, eds., *Readings in Social Psychology* (New York: Holt, 1975), pp. 169–178.

[65]White; Richard G. Gelles and Murray A. Straus, "Family Experience and Public Support of the Death Penalty," in Hugo Adam Bedau and Chester M. Pierce, eds., *Capital Punishment in the United States* (New York: AMS Press, 1975); Charles W. Thomas and Samuel C. Foster, "A Sociological Perspective on Support for Capital Punishment," in Hugo Adam Bedau and Charles M. Pierce, eds., *Capital Punishment in the United States* (New York: AMS Press, 1975).

[66]Ann Marie Cunningham, "Is There a Seismograph for Stress?" *Psychology Today* 16 (October 1982), pp. 46–52.

Social science data can tell us of community consensus or community standards on an issue. It can tell us what groups have what attitudes and how these attitudes change over time. It can tell us something about why people hold the positions they do. Social science data has been used to establish community standards of justice and cruelty vis-à-vis the death penalty. It is partly through changing community standards that we have come to declare child abuse and spouse abuse as unacceptable practices. Social surveys are valid ways of assessing these standards.

But a reliance on community consensus for social policy introduces a relativistic element into public policy. Many public issues are moral issues of a sort we intuitively feel should not depend on majoritarian sentiment. The example of slavery is often cited. The example of the death penalty might be another, as public support for its abolition has dropped off in recent years so that a majority now favors the death penalty. I would find slavery and the death penalty immoral regardless of public opinion, and as a citizen would want public policy to reflect these moral convictions.

We cannot base moral judgments on public opinion. Rather, moral judgments properly emerge from the religioethical value systems to which individuals subscribe. But in the long run, are these not the same? As a sociologist, I am committed to the proposition that religious value systems and their applications in codes of morality are grounded in society.[67] The field of hermeneutics recognizes the culturally shaped forms of religious truth. Since Durkheim, we have recognized the social as well as the spiritual character of religion and morality, the subjective nature of religion and truth.

Furthermore, in a pluralistic society, we do not share absolute moral standards. Here, I believe, we must differentiate personal and group morality from law and public policy. Ultimately, in a pluralistic democracy, the social distribution of moral convictions (public opinion, in other words) will and should affect public policy through the political process in legislative bodies or through judicial judgments influenced by social values. Such is the nature of society.

At a minimum, I assert that ethical formulations and public policy must be grounded in the real world and must come to grips with the real world as reflected in empirical data. Moral positions in any ethical-religious system may, in fact, not be as absolute as we maintain but may change with culturally shaped changes in the interpretation of basic canons. Morality is defined in part within the con-

[67]Émile Durkheim, *The Elementary Forms of Religious Life* (New York: Free Press, 1912, 1965).

text of a particular society at a particular time and in terms of the possibilities of that society. Our discovery of child abuse and neglect in an era when children experience less direct abuse and better material conditions[68] illustrates this point.

The possibilities of the society reside in its deep values, not only in public opinion at a particular time on a particular policy issue. Thus, the argument of this paper depends on my perception of our societal values as well as on poll data. Claims based on values are one route to the correction of morally wrong practices, such as slavery, as the abolitionist movement reminds us.

Coming to grips with value contradictions has in the past produced social change that most of us would view as moral. Gunnar Myrdal long ago (1944)[69] pointed out that many racially discriminatory practices were accepted; our value of "racism" (acknowledged by Williams in 1951)[70] was in conflict with our value of "equality." We resolved this "American dilemma" through the civil rights movement and continued efforts to remove racial discrimination.

Faith (that a society is based on sound moral values that will ultimately assert themselves) as well as reality (that social forces—such as public opinion—will probably determine public policy and law) lead us back to the necessity to take public attitudes into account in policy formation.

## CONCLUSION

The issue of abortion is tied into our basic social structure and values, which appear to call for a resolution in terms of individual rights. The legal system is fixed in this form and seems likely to grind on to produce such an individual rights solution. Much dissatisfaction with this individualistic perspective has been expressed in the other papers in this volume. Much dissatisfaction will likely be expressed with any moral relativism. However, as a sociologist, I do not believe that we can escape the social structural shaping of values. In consequence, I believe that it is incumbent on us to survey the social world and to take it into account in moral and legal decision-making.

With regard to abortion, we have a situation in which few can

---

[68]Lloyd DeMause, "Our Forbears Made Childhood a Nightmare," *Psychology Today* (August 1975), pp. 85–88; Murray A. Straus, Richard J. Gelles, and Suzanne K. Steinmetz, *Behind Closed Doors: Violence in the American Family* (Garden City, N.Y.: 1981).

[69]Gunnar Myrdal, *An American Dilemma* (New York: Harper and Row, 1944).

[70]Williams.

agree on the particular situations in which a woman may abort. But at a higher level of generality, a large majority can agree either that abortion should be forbidden in some circumstances or that it should be permitted in some circumstances. Which way the middle group goes will determine the politically effective consensus. I believe that it will move toward the permissive solution, because that solution is more compatible with some basic American values.

CHAPTER 2

# Abortion and the Meaning of Life

KRISTIN LUKER

## AUTOBIOGRAPHICAL STATEMENT

*As a social scientist who has spent the last seven years probing the whys and wherefores of how people come to feel the way they do about abortions, I am embarrassed to say that I am not entirely sure where my own interest in the topic comes from. I myself have never had an abortion, and my mother underwent lengthy and painful fertility treatments in order to have her three children.*

*Of course, as I am in my late 30s and have lived for many years in California, abortion is very much a part of my life: Almost all my friends have had abortions, a predictable number of my students have abortions every year, and many of those closest to me have faced the abortion dilemma. In addition, because most of my professional life has focused on abortion, people who know of my research interest often feel compelled to tell me about their experiences with abortion, partly because they feel that I will take a professional interest and partly because they have never been able to discuss this intimate event with anyone else. (Although it may be hard for people in their 20s to imagine, until the latter part of the 1960s, abortion was simply not discussed in polite company. I lived through the period when women suddenly felt the opportunity for the first time to speak freely about abortion.) My elderly Berkeley landlady once told me shyly of an abortion she had had in 1926; my best friend's mother told me of going to Mexico during World War II. Thus I, more than most, have come to see what abortion means to women, and to the men who care about them.*

*If I had to choose a single event that triggered my interest in abortion, it would probably be my college roommate's illegal abortion in the early*

KRISTIN LUKER • Department of Sociology, University of California at San Diego, California 92093.

*1960s. As a loyal friend, I accompanied her for her pregnancy test (she, demurely attired with a borrowed wedding ring on her finger, which she twisted nervously throughout). Once the pregnancy was confirmed, her choices seemed stark: Her boyfriend had left her, the shame and stigma of a home for unwed mothers seemed out of the question, and an illegal abortion seemed the only remaining option. Like the activists I studied, my roommate and I were drawing on tacit beliefs about the nature of the embryo, women's roles, and the role of human control over unforeseen events. The abortion was a nightmare, as were so many in that era. She was met on a street corner in Mexico by a taxicab driver, aborted without anesthesia, and unceremoniously dumped, shivering and retching, on still another street corner. This was my introduction to abortion and—when I realized how totally a woman's life can be changed by one microscopic, wayward sperm— my introduction to feminism, although it took me years to make the connection.*

*My personal and professional experiences have convinced me of several inescapable conclusions. First, there is no reason to assume that the answer to the abortion problem is contraception. Americans smoke, drive when they've been drinking, and steadfastly refuse to fasten their seat belts. Why should we expect contraceptive behavior to be of a higher standard, when everyone agrees that correct behavior in these other areas can literally save lives? Unintended pregnancies, like lung cancer and automobile deaths, are a fact of life. The only real policy choice that confronts Americans is whether a significant portion of those pregnancies will be ended legally or illegally. (My conversations with elderly women make it clear that many unintended pregnancies will be ended, no matter what law or social policy says.) Finally, I am convinced that this policy choice cannot be made rationally. Feelings about abortion draw too much on deeply held, tacit values about the meaning of life for people to admit of any compromise.*

Abortion polarizes. Much like abolition, civil rights, and the prohibition of alcohol, abortion is an issue whose advocates see little in the way of nuances. People who care about the issue of abortion care intensely, and the abortion debate is marked by passionate heat and very little light.

This paper argues that the opportunities for a rational resolution of this issue appear to be dim. Drawing on a five-year study of prolife and prochoice activists,[1] I argue that prolife and prochoice people come from very different parts of the social world, have very different sets of resources with which to confront that world, and have visions

---

[1]The full report of this research is contained in Kristin Luker, *Abortion and the Politics of Motherhood* (Berkeley: University of California Press, 1984).

of the world that both ratify and shape their own places in it. For these activists to examine closely their own beliefs about abortion, much less to change those beliefs, would mean calling into question everything in which they believe.

In the course of this research, 212 activists were interviewed on both sides of the issue[2] and were routinely asked about a number of "background variables," sociodemographic characteristics such as where they were born, their education, their income, the number of their children, and their occupation. When these activists were compared with one another (and with their opposite numbers on the other side of the debate), certain broad characteristics of status, style, and values unified those on a given side of the issue and simultaneously differentiated them from their opponents.

As one crude measure, the prolife and the prochoice activists lived in very different financial worlds. Whereas one third of all prolife people made less than $20,000 a year, only one prochoice person in five made that little, and some considerable portion of them were accounted for by young, single women just starting out on a career. Conversely, whereas a little over a third (35%) of prolife people made more than $30,000 a year, over half of the prochoice people made that much. Prochoice income was, in fact, clustered in the upper end of the income scale: Almost one prochoice person in four in this study made $50,000 a year or more.[3]

This discrepancy was in large part due to the different educational and occupational levels attained by the two sides. More than half of the prochoice people had gone on to further education after finishing college: 37% had undertaken some graduate work beyond the B.A., and another 18% had an M.D., a law degree, a Ph.D., or a similar postgraduate degree. Prolife people were by comparison less well educated: 8% of the prolife people in this study had only a high-school degree or less education, and another 22% had not finished college. In comparison, only 2% of the prochoice people were high-school graduates, and only 8% had not finished college.

[2]These activists were those who met the strict criteria of the term *activist*, and who were located in the state of California. Comparative interviews were undertaken in six other states, but those data are not reported here. For details, see "Methodological Appendix" in Luker, *Abortion and the Politics of Motherhood*.

[3]Note that this is *family* income in large part. Prochoice people are more well-to-do than prolife people because, if they are women, they are better educated than their prolife counterparts, are far more likely to work, are more likely to work in well-paid jobs than those few prolife women who do work, and are also more likely to be married to elite professionals. Thus, their family income typically represents the conjoined incomes of two elite professionals, whereas prolife family incomes typically represent the income of one upper-blue-collar or lower-white-collar worker.

Also, 22% of the prolife activists had a college degree, whereas 27% of the prochoice people did. These differences were in large part a product of differences among women activists, and they became even more dramatic when women activists alone were examined (see Table 1).

These educational differences were reflected in occupational differences as well. Because of the past history of the two movements, in which elite professionals predominated, both sides had a roughly equal number of people engaged in the major professions: 14% of the prochoice people were doctors, lawyers, and the like, whereas 13% of the prolife people were. However, even here, the differences among *women* were striking. Most of the pro*choice* doctors, lawyers, and Ph.D.'s were women, whereas most of the pro*life* professionals were men. The occupations of the remaining prolife and prochoice people were also quite different. Of the prochoice people, 20% were executives in large businesses, or managers, as compared to 12% of the prolife people, and 51% were small-business people, or administrators, in contrast to only 34% of the prolife people. Perhaps most dramatically, 31% of the prolife people described themselves as primarily homemakers, in contrast to none of the prochoice people.

These economic and social differences had their counterparts in the choices that the two sides had made with respect to marriage and family life. Although both prolife and prochoice people were almost equally likely to have never been married (19% and 22%, respectively), only 3% of the prolife people had ever been divorced, compared to 10% of the prochoice people. Similarly, 5% of prochoice people described their marital status as "living together," whereas none of the prolife people did so. The prochoice families were also on the whole smaller than the prolife families: The average prochoice

### TABLE 1. Education

|  | All prolife (%) | All prochoice (%) | Female prolife (%) | Female prochoice (%) |
|---|---|---|---|---|
| Less than high school | 2.2 | 0.0 | 1.7 | 0.0 |
| High-school graduate | 6.6 | 2.0 | 8.6 | 2.9 |
| Some college | 22.0 | 8.2 | 29.3 | 8.6 |
| College graduate | 28.6 | 26.5 | 31.0 | 31.4 |
| Graduate/professional | 16.5 | 36.7 | 13.8 | 37.1 |
| M.D., Ph.D., J.D. | 18.7 | 18.4 | 6.0 | 17.1 |
| Technical training | 5.5 | 2.0 | 8.6 | 2.9 |

family had between one and two children (and was more likely to
have one); the prolife families had between two and three and were
more likely to have three. (One prolife woman in five had six or
more children.) The prolife people had also married at a slightly
younger age than did their prochoice counterparts and were likely
to have had their first child earlier.

In terms of religious affiliation, almost 8 of every 10 people
active in the prolife movement in this study were Catholics, but 2
of these 8 were converts. The remainder were Protestants (11%), a
scattering were Jewish (1%), and a few said that they had no religion
(5%). Prochoice people, in contrast, did not consider themselves
religiously affiliated. Over half (55%) said that they had no religion,
22% thought of themselves as vaguely Protestant, 6% were Jewish,
and 8% had what they called a "personal" religion. There were in
this group of prochoice activists none who currently described themselves as being Catholic, although 20% of the prochoice activists in
this study were raised in that religion. These differences in orientation were buttressed by differences in behavior. Prolife people
found their religion vital to their daily lives: half of them attended
church once a week, and 13% attended more often. Only 2% of all
the prolife activists never attended church. Conversely, only 20%
of the prochoice people *ever* attended church, and the overwhelming
majority said that organized religion was not an important part of
their lives.

If we keep in mind the inherent difficulties in the statistical use
of averages, who were the "average" prochoice and prolife advocates?
When the background data of the two sides are considered carefully,
two very different "average" activists emerge. The average prochoice
activist is a 44-year-old married woman who grew up in a large,
metropolitan area. She was married at 22, has one or two children,
and has had some graduate or professional training after the B.A.
Education was a tradition in her family: Her father graduated from
college. This average prochoice activist is married to a professional
man and is herself employed in the paid labor force, and her family
income is more than $50,000 a year. She is not religiously active,
feels that religion is not important to her, and attends church very
rarely, if at all.

The average prolife activist is also a 44-year-old married woman
who grew up in a large, metropolitan area. Unlike her prochoice
counterpart, she married at 17 and has three children (and a substantial minority have six or more children). Her father was a high-
school graduate, and she herself either did not finish college or has
only the B.A. She is not employed in the paid labor force, she is

married to a small-business man or a lower white-collar worker, and her family's income is $30,000 a year. She is Catholic (and may have converted to Catholicism), and her religion is one of the most important aspects of her life: She attends church at least once a week, and occasionally more often.

## INTERESTS AND PASSIONS

To the social scientist (and perhaps to most of us), these social background characteristics connote lifestyles and values as well. We intuitively clothe these bare statistics with assumptions about these activists' beliefs and values. The prochoice women, for example, emerge as educated, affluent, liberal professionals, whose lack of religious affiliation suggests secular, "modern"—or, as prolife people would put it, "utilitarian"—outlooks on life. Similarly, prolife people's income, education, marital patterns, and religious devotion mark them as traditional, hard-working people who hold conservative views on life, "polyester-types" to their opponents.

These assumptions, as I shall show, are in large part true. But their relationship to the abortion issue, and to the world of resources in which these activists find themselves, is more complicated than one might think at first glance. Because prochoice activists live with certain kinds of resources (education, occupation, income, and "status"), it is true that they tend as a group to hold beliefs and values that are consonant with these resources. Highly educated prochoice women, for example, feel that it is important to "get ahead," and their feelings about abortion are intermingled with beliefs that parents should have children only when they can give those children the best educational, emotional, and financial opportunities. Similarly, prolife women, whose economic fate rests not in their own hands but in those of their husbands, and who are, in turn, relatively less well equipped to get ahead, reject in principle the idea that individuals are in control of their own fates. Moreover, this is a dynamic and on-going process. Individuals are constantly reshaping both the world in which they live and their beliefs about that world, and their beliefs about the way the world is organized shape how much of it they see as open to change, as well as determining how active they choose to be in molding it.

Thus, individual attitudes about abortion do not exist in a vacuum. On the contrary, beliefs and attitudes about motherhood; about sexuality; about men and women; about the role of children; and, more broadly, about such global things as morality and the role of rational planning in human affairs—all are intricately related, and all shape an individual's attitudes toward abortion. At issue is an attitude not only about a single issue—abortion—but about an entire view of the world. On almost every relevant dimension of life, prolife and prochoice values are internally coherent, vigorously defended, and mutually antagonistic.

## PROLIFE VIEWS OF THE WORLD

Regarding the proper roles in life for men and women, for example, prolife activists as a group believe that men and women are intrinsically different, and that this difference is both a cause and a product of the fact that they have different roles in life:

> MRS. OSPREY: [Men and women] were created differently and we are meant to complement each other, and when you get away, speaking on a purely natural plane, when you get away from our roles as such, you start obscuring them. That's another part of the confusion that's going on now, people don't know where they stand, they don't know how to act, they don't know where they're coming from, so your psychiatrists' couches are filled with lost souls, with lost people that for a long time now have been gradually led into confusion and don't even know it.

Consequently, prolife activists concur that men and women, as a result of these intrinsic differences, have different roles to play: Men are best suited to the public world of work, whereas women are best suited to rearing children, managing homes, and loving and caring for husbands. Because of this view of the nature of men and women, most prolife activists believe that motherhood—children and families—is the most fulfilling role that women can have. To be sure, they, like the rest of us, live in a world where over half of all women work, and they do acknowledge that some women are employed. But although almost all of them say they believe that women who do work should have equal pay for equal work, this belief does not necessarily translate into a belief that women *should* work. On the contrary, they subscribe quite strongly to the traditional belief that women should be wives and mothers *first*, and that if women *must* work, they should do so only as an adjunct to their primary role. Mothering, in their view, is itself a full-time job, and any woman who cannot commit herself fully to mothering should eschew it entirely. In short, working and mothering are either-or choices; one can do one or the other, but not both:

> MRS. KESSEN: Well, if that's what you've decided in life, I mean I don't feel that there's anything wrong with not being a wife or mother. If

> someone wants a career, that's fine. But if you are a mother, I think you have an important job to do. I think you're responsible for your home, and I think you're responsible for the children you bring into the world, and you're responsible for, as far as you possibly can, to educate and teach them; obviously, you have to teach them what you believe is right. Moral values and responsibilities and rights and I think . . . it's a huge job and you never know how well you're doing until it's too late.

As Mrs. Kessen suggested, because prolife activists see having a family as a demanding (and in particular an *emotionally* demanding), labor-intensive job, they find it hard to imagine that a woman could put 40 hours a week into her job and still have time for her husband and children. Equally important, they feel that different kinds of emotional "sets" are called for in the workplace and in the home place.

Because prolife people see the world as inherently divided both emotionally and socially into two separate spheres, a male sphere and a female sphere, they see the loss of one of those spheres as a very deep loss indeed. If tenderness, morality, caring, emotionality, and self-sacrifice are the exclusive province of women, when women cease to be traditional women, who will provide the caring and the tenderness? Dr. Ulrich made the point that although women may have suffered from the softening influence they provide for men and for the society as a whole, they have much to gain as well:

> I think women's lib is on the wrong track. I think they've got every gripe and they've always been that way. The women have been the superior people, they're more civilized, they're more unselfish by nature, but now they want to compete with men at being selfish. And so there's nobody to give an example, and what happens is that men become *more* selfish. See, the women used to be an example, and they had to take it on the chin for that then, but civilization was due to them, but they also benefited from it because we don't want to go back to the cavemen where you drag the woman around and treat her like nothing. Women were to be protected, respected, and treated like something important.

In this view, everyone loses something when traditional roles are lost. Men lose the nurturing that women offer, and this nurturing is what gently encourages men to give up their potentially destructive and aggressive urges. Women, by extension, lose the protection and the cherishing that men offer. And children lose full-time loving by at least one parent, as well as clear models for their own future. Thus, abortion is offensive to these people not only *per se*, but because it implicitly challenges their visions of maleness and femaleness.

By the same token, these different views about the intrinsic nature of men and women also shape prolife views about sex. The nineteenth century introduced new terms to describe the two faces of sexual activity, distinguishing between *procreative love* and *amative love*. As the names imply, *procreative love* was used to describe sexual activity whose main goal was reproduction, and *amative love* was used to describe sexual activity whose goal was sensual pleasure and mutual enjoyment. Borrowing these two terms permits us to encapsulate the differences between the prochoice and the prolife points of view on sex.

For the prolife people in this study, most of whom were ideologically committed to the idea that women should be wives and mothers first, the relative worth of procreative and amative sex was clear, in part because many of them, being Catholic, accepted some version of a natural law theory of sex that holds that a body part is destined to be used for its physiological function:

> MR. ESTER: You perceive a certain purpose to sexuality. It must be there for some reason. You're not just given arms and legs for no purpose; it's not just an appendage that just floats around. So there must be some cause [for sex] and you begin to think, well, it must be for procreation ultimately, and certainly procreation in addition to fostering a loving relationship with your spouse.

But more important, these views are intimately related to the fact that prolife people have chosen a lifestyle based on traditional roles, and a commitment to amative sex is at odds with a primary commitment to mothering.

Because many prolife people see sex as literally sacred, *and because, for women, procreative sex is a fundamental part of their "career,"* they are disturbed by values that seem to them both to secularize to and profane sex. That whole constellation of values that supports amative sex (sometimes, in modern times, called *recreational sex*) is seen by them as doing just that. Values that define sexuality as a wholesome physical activity, as healthy as volleyball but somewhat more fun, call into question everything that prolife people believe in. Sex is sacred because in their world view it has the capacity to be transcendent—to bring into existence another human life. To routinely eradicate that capacity with premarital sex (where very few people seek the opportunity to bring a new life into existence), contraception, or abortion is, from their point of view, to turn the world upside down.

As might be imagined, given the discussion so far, prolife attitudes about contraception are rooted in these views about the inherent differences between men and women and about the nature and purpose of sexuality. Although the prolife activists in this study often pointed out that the movement is officially neutral on the topic of contraception, their interviews suggested that this statement does not fully capture the complexity of their views and feelings. Virtually all of the activists in this study felt very strongly that the pill and the IUD were abortifacients (that is, that they cause the death of a very young embryo, at least sometimes) and were entirely confident that both the pill and the IUD would be banned by any law that banned abortion. Most of them, furthermore, did not themselves use contraception, basing their nonuse on moral grounds:

> DR. IVY: I think it's quite clear that the IUD is an abortifacient 100% of the time, and the pill is sometimes an abortifacient and it's hard to know just when, so I think we need to treat it as an abortifacient. It's not really that much of an issue with me, even if it weren't. I think there's a respect for germinal life that is in my mind equivalent to a respect for individual life, and if one doesn't respect one's generative capacity, I think one will not respect one's own life or the progeny that one has. So I think there's a spectrum there that begins with oneself and one's generative capacity.

The stance of prolife activists toward other people's use of contraception is therefore ambivalent. They are confident that should a human life law pass, pills and IUDs would no longer be available, so that when they discuss "artificial" contraception, they in fact mean the condom, the diaphragm, and vaginal spermicides. But many of them feel that the answer to the problems of contraception—not only for people with their moral views, but for others as well—is natural family planning (NFP), the modern version of the rhythm method.

When prolife people use natural family planning as a form of fertility control, not only is the underlying moral rationale different from the prochoice side's use of contraception, so is the goal. Although prolife people support "natural" methods that do not "frustrate" the procreative function, they are using these methods to *time* the arrival of children, *not to foreclose entirely the possibility of having them.* Thus, the risk of pregnancy with natural family planning is not only *not* a drawback, but prolife people see it as a positive force that can enhance the marriage:

> MR. APPLE: I'll tell you, when you're using a so-called natural method, if you try to be perceptive you can be incredibly perceptive as to when the fertile period is. But you're not going to be so perceptive that you're going to shut off every pregnancy. You know, there are a lot of things that people are just—in my opinion, add this note—simply do not understand because they've had no experience with it. It's like somebody who eats in restaurants all the time, and they've never been on the farm and had a natural meal—you know, where the food comes

from the freshly killed animals the same day, from the fields. They don't have any concept of what a natural meal is like, and I think the same thing is true in the sexual area. I think that when you begin, when you take the step of cutting off all possibility of conception indefinitely, that it puts emotional and physical restraints on a relationship which divest or remove from it some of its most beautiful values, and it's hard— How do you share that kind of information? The frame of mind in which you know there might be a conception, in the midst of a sex act, is quite different from that in which you know there could not be a conception, and it's the difference between eating this processed prepared food in a restaurant and eating a natural meal on the farm. Now, I don't know how meaningful that comment is, but I don't think that people who are constantly using physical, chemical means of contraception really ever experience the sex act in all of its beauty. That's my opinion.

Ironically, therefore, the one thing it is commonly assumed that everyone wants from a contraceptive—that it be 100% reliable and effective—is precisely what prolife people do *not* want from their method of fertility control.

Prolife values on the issue of abortion—and, by extension, on motherhood—are intimately tied to these preceding values. But they also draw more directly on notions of motherhood (and fatherhood) that are not shared by their prochoice opponents. In part, this might seem obvious; after all, prolife people account for their own activism by referring to the notion that babies are being murdered in their mothers' wombs. But prolife feelings about the nature of parenthood draw on other, more subtle dimensions as well.

Prolife people feel that one becomes a parent by being a parent. Parenthood is for them a "natural" rather than a social role. One is a parent by virtue of having a child, and the kinds of values implied by the in-vogue term *parenting* (as in "parenting classes") are alien to them. By extension, the preparations one makes for parenting are decidedly secondary. The kind of material and educational preparations that prochoice people see as necessary achievements before one can even consider the idea of becoming a parent are seen as a serious distortion of values by prolife people. When life focuses on job achievement, home owning, and money in the bank *before* one has children, then prolife people fear that children will be seen as a barrier. Interestingly, in this context, a number of prolife people made the point that few people actually *enjoy* the state of being pregnant:

MRS. NEHR: You know, which reminds me, I never wanted to have a baby, I never planned to have five children, I never felt the total joy that comes from being pregnant. Oh I was sick, I mean *sick*, for nine months. I mean my general attitude was "Hell, I'm pregnant again."

> But I thought pregnancy was a natural part of marriage, and I believed
> so much in the word *natural*, and so I loved the babies when they were
> born and I realized that a lot of women have abortions in that first
> trimester out of the fear and sense ... it's a physical as well as a psy-
> chological fear that they experience, the depression, whatever, the changes
> that are happening to your body that I mean a lot of them will regret
> having that abortion later on. They work too fast, the doctors advise
> them too fast. They can outgrow that feeling of fear and reaction if
> they give themselves a chance.

Prolife activists are concerned, therefore, that women will seek
abortions before they have had a chance to accommodate themselves
to what they see as the admittedly unpleasant reality of being pregnant.

Prolife values on children, therefore, represent an intersection
of a number of the values already discussed. Because they feel that
the point of sexuality is to have children, they cannot plan the exact
number and timing of children with total confidence. As they cannot
plan the exact number and timing of children, they feel that it is
wrong (and foolish) to make entirely detailed life plans predicated
on exact control of fertility. Given that children will influence one's
life plans more than life plans will influence the number of one's
children, it is also wrong to value those things—primarily money
and what it will buy—over the intangibles that children can bring.
Thus, reasoning backward, prolife people object to every step of
prochoice logic: If one values material things overly much, one will
be tempted to try to plan stringently in order to achieve those material things. If one tries to plan overly stringently, one will be tempted
to use highly effective contraception, which removes all potential of
childbearing from a marriage. Once all potential for children is eliminated, the sexual act is distorted (and for religious people, morally
wrong), and husbands and wives lose an important mutual bond.
Finally, should contraception fail, a husband and wife who have accepted the logic of all of these previous steps are ready and willing
to resort to abortion in order to achieve their goals.

This is not to say that prolife people do not approve of planning.
They do. But because of their world view, their religious faith, and
the concrete circumstances of their lives, they see human planning
as having concrete limits. To them, it is a matter of priorities: If
individuals want fame, money, and worldly success, they have every
right to achieve them. But if they are willing to take a chance on the
roulette wheel of the sexually active, they have an obligation to
subordinate all other parts of life to the responsibilities that such
activity entails.

Prolife values with respect to sex and contraception are also
located in still deeper feelings—strongly felt, but rarely articulated

beliefs about the nature of morality. Prolife people as a group subscribe to explicit and well-articulated moral codes. (After all, many of them are veterans of childhood ethics and religion classes.) Morality for them, therefore, is a straightforward and unambiguous set of rules that specifies what moral behavior is.

Because prolife people believe that these rules originate in a divine plan, they believe that these rules are in principle true and valid across time, across cultural settings, and across individual values. "Thou shalt not kill," they argue, is as true now as it was 2,000 years ago, and the cases to which it applies are still the same. Thus, they tend to locate their morality in traditional, ancient codes (the Ten Commandments, the "Judeo-Christian" law) that have stood the test of time and that exist as external standards against which behavior is measured.

Moreover, a clear-cut moral code leaves little room for nuances in the reasoning of prolife people. Either the embryo is a human life or it is not, but the idea of an intermediate category—a *potential* human life—is one that is incomprehensible to prolife people. Also, the prochoice concept that individuals should personally decide on the moral status of this intermediate category is strange to the average prolife person, given their view of morality. Moral codes dictate, humans obey. The concept of an individually negotiated moral code is simply not a part of their moral repertoire.

This lack of nuances in a strict moral code also has its repercussions in private life: Prolife people, their rhetoric notwithstanding, do have abortions. In the present study, prolife people active in "life centers" volunteered information about the fact that other prolife people had been known to seek abortions. Life centers are organizations staffed and funded by the prolife movement, located in hospitals or other medical settings. They offer free pregnancy tests and pregnancy counseling, should the pregnancy test prove positive, although counselors in life centers, of course, actively encourage women to continue their pregnancies. Because most places that offer free tests and counseling are also abortion referral centers, many women come to life centers in the mistaken belief that they can get a referral for an abortion, and life center counselors estimate that as many as a third of the women they see go on to have an abortion, even after prolife counseling. Because life centers are, by definition, prolife, when employees reveal that prolife people (and in particular, the children of prolife people) have come to these centers seeking abortions, this is persuasive. Prolife people, after all, have something to lose in admitting that their own members (and their own children), like the rest of us, have trouble in always living up to their ideals.

## PROCHOICE VIEWS OF THE WORLD

On almost all of the dimensions just considered, the values and beliefs of prochoice people are very different from those of prolife people. Prochoice men and women live in very different social worlds from those of prolife men and women, and their values reflect that fact. For example, in contrast to the prolife view that men and women are inherently different and therefore have different "natural" roles in life, prochoice people believe that men and women are substantially equal. As a result, they see women's reproductive and family roles not as a "natural" niche, but as a two-sided category: on the one hand, a satisfying option when freely chosen; on the other, a barrier to full equality when coerced. The organization of society, they argue, means that motherhood, as long as it is involuntary, is always potentially a low-status, unrewarding role to which women can be banished at any time. Thus, from their point of view, *control* over reproduction is an essential part of women's being able to live up to their full human potential:

> MS. ELAN: I just feel that one of the main reasons that culturally women have been in a secondary situation is because of the natural way things happen, that women would bear children; they had no way to prevent this, except for, you know, nonsexual involvement. And that was not a practical thing down through the years, so without knowing what to do to prevent it, women would continually have children. And, then, if they were the ones bearing the child, nursing the child, it just made sense that they were the one to rear the child where they would be in that situation. I think that was the natural order. When we advanced and found that we could control our reproduction, we could then choose the size of our families, or if we wanted families. But that changed the whole role of women in our society. Or it opened it up to change the role. To allow us to be more than just the bearer of children and the homemaker. It's not to say that we shouldn't continue in that role, but that it's a good role, but not the *only* role for women.

Although prochoice people agree that women (and men) do find children and families a satisfying part of life, they also believe that it is foolhardy for women to believe that this is the only life role that they will ever have. They argue, in essence, that prolife women who do not work outside of the home, who do not wish to, and who try to limit other women from doing so are just one man away from disaster. A death, a divorce, desertion, or disability can plunge a woman with no career skills or experience perilously close to the edge. Pointing to the ever-increasing numbers of "displaced homemakers"—women who have spent a life in a marriage and find themselves suddenly divorced or widowed, in penury with virtually no financial or employment resources—the prochoice activists argue that the prolife women, who in both their values and their lives put work in the paid labor force secondary, live in a precarious world of wishful thinking.

At the same time, prochoice people value what I have earlier called *amative sex*. Prolife values that hold that sex is important—and indeed sacred—because of its inherent reproductive capacity strike many prochoice people as absurd. From their point of view, if the purpose of sex were reproduction, no rational Creator would have arranged things so that people have literally hundreds of acts of intercourse over their lifetimes and literally thousands (and in the case of men, millions) of sex cells—egg and sperm—at the ready. More to the point, if sex is basically procreational in nature, then it *must be highly socially regulated*, lest a baby be created when none is intended. In particular, *women* must be protected—and, in their viewpoint, repressed—because an otherwise free and uninhibited expression of sexual wishes might land individual women "in trouble" and overpopulate the species. In prochoice values, both the "double standard" and "purdah"—the ancient custom of veiling women and keeping them entirely out of the public eye, lest they be too sexually arousing to men—are the logical outcomes of focusing too intensely on the protection of women's reproductive capacities.

Significantly in this context, many of the prochoice people describe themselves as having grown up in families with very traditional sexual values that they now see as "sex-negative" because they focus on the dangers of sexual feelings let out of control. They see themselves as adults now seeking a set of "sex-positive" values for themselves and for the society as a whole, values that emphasize the pleasure, beauty, and joy of sex rather than its dangers. When prochoice people speak of sex-negative values, they mean that in their families sex was not openly talked about, that it was not portrayed as something to be enjoyed for its own sake, and that budding childish sexuality—masturbation, adolescent flirting—was often treated harshly. Premarital sexuality, especially when pregnancy ensued, was a "fate worse than death."

Such harsh treatment of sex makes sense if there is a presumption that sexuality can lead to genital expression and that pregnancy can (and indeed *should*) result from such genital expression. But for people who plan anyway to have small families, who have no moral opposition to contraceptives, who value rational planning in all realms including pregnancy, and whose other values focus them on the here and now and on other people rather than on the future and God, treating sex as a taboo seems irrelevant at best and potentially damaging at worst.

Prochoice people, therefore, believe that sexual activity is good as an end in itself, and they therefore see sex as primarily amative. The main role of sexuality for them is not the possibility of children— at least, for much of a lifetime—but pleasure, human contact, and, most important perhaps, intimacy.

Despite Mr. Ester's claims earlier, prochoice people *do* believe that sex can be sacred, but it is a different kind of sacredness that they have in mind. For them, sex is sacred when it is mystical, when it dissolves the boundaries between the self and the other, when it brings one closer to one's partner, and when it conveys a sense of the infinite. Transcendent sex for them is rooted in present feeling, rather than in something that may happen in the future.

An important corollary is that, whereas sex for prochoice people has the *capacity* to touch on the sacred, sacredness is a goal to be attained, not an intrinsic part of the situation. That kind of sex can be achieved only when people feel security, trust, and a love for themselves and for their partner. As the spiritual aspect of sex is something to be attained rather than a given (although sometimes, like a state of grace, it just occurs), it follows that prochoice people do not denigrate sexuality that does not achieve this goal. After all, sex is something that needs practice if it calls on such delicate social and emotional resources as trust, caring, and intimacy. As a result, premarital sex, contraception, and infidelity are evaluated by prochoice people according to their ability to enhance or detract from these conditions of trust and caring. In their value scheme, something that enables people to be closer to one another—to create opportunities for intimacy—simply cannot be wrong.

These attitudes about the nature and the meaning of sex also shape prochoic views on contraception. To be sure, contraception *per se* is not a salient issue for most prochoice people. Like vaccines and dental hygiene, it is a necessary, straightforward, and not very controversial part of life. (Indeed, they find prolife objections to contraception mysterious and dismiss them by assuming that such objections are merely medieval—or "religious"—in nature.) Although prochoice people have some pragmatic concerns about contraception—how unpleasant some methods are, how safe other methods may be—they make no moral associations with contraception *per se*. Because their primary moral value in sexuality is amative, focusing on attaining intimacy with the self and the other, then a good (and hence, moral, if one can stretch the term) contraceptive is one that is safe, undistracting, and pleasant to use. Because their moral concerns do focus on intimacy and caring, and because they furthermore *do* use contraception to postpone childbearing for long periods of time, their ideal contraception is easy to use, *highly effective*, and not a risk to their health.

The one moral concern that prochoice people do have about contraception (or, more precisely, birth control) is that many of them feel uncomfortable with the use of abortion as a routine way of controlling fertility, when abortion is used in place of, rather than as a backup for, traditional methods of contraception. In part, such opposition is pragmatic: Repeated abortions have their own set of health risks.

> INTERVIEWER: Who are the "extremists"?
> REV. OWENS: Those people who are happy to use abortion as a means of birth control, who are advocates of using no form of contraception and relying upon abortion. I cannot agree with that position for physical reasons; I believe it's unhealthy.

But physical risks are not the whole story. The interviewer pursued the question with this respondent:

> INTERVIEWER: Do you have some moral concerns about that, too?
> REV. OWENS: Yes, and they're vaguer. Last time at my class in human sexuality, a young woman brought this up, and I was grateful to her because I seldom bring it up myself because it's a spiritual issue. There's a spiritual force within a woman when she's pregnant and people of great spiritual sensitivity have to deal with the reality of that potential life, and a lot of people don't think there's this kind of subtlety, and when they do, I'm very supportive of them. Yes, there's a spiritual issue involved. I take the idea of ending the life of the fetus very, very gravely. I'm troubled by that, but this doesn't in any way diminish my conviction that a woman has the right to do that, but I become distressed when people regard pregnancy lightly and ignore the spiritual significance of a pregnancy.

As the Reverend Owens's response suggests, opposition to abortion as a routine form of birth control is based on a very complex and subtle moral reasoning. For most prochoice people, the personhood of the embryo does not exist at conception but develops at some later point. (Some activists choose viability as the point when personhood begins; others choose birth itself.) Unlike the prolife stand, however, which sees personhood conferred at the moment of conception, the prochoice view of personhood is a *gradualist* one. Thus, although an embryo may not be a full person until viability, it has the rights of a potential person at all times, and those rights become more morally compelling over the length of the pregnancy. (Therefore, wearing an IUD is morally acceptable to all prochoice people, as in their view very early embryos are little more than fertilized eggs.) Prochoice people accept that sometimes the potential rights of the embryo have to be sacrificed to the actual rights of the mother. But a woman who arbitrarily or capriciously brings an embryo into existence, *when she had an alternative*, is seen as usurping even the potential rights of the embryo by trivializing them, and this attitude offends the moral sense of the prochoice activists.

Because they see at least three categories during pregnancy—a fertilized egg without much moral significance (whose life can be ended by wearing an IUD, for example); an embryo, which is a transitional state; and a baby, who makes full moral claim on the human community—prochoice people make sense of the embryo by referring both backward and forward in time. A "menstrual extraction," which is a very early abortion performed within the first three weeks of pregnancy, is less morally troubling than a later, second-trimester abortion, and the moral justification for the later abortion must therefore be correspondingly stronger.

It is in this context that prochoice values about parenting—about the kind of life that the baby-to-be might reasonably expect to have—play such an important role. Prochoice people, for example, have very clear standards about what parenting entails: It means giving a child the very best set of emotional, psychological, social, and financial resources that one possibly can as preparation for future life. Prochoice people feel that it is the duty of a parent to prepare the child for the future, and good parents are seen as arranging life (and childbearing) so that they can do this most effectively:

> Ms. MORRIS: Well, I think that there's a difference between saying that a family should have *all* the children that whoever, the Lord or someone, sends them. And to me, caring about your family means not to have more children than you can give—than you have enough to give them . . . nurturing and . . . not just financially, but in all ways. And I really believe that more families are broken up by unwanted pregnancies and unplanned pregnancies than are ever held together by them.

These values about what a good parent is support and shape prochoice attitudes toward children and the timing of their arrival. Because children demand financial sacrifices, for example, couples should not have them until they are in a financial position to give their children the best. Otherwise, under pressure, parents will come to resent a child, and the lack of emotional and financial resources available to the parents will limit their ability to be caring, attentive, and nurturing to their children. As a corollary, prochoice people want children who feel loved, who have self-esteem, and who "feel good about themselves," and they feel that parents should postpone childbearing until they have the proper *emotional* resources to do the intense one-to-one psychological caring that good parenting takes. (The combination of financial and emotional considerations is what they have in mind when they make the statement that prolife people find unfathomable, that they are not "ready" for childbearing.)

Because prochoice people see the optional raising of children as requiring financial resources, large amounts of "human capital" skills, and emotional maturity, they often worry about how easy it is to have children. In their view, people stumble into parenthood without appreciating what it takes:

> Ms. NEWSOME: I would say that the tip of the iceberg is purposeful parenthood, yes, I am interested. I think life is too cheap. I think we're too easy-going. The automaticness that everybody shall be a mother, that's Garrett Hardin's "compulsory motherhood" concept. Hell, it's a privilege, it's not special enough. The contraceptive agent affords us the opportunity to make motherhood real, real special, and I think again, we have a moral obligation, in the sense of Emerson: New occasions teach new duties. In that sense, with new technology, when you can go to the moon, you can no longer be casual about going to the moon because now it's an act of commission rather than omission. And the same is true—motherhood used to be an act of omission, I mean, you just didn't have any choices, philosophically speaking. You did it because there wasn't anything else to do. And now we have to change the question. We used to say, Why not have a baby? And now we say, Why? So that things have changed just plain philosophically about parenthood, and that's just one part of it.

Because prochoice activists feel that abortion in the long run will enhance the quality of parenting by making it optional, in this respect they see themselves as being on the side of children when they advocate abortion. Consequently, in contrast to prolife people, who feel that parenthood will be enhanced by making it *inclusive* and that all married people should be open to the arrival of children, prochoice people feel that the way to upgrade the quality of parenthood is to make it more *exclusive*:

> REV. OSTER: It stems out of, I think, the same basic concern about the right to share the good life and all these things; that children, once born, have rights which we consistently deny them. I remember giving a talk, that I thought that one of my roles was to be an advocate for the fetus, and for the fetus's right not to be born. I think the right-to-lifers thought I was great until that point. . . . In this sense, that I think if I had my druthers I would probably pursue a course which would, as I do advocate verbally, the need for licensing pregnancies, which seems to contradict what I've just said, but I don't think it really does.

In part, this view is connected to prochoice views about planning. A planned child is a wanted child, and a child who is wanted starts out on a much better footing than one who is not. Not that the prochoice activists necessarily accept a narrow view of "wantedness":

> Ms. HOLMES: Yes, I think that raising a child is a contract of 20 years at least, and I've still found it going on after 30 some, so I think that if you're not in a life situation where you can possibly undertake the commitment to raising a child, you should have the choice of not doing so at the present time. Maybe I'm not being logical, and I don't mean to say that every child is initially unwanted, would remain unwanted, and becomes a social problem. Of course, many people don't want the child when they find out that they're pregnant but they resolve negative feelings, and by the time the child is born, they do want it, and that's probably far more common. But if they don't want it enough to seek an abortion, then probably they shouldn't have [that child]. And I'm as much concerned with the child as the rights of the woman, but I am also concerned with the rights of the woman.

Not surprisingly, the values that prochoice people hold about sex, contraception, and abortion have their roots in deep values about the nature of morality, as was exactly the case for their opponents. Either implicitly or explicitly, prochoice people believe in "situation ethics." Partly because they are pluralists, they seriously doubt whether any one moral code can serve everyone. Partly because they are secularists, they see the traditional Judeo-Christian codes note as absolute moral rules, but as ethical guidelines that emerged in a specific historical time and that may or may not be relevant now. Perhaps most centrally, morality for prochoice people is not a blind "take it or leave it" set of rules, like the Ten Commandments, but the application of a few general ethical principles to a vast array of cases. All of these factors, combined with their staunch belief in the rights of the individual, lead to a belief that only individuals, not governments or churches, can ultimately make ethical decisions. It is tempting to describe their moral positions as quintessentially "Protestant," if one takes this term as being descriptive of a style rather than a religious history. In other words, prochoice people tend to see ethical issues as matters of individual conscience, guided by moral principles, rather than as moral codes *per se*. Hence, the emphasis that prochoice people put on abortion as an *individual, private* choice:

> Ms. HOLMES: Well, of course you can't deny that [abortion] is ending something that's alive, but we took the position that the decision to bear a child, to raise a child, is a private decision between—it's a private decision, an ethical private decision, and the state has no interest in regulating it. Now if this is a matter of conscience, and if your beliefs would be contrary to abortion, then of course you can decide not to have an abortion, even if it meant some other sacrifice.

This quote illustrates three key features of prochoice moral logic. First, there is the implied distinction between an embryo and a child, which all prochoice people take for granted. Second, and perhaps more interesting, is the idea already noted that the embryo, although not a child, is nonetheless "alive" and thus has some implicit moral rights. Finally, there is a pluralist view: If a person has a different moral view of abortion, she should follow her conscience, "even if it meant some other sacrifice." These three features summarize the core of prochoice morality: Morality consists of weighing a number of competing situations and rights and trying to reconcile them under general moral principles, rather than explicit moral rules.

To use a religious metaphor again, the prochoice activists seem to have a New Testament approach to morality. Although relatively few mention either the New Testament or Joseph Fletcher's situation ethics by name, they do call on the moral principles associated with these two sources. That is, when trying to decide what is the moral thing to do, prochoice people ask what is the *loving* thing to do. The choice of the word *loving* emphasizes the fact that moral judgments rely on a subjectively reasoned application of moral principles, rather than on an externally existing moral code.

## THE FORESEEABLE FUTURE

This study suggests that the abortion debate will continue to be a bitter one for the foreseeable future. At stake are not only two different definitions of the embryo, but also two different definitions of the world: Motherhood, the appropriate roles of men and women, and the nature of morality. Because individual values about these related issues run so deep and literally so close to home, reasoned discussion, calm dialogue, and compromise are all equally unlikely. Individuals are unwilling to discuss, much less compromise, their views on abortion. For all of the activists in the study, abortion was merely the tip of the iceberg.

## CHAPTER 3

# Reflections on Abortion, Values, and the Family

## JEAN BETHKE ELSHTAIN

### AUTOBIOGRAPHICAL STATEMENT

*My position has emerged complicatedly, first through familial and religious influence. As a child, I was taught the importance and integrity of life and the need to protect it. I remember my sisters and me doing our best to rescue fallen birds and nurse them back to health. We laboriously mixed an earthworm paste to feed to the birds through eye droppers. We mourned the deaths of baby chicks, ducks, and calves. Life was valuable, we were taught, not for instrumental reasons but in itself. The part of "me" that remains importantly the child that I was reasons thus: If a baby chick deserves respectful "tending to," does not a vulnerable, wholly dependent human life? Is that not what we are talking about if we talk ordinary language and refuse to retreat behind a screen of distancing, "medicalized" abstractions ("products of conception," "fetal matter," and so on)?*

*There are ways in which this direct and beautifully simple moral response has been both challenged and affirmed in my adult life. It has been challenged by my recognition of the desperate circumstances and situations in which many women find and have found themselves, for it is women who bear the most direct and inescapable brunt of human procreation. I do not call to mind here the desperate teenager alone but, say, the menopausal woman in her 50s who has every reason to believe that she is past reproductive age but finds, to her astonishment, that she is not. If one is a merciful and*

JEAN BETHKE ELSHTAIN ● Department of Political Science, University of Massachusetts, Amherst, Massachusetts 01003.

*compassionate being, then one's mercy and compassion must go out to these women and must not limit itself to the unborn. So I cannot accept an absolute prohibition on abortion. But I do not—and cannot—see that "right" as absolute. Here, I can draw on political and theoretical imperatives that are confirmatory of a* respect-for-life *position.*

*I am also influenced in my present position by a particular sort of social theory and philosophy—interpretive, reflective, and critical—together with my political concern that the white, middle-class or upper-middle-class majority has, all too often, presumed to legislate in behalf of, or undercover of, others, claiming that these others (the poor or the minorities) require reforms that they might not be in a position to "see" for themselves. I believe that people must speak for themselves, in their own language, to their most urgent concerns. This belief introduces immediate ambiguity into the abortion debate—and deepens the ambiguity of my own position. For I am in fact part of a large majority that opposes both* abortion on demand *and an* absolute restriction *on abortion. This position suggests to me that my autobiographical history—though confirmed by a later commitment to a certain mode of social theorizing—is not mine alone but is shared by many Americans who are irrepressibly pragmatic yet stubbornly ethical and moral in their concerns. We should acknowledge, not quash, these moral sensibilities. The abortion debate is vital, for it means that we are still concerned about the sort of people we are and the kind of lives we are living.*

We live in a society marked by moral conflict. This conflict has deep historical roots and is reflected in our institutions, practices, laws, norms, and values. The abortion debate taps strongly held, powerfully experienced moral and political imperatives. These imperatives, in turn, are linked internally to a cluster of complex concerns and images evoking what sort of people we are anyway and what we aspire to be. The abortion debate won't "go away," nor should it. For we are, after all, talking about matters of life and death, freedom and obligation, rights and duties: None of us can dispute that, and none of us can be nonplussed when we face the dilemmas that the abortion question poses.

In this essay, I hope to jog our thinking on abortion, values, and the family by showing how, importantly, the positions we hold are shaped by our prior (if, at times, tacit) acceptance of one of a pair of contrasting images of the human community and of the nature and "good" of that community and the human beings who comprise it. In my introductory section, I offer some general observations on language and the abortion debate. The second section sets up two alternative frames—the social contract and the social compact—within which I situate reflections on abortion and the family. In the third section, I proffer some mordant reflections on the "clear and present dangers" that I believe we face *if* we remain tied to a utilitarian ethic and to a perspective that absolutizes choice and exalts control at the expense of principles of obligation, human interdependency, and caretaking.

## LANGUAGE AND THE ABORTION DEBATE

The resources of ordinary language are supple, and they are available to all within a linguistic community. Language importantly constitutes social reality and frames available forms of action. We are all interlocutors in a language community and hence participants in a project of theoretical and moral self-understanding, definition, and redefinition. We can never leap out of our linguistic skins. Our values, imbedded in language, are not icing on the cake of social reasoning but are instead part of a densely articulated web of social, historical, and cultural meanings, traditions, rules, beliefs, norms, actions, and visions. In a society that lacks a moral consensus—our own—the differences that emerge in the language of moral debate take us, if we probe beneath the surface, to the heart of competing understandings of human life. A way of life, constituted in and through language, is a complex whole. One cannot "seal off" attitudes toward the unborn and their fate from other features of the culture. Abortion is not an isolable "variable": It does not exist apart from everything else.

My reflections on abortion, values, and the family emerge, therefore, from a standpoint *within* our culture, not from some Archimedean point of neutral and abstract observation outside it. I try to see through the eyes of others, but always with an eye to critical reflection on the understandings and arguments of others, as well as my own. Interpretive theory of the sort exemplified in this essay probes individual and social meaning. The theorist takes the measure of a culture's reigning symbols of life and death, its unifying or disunifying tendencies, and its sense of purpose or of drift.

Briefly, I shall deepen the discussion of language and moral life by drawing on debates in theories of language and morality as I move to an explicit treatment of the problem at hand. There is no simple test, no easy calculus, by which to assay whether the language and the terms of discourse that we are using help us to see clearly or blind us to important features of moral existence. Language that is inadequate to its task may creep up on us unawares, over time, as social norms evolve or as terms drawn from one sphere—law or medicine, for example—are deployed to "cover" broad areas of moral and political life on the grounds that our ordinary linguistic resources won't serve. As one turns to the question of language and the abortion debate, one confronts a problematic scene. The morally distancing language in that debate—particularly on the part of those who might be called "extreme" or "ultra" liberals or prochoice absolutists—is deeply troubling. I shall offer a few examples drawn from a group of prochoice analysts and philosophers whose implicit aim is to sever our stance on abortion from our emotions altogether. Human emotions are construed, within this abstract, analytic scheme of things, as irrational, serving only to muddy the water.[1]

Examples of discourse that aim to distance us, to throw up a linguistic barrier between us and the reality and conflict of abortion, include arguments that construe the fetus, variously, as a "parasite," a "tenant," an air-borne "spore," or "property." The biologically human status of the fetus is covered up. If an adult human is to be prevented from recognizing in the developing fetus some shared humanness, the fetus must first be dehumanized. Reviewing the arguments of extreme prochoice advocates Michael Tooley and Mary Anne Warren, Philip Abbott recalled the examples that these philosophers (and others) have deployed to make their case. Not one is drawn from everyday human social existence; not one makes contact with ordinary life, language, and moral conflict in a way that I hope to do in this essay. Abbott writes:

> Sixteen examples (and there are variations) are used to analyze the morality of abortion. But what examples! The world of the philosopher is filled with people seeds, child missile launchers, Martians, talking robots, dogs, kittens, chimps, jigsaw cells that form human beings, transparent wombs, and cool hands—everything in fact but fetuses growing in wombs and infants cradled in parents' arms.[2]

Challenged, such prochoice philosophers would respond that we cannot confront the human condition directly, for our minds are too muddled by emotional debris. As proof of this debility, Tooley cited our revulsion to infanticide, seeing it as an irrational taboo "like the

[1]One irony in arguments against emotionalism in moral debate lies in the fact that it is precisely views that sever reason from passion and mind from body that have provided the philosophical soil that yields sexist presumptions, given women's ostensible incapacities for rational reflection and tendencies to be overrun by feeling.
[2]Philip Abbott, *The Family on Trial* (University Park: Pennsylvania State University Press, 1981), p. 138.

reaction of previous generations to masturbation or oral sex."[3] Feminist philosophers Elizabeth Rapaport and Paul Sagal noted that this extreme liberal position is extremely vulnerable; if one accepts it, one also endorses the right to infanticide. Tooley's position, they declared, "permits unrestricted infanticide."[4]

With Abbott, Rapaport and Sagal, and other critics, I reject easy liberal solutions and refuse to strip our language of moral evaluators as the absolute prochoice position requires. It seems to me that Jane English, another feminist thinker, was correct when she said that "anti-abortion forces are indeed giving their strongest arguments when they point to the similarities between a fetus and a baby, and when they try to evoke our emotional attachment to and sympathy for the fetus." The 24-week-old aborted fetus, for example, is so much like a premature infant that "no one can be asked to draw a distinction and treat them so very differently."[5] So I shall avoid all the euphemisms deployed to avoid thinking clearly about what is going on when abortion is going on. I shall not supplant images of the unborn with medicalized talk of "fetal matter" or "products of conception." One must be wary of attempts to constrict the vitality of moral discourse in any area of human life, for once benumbed in one area, one's emotions may continue to be suppressed, and a pervasive and unreflective mode of denial and suppression may evolve.[6]

On the other hand, the occasional use of hyperemotional language by some right-to-life proponents and activists—calling all abortions cases of "murder," making of the woman who aborts and those who abort her murderers or accomplices to murder—is too strong. This language, too, washes out all ambivalence and precludes reflection on the deeply troubling ambiguities of abortion. The minimal point of these reflections is that words matter. The words with which we characterize our daily lives and our moral conflicts count for

[3]Michael Tooley, "Abortion and Infanticide," in Marshall Cohen, Thomas Nagel, and Thomas Scanlon, eds., *The Rights and Wrongs of Abortion* (Princeton, N.J.: Princeton University Press, 1974), pp. 54–55.
[4]Elizabeth Rapaport and Paul Sagal, "One Step Forward, Two Steps Backward: Abortion and Ethical Theory," in Marty Vetterling-Braggin, Frederick A. Elliston and Jane English, eds., *Feminism and Philosophy* (Totowa, N.J.: Littlefield Adams, 1977), p. 410.
[5]Jane English, "Abortion and the Concept of a Person," in Vetterling-Braggin et al., p. 426.
[6]Surely, it is fair for opponents of abortion to conjure up images of aborted fetuses even as it was fair for antiwar activists to react to pictures of napalmed Vietnamese children. Our emotions are complex, threaded through and through with thought, and should be engaged by moral debate lest we try to be, and perhaps succeed in becoming, monsters of abstract systematization.

something. Were our language to be stripped of its moral dimension, as in extreme prochoice positions that grant the fetus no moral weight, nor even a human reality, we would be denied our power as speaking subjects to reflect and to "see" what is going on. But an absolutist moral language also blinds us to ambivalence and complexity. I shall try to steer between these two unacceptable alternatives. I shall try to stay on the ground of practical reasoning, eschewing fanciful and extreme examples, and within terms of ordinary discourse.

## ALTERNATIVE FRAMEWORKS FOR REFLECTION ON ABORTION AND THE FAMILY

I have pointed out that one intrinsic feature of our moral life is the pervasiveness of moral conflict. These conflicts are infused with morally particular ties of obligation, on the one hand, and abstract right and the free choice of the rational individual, on the other. Some of us tend to stress one side of this ledger, the rest of us the other. Situating debates on abortion and the family *inside* the universe constituted by these moral poles means one's case will be pushed one way or another, depending on one's own moral location. Unless one has fully opted for abstract right and individualism or, alternatively, for full absorption of the individual in a web of obligations to others, one's perspective will be touched by the overlap and tension between these broad frameworks. For the purpose of this essay, I am less interested in the way in which these frameworks shade into one another than I am in the postures and the possibilities that each, defined as distinct from the other, nourishes, sustains, or denies.

If social theory, in some sense, makes explicit a society's institutions and practices, the distinctly *atomistic* turn of much prochoice theorizing expresses an important truth about our society: The current order of things, under the radicalizing forces of liberalism, capitalism, and technology, tends increasingly to constitute its members as sovereign selves or consumers, our contemporary variant on the abstract individual of classical atomistic theory.[7] Atomistic theory grounds the notion of a *social contract*. The contract model has its historical roots in seventeenth-century social contract theory, and it incorporates a vision of society as constituted *by* individuals *for* the fulfillment of individual ends. "The term is also applied," wrote Charles

---

[7]One question for feminists and other social critics is whether they should challenge the atomistic construal of the social world or, instead, make their case in and through its reigning presumptions.

Taylor, a political philosopher, "to contemporary doctrines which hark back to social contract theory, or which try to defend in some sense the priority of the individual and his rights over society, or which present a purely instrumental view of society." The central feature of this tradition, which cannot be eliminated, is an "affirmation of what we could call the primacy of rights."[8] Rights are primary and fundamental, but the same status is denied to any principle of belonging or obligation. Primacy-of-rights theory has been one of the most important formative influences on the political consciousness of the West; indeed, we are so immured in the world that this notion has wrought that most of us most of the time grant individual rights *prima facie* force. Atomism makes this doctrine of primacy plausible, by insisting on human self-sufficiency and on the absolutely central importance attached to "freedom to choose one's own mode of life."[9] The view that makes freedom an absolute perforce

> exalts choice as a human capacity. It carries with it the demand that we become beings capable of choice, that we rise to the level of self-consciousness and autonomy where we can exercise choice, that we not remain mired through fear, sloth, ignorance, or superstition in some code imposed by tradition, society, or fate that tells us how we should dispose of what belongs to us.[10]

These presuppositions set the frame for prochoice arguments grounded in the language of rights. But they also provide the base for ultra-liberal or extreme liberal positions for abortion on demand as the woman's absolute right to choose and control.

Let me explain the difference between modified arguments from rights and an extreme atomist position. Classical liberalism, remember, affirmed rights and choice. The liberating vision was one of a person, a transcendental self, freed from nature, from the irrational constraint of tradition, and free to construct a new order. This bracing vision of the free individual, antecedent to social conditions, is subject to particular forms of dissolution, however. As Rapaport and Sagal pointed out, "Simply to employ the language of moral and legal rights . . . is to inherit all the ambiguities associated with this language."[11] These ambiguities elide into a deformation implicit in atomistic and rights theory: the vision of the possessive individual.

It is the contention of C. B. Macpherson that seventeenth-century liberal contract theory contained a "possessive quality," by which

[8]Charles Taylor, "Atomism," in *Power, Possessions and Freedom: Essays in Honor of C. B. Macpherson*, pp. 39–61.
[9]Ibid., p. 48.
[10]Ibid.
[11]Rapaport and Sagal, p. 408.

he meant that it conceived "of the individual as essentially the proprietor of his own person or capacities, owing nothing to society for
them. The individual was seen neither as a moral whole, nor as part
of a larger social whole, but as owner of himself."[12] Society consists
of an aggregate of such contracting, proprietary persons. As liberal
argumentation fused with market images, the *terms* under which individuals came to act in public got construed as wholly instrumental.
In this picture, others become means to my end or barriers in my
way. As social protest or self-advancement, the point is to "get yours."
Any constraint on individual consumerist "wants" or "demands" is
seen as coercive. The language of want and demand in our time
signifies the particular shape that liberal discourse takes within a
consumerist order. Individuals are stripped of a social matrix; hence,
questions of the responsibility that freedom entailed in classical liberal doctrine are also lost. Evocations of choice conjure up images
of a social atom getting, acquiring, and keeping. This image is powerfully reflected in the liberal argument for abortion, locating those
arguments squarely inside the contract frame. As Rapaport and Sagal
noted, argument for abortion couched exclusively in the language of
rights focuses "on individual persons" and neglects

> relationships involving family, class, race, and humankind—relation-
> ships which might prove crucial to the resolution of a problem like
> abortion. Even if the extreme liberals could make good their claim for
> the nonpersonhood of the fetus, obligations involving other social re-
> lations would still require careful attention, for these factors might yield
> restrictions on the extreme liberal position.[13]

Under the tacit terms of atomism and contract doctrine, abortion
gets cast as the right of a possessing and choosing self—some even
claim an absolute right having *prima facie* force. In choosing to abort,

---

[12]C. B. Macpherson, *The Political Theory of Possessive Individualism* (Oxford: Oxford
University Press, 1963), p. 3. Macpherson laid out seven premises of possessive
individualism. These are (1) what makes a person human is his or her freedom
from dependence on the will of others; (2) freedom from dependence on others
means freedom from any relations with others except those that the individual
enters voluntarily with a view to his or her own interest; (3) individuals are
essentially proprietors of their own person and capacities, for which they owe
nothing to society; (4) although an individual cannot alienate the whole of his
property in his person, he may alienate his capacity to labor; (5) human society
consists in a series of market relations; (6) since freedom from the will of others
is what makes us human, each individual's freedom can rightfully be limited only
by such obligations and rules as are necessary to secure the same freedom to
others; and (7) political society is a human contrivance for the protection of
property in person and goods.
[13]Rapaport and Sagal, p. 414.

the woman demonstrates her freedom from the chains of nature and tradition and takes her stand on the same ground as the male sovereign, rational self. I shall explore this devolution from "rights" to "wants" in the ultraliberal prochoice argument, showing how this position grants all the weight of moral argumentation to a particular understanding of an atomized self. Then, I shall examine, briefly, how the family fares within this scheme of things. I mentioned in the first section some of the arguments from respected abortion philosophers. But in more popular forms of prochoice argumentation, one finds the same presumptions, less abstractly couched, at work. For example, Ti-Grace Atkinson, a radical feminist, defined the fetus as a woman's property, along with what she called the woman's "reproductive function."[14] Recalling Macpherson's notion of possessive individualism, within which the individual is construed as the sole proprietor of self, Atkinson claimed that the woman may

> decide to permit the one, i.e., the special function, her function, to operate upon her raw material gift . . . or the woman may decide to stop the process; the embryo is destroyed. . . . It is only when the fetus ceases to be the woman's property . . . that the choice to exercise or not her reproductive function or that the fetus can be interfered with.[15]

Translating proprietary and market language into the abortion debate, Atkinson assumed the power to confer or to deny "personhood" on another. Jane English challenged this ultraliberalism because, as she puts it, "you cannot do as you please with your own body if it affects other people adversely." Even if one decides that the fetus is not a person (in the full-blown, legal sense) "that does not imply that you can do to it anything you wish. Animals, for example, are not persons, yet to kill or torture them for no reason at all is wrong."[16] But the hard-line version of atomistic contractualism will admit of no such possible constraints or brakes on absolute choice.

The fusion of "rights" with "wants" and market language is evident in Garrett Hardin's justification for abortion. He argued that the "unwanted" should not be brought into the world because "they are more likely than others to be poor parents themselves and *breed another generation of unwanted children*."[17] Or, the unwilling pregnant woman *threatens* society, he said, with her unwanted child. Hardin conjured up the image of a society overrun by the "unwanted," most

---

[14]She is radical to the extent that we accept ultraliberalism as radical.

[15]Quoted in Daniel Callahan, *Abortion: Law, Choice and Morality* (New York: Macmillan, 1970), p. 462.

[16]English, p. 417.

[17]Cited in Lawrence Lader, *Abortion* (Indianapolis: Bobbs-Merrill, 1966), p. 156. (Italics added.)

of them poor. We are made to be fearful of the threat posed by the pregnant woman—just as Thomas Hobbes, in his classic *Leviathan*, aimed to make us so fearful of our fellows that we opted for a political world of absolute, authoritarian controls. Lawrence Lader went on to compound our fears by warning that "unwanted children" (most, again, belonging to minority groups) pose a threat to social order. He wrote, "Above all, society must grasp *the grim relationship between unwanted children and the violent rebellion of minority groups.*"[18]

The crassness of market standards is also evident when pro-abortion thinkers make their case from "value" theory, a spin-off of neoclassical market economics. For Hardin, the fetus's value is "entirely dependent" on the social value attributed to it by society. Daniel Callahan, in a critique, pointed out that the implications of arguments from value, within the contractual frame, are straightforward and dire: The fetus has no value; "it awaits someone's wanting it"; then, and only then, "is it of moral interest or human worth."[19] Hardin's insistence that the fetus is entirely dependent on social "value," on that value attributed to it by a market society at the going price, preserves consumer sovereignty and untrammeled choice but strips us of our terms of moral evaluation.

The narrow rationalism implicit in the atomist ideal—one that locates us, remember, as so many choice-making Robinson Crusoes on islands disconnected from essential ties with others—emerges in Lawrence Lader's arguments for liberalized abortion. He stigmatized women without the "abortion option" as creatures stuck "at the level of brood animals." Human birth at this level, he insisted, is often "the result of *blind impulse and passion*," the children born are "little more than the *automatic reflex* of a biological system."[20] Lader's fear of impulse and passion is instructive, for the ultraliberal rationalist can see passions and emotions only as bestial or potentially anarchic. The answer to what is seen as woman's animal-like and irrational state—the "one just and inevitable answer"—becomes abortion, "the final freedom." Lader quoted an associate editor of *Harper's* with approval when she noted, with reference to Aid to Dependent Children, "It is a bitter irony that here in New York, where some of the *most enlightened efforts* of the Planned Parenthood movement are based, hundreds of thousands of mothers still live in *as dark ignorance*

---

[18]Ibid., p. 156. (Italics added.)
[19]Callahan, p. 457.
[20]Quoted in Callahan, p. 540. (Italics added.)

*as the peasants of a remote Pakistani village.*"[21] This quotation suggests how a position grounded in rationalist choice-making can see those who do not fully share that position as only unenlightened, ignorant, or backward, either deliberately or through no fault of their own.

The U.S. Supreme Court's 1973 decision in *Roe* v. *Wade* borrowed from classical liberalism the notion of an autonomous self having the right to privacy and fused that with state interest. That is, the decision, a perfect mimesis of liberal society, was pitched to the unequally matched poles of sovereign individual and sovereign state, with no mediating social relations, institutions, ideals or practices between. The court pushed this liberal/state dichotomy by denying that husbands or anybody else had any right in the matter of deciding the fate of fetal life in the first six months of that life, thereby declaring that family and community considerations could and should be stripped from the adjudication of the rights of a sovereign self.

This decision gives us important clues to how the family fares in the world of atomism and the social contract. If the preceding discussion has any force, the answer flows rather predictably. The family is an anomaly within a world bounded by the sovereign self, the primacy of rights, free choice, and contractual obligation as the only acceptable form of obligation. Historically, liberal voluntarism and family, kin, and communal ties have never made for an easy mix. One serious problem lay in the fact that the woman's legal subordination to her husband constituted an authority relationship that did not square with the terms of the liberal public sphere. Questions of women's continued immersion in the familial web still haunt feminist discourse and color approaches to the abortion debate—as they should. But in our era, the tension between particular rights and

---

[21]Lader, p. 159. (Italics added.) An analogous disquieting manichean disjuncture between the forces of light and darkness appears in Rosalind Pollack Petchesky, "Antiabortion, Antifeminism, and the Rise of the New Right," *Feminist Studies* 7, no. 2 (Summer 1981), pp. 206–246. Petchesky gave a long recitation of good guys versus bad but failed to deal with the fact that the "right-to-life" movement is, as the work of Kristin Luker demonstrates, grass roots—not a conspiracy launched by the Catholic Church as she suggests. Moreover, her piece condemns the antiabortion forces for doing politics, for working to pass or repeal laws, "engage in political education and struggle, establish networks, support sympathetic candidates," and so on. Apparently meaning to condemn them, she stated: "In other words, from the outset, the 'right-to-life' movement was set up to be a political action machine to influence national and local elections" (pp. 213–214). Would she attack the nuclear freeze or feminist organizations on similar grounds? Is politics an option only for those with whom we agree?

abstract right has shifted to children as well, and one hears arguments for children's liberation in ultraliberal discourse.

Such arguments eliminate childhood as a distinctive and dependent period in the human life cycle, seeing that dependency as being imposed by illegitimate adult authority. Children are urged to take their place as atomistic individuals in society, with a paternalistic welfare bureaucracy supporting a lifestyle liberated from oppressive parents. In the words of Abbott, all this comes down to

> a rights model that takes as its basis self-sufficient rational human beings. A good portion of humanity at any given moment does not fit that criterion and children and those who are about to become children make up the bulk of the segment of that population. Since a rights model is designed to make us aware of our self-sufficiency as moral agents, it says little about solidarity among human beings.[22]

Women, then, and children are to join ranks with males as sovereign, free, rationally choosing agents. In more complex evocations, the case gets made that women have yet to enjoin the full dignity of classical personhood. But the extreme liberal also sees in women's links to biology, birth, and nurturing only the vestiges of our "animal" origins, the residues of our preenlightened history. Women, long suspect as emotional, embodied beings, can become "persons" only if they, too, embrace and act on sovereign choice and sever their links with nature. Within the frame of the atomistic construal of the social world and a rationalist conception of human choice and action, proabortion arguments are *not* cast as occasionally necessary but regrettable, and sometimes tragic, responses by particular women to desperate necessity; instead, they become *essential* to women's freedom. Abortion is turned into the technological resolution to what might be called the woman's *control deficit* in the extreme liberal scheme of things—her lesser capacity to control all aspects of life, given her continuing links to nature. The "final freedom" increases that control, and control is a good thing by definition. There is a prior power move here, however, for absolute freedom to abort presumes a female subject to whom

> dependency entails absolute control. If something is within our power, i.e., the fetus, we have the right to control, even destroy it. Humanity gets defined by self-sufficiency. This is a very different sensibility from one that links dependency with responsibility, with care not control.[23]

---

[22]Abbott, p. 142.
[23]Carol McMillen, *Women, Reason and Nature* (Princeton, N.J.: Princeton University Press, 1982), p. 127.

There is an interesting sociological footnote to this form of theoretical and moral argumentation, particularly for the feminist analyst. Polling data from the early 1970s through the present show that abortion-on-demand is more highly favored by men than by women. The single group most consistent in favoring an extreme liberal position on abortion is white upper-middle-class males. In trying to explain this phenomenon, Judith Blake concluded that "upper class men have much to gain and very little to lose by an easing of legal restrictions against abortion."[24] For such men, relaxed abortion promises fewer restrictions on sexuality and lowers financial responsibility and dependency.[25] Abortion-on-demand has also been a linchpin in Hugh Hefner's pathetic playboy philosophy, from its beginnings through the present. So it is a bit difficult to see why some feminists construe abortion rights as pitting men (seeking to keep women enchained) against women (demanding liberation). Clearly, the picture is more complex. What does seem evident, however, is that the atomistic argument can readily accommodate feminist dissent cast within the terms of its animating ethos.

To summarize briefly, the atomistic, contractual frame exudes a politics of self-interest undertaken by a freely choosing, rational agent who, within the present order, is reborn as a sovereign consumer. Liberalized abortion poses no serious challenge to this order; indeed, the force of the doctrines of *prima facie* rights, free choice, and self-interest promotes and sustains abortion imperatives, which are seen as part of woman's freedom and as one way to free all of us from the last vestiges of bondage to nature and to the past. In the world of the social contract, it is difficult to accommodate the family as something other than a "nonbinding commitment" (the modern oxymoron). But the traditional family, an institution grounded in obligation, not rights, poses great difficulties for liberalism. Indeed, the very notion of *traditional* derives from the Latin *traditio* or *tradere*, meaning "to give order," to transmit belief and custom, to hand down and hand over, and this derivation lies at the base of notions of the "traditional family." As I have argued, extreme liberalism would effect a break with all precontractual tradition.

I shall now turn to the second broad frame, the social compact, asking what images of the human self, what values and notions of

[24]Judith Blake, "Abortion and Public Opinion: The 1960–1970 Decade," *Science* 171 (12 February 1971), p. 544.
[25]Rosalind Pollack Petchesky, "Reproductive Freedom: Beyond 'A Woman's Right to Choose,'" *Signs* 4, no. 4 (Summer 1980), pp. 661–685, discounts the empirical evidence from Hilda Scott and Kristin Luker, who have shown how abortion policy encourages male disengagement.

family it calls forth. The issues at stake between the more rooted social and historical beings of the social compact and their atomistically understood opposites are serious and go very deep. Beings who see themselves primarily through the social compact idea do not find at all self-evident the atomist starting point in primacy of rights and absolutizing of choice. In contrast to the standpoint of modern individualism and its rationalist, thin view of self, the compact self is "thick," more particularly situated, a historical being who acknowledges that he or she has "a variety of debts, inheritance, rightful expectations, and obligations" and that these "constitute the given of my life, the moral starting point."[26] Rejecting modern detachment and deracination as primarily defining the self and moral life, the compact being understands or believes that if she cuts herself off from the past, as required by the ultraindividualist mode, she deforms present relationships. The argument here is not that the compact self is totally imbedded within and defined by particular ties and identities, but that she recognizes that without *that* beginning there is no beginning at all.

The world of the social covenant or compact is in tension with the dominant liberal surround, and it must also be supple enough to provide for rebellion and dissent from within. Tradition is not of a piece. The past presents itself as the living embodiment of vital conflicts. Rebellion against one's particular place is one way to forge an identity with reference to that place. But there is little "space" in the compact frame for rebellion to take the form of an atomism that excises all social ties and relations as the individual freely chooses. The familial base of the social compact cannot be understood from the standpoint of contract theory. The compact is an ideal that bears within it intrinsic notions of "good" not reducible to the functional requisites of some "higher" order. In the contract model, the family gets bracketed or severed, and women's traditional roles and identities are, and have been, devalued. Within the social compact, women's identities as wives, mothers, community benefactors, and social activities are not sealed off and are less likely to be devalued.

The contract model leaves no space for, nor does it allow symbolic force to, those contributions of women that have been linked to the human life cycle, to the protection and nurturance of vulnerable human existence. In atomistic construals, women's partial contributions cannot stand, symbolically, for social regenesis as a whole;

---

[26] Alasdair MacIntyre, *After Virtue* (South Bend, Ind.: Notre Dame University Press, 1981), p. 205.

they do not get writ large on the social screen. Indeed, they cannot because the predominant force of images in the contractual world is an ontology of extrinsically sundered atoms rather than intrinsically linked beings. Within the compact vision, however, what women do, what women, in some sense, are, can be seen—there is at least the possibility—as presenting a picture of human society overall as a caring society. By a caring society, I mean one that renounces a technological politics in favor of a sense of history and community; that repudiates a narrow rationalism contemptuous of the values of diverse forms of life that do not fit the rationalist model; and that promotes a reconciliation with nature rather than its continued despoilment.

Any ongoing way of life must have in its number an important segment devoted to the protection of vulnerable human existence. Historically, that protection has been seen as the mission of women. The pity is *not* that women have reflected an ethic of social responsibility but that the public world of ultraliberalism has, for the most part, either repudiated such an ethic or offered us deformed versions in welfare-state bureaucracies.[27] It is my conviction that both feminism and family are jeopardized by moves to disarticulate women altogether from this compact world and its animating ethos. I realize, of course, that historically family and community have been enormously constraining and burdensome for women in particular ways. But what I shall here call the *modern traditional family* cannot be the unconsidered, unreflective family of old that placed all the responsibility for nurturing on women. I shall have more to say on this modern traditional family below, but first, I want to explore the historical roots of my image of a social compact world within which obligations and duties have great, at times overriding, force.

One historical root is the Christian vision of community. Early Christians viewed the Church as an artificial kin group; its members "were expected to project onto the new community a fair measure of the sense of solidarity, of the loyalties, and of the obligations that had previously been directed to the physical family."[28] There was never, nor can there be, some final resolution of the tension between the individual and the community. But the early Church, seen symbolically as mother (*pia mater communis*), exerted a powerful depri-

---

[27] What I have in mind here is not the usual conservative lament but the emerging radical critique of welfarism and a politics of social control.

[28] Peter Brown, *The Cult of the Saints: Its Rise and Function in Latin* (Chicago: University of Chicago Press, 1981), p. 30.

vatizing imperative. Most important, the Christian redefinition of the classical city was radical: "It included two unaccustomed and potentially disruptive categories, the women and the poor."[29] As members of this new community, women assumed a vastly expanded public role—documented by the historian Peter Brown—as they visited the sick, gave alms, founded shrines and poorhouses in their own names, participated in religious ceremonials, and so on. The classical political division (citizen/noncitizen) was supplanted with a model that embraced rich and poor, male and female, and put the rich under a duty to support the poor.

From such beginnings flowed centuries of by no means consistent institutional growth and change. With the victory of the Machiavellian power-politics paradigm and the subsequent emergence of the atomistic doctrine that I have already explored, the link between women and an ethic of caring, succor, endurance, grace, and so on went underground, as it were, and became a submerged discourse, devalued by the dominant male public voices and sphere. To be sure, the historic accretion of all those images of goodness bore heavily on women and sometimes squashed them or forced them into self-abnegation.[30] But the historical and symbolic link of women, their lives, and their embodiment to notions of empathy and compassion lingered and animated generations of female activists and reformers.

Women's worlds and identities could not remain untouched by liberal individualism and the capitalist market. I suggested above a few of the problematic effects, as well as the promises, of these developments. Clearly, the pressure put on the traditional family, community, and female identity by the presumptions of the liberal, rationalist frame compels those who see in the idea of the social compact one locus of resistance to our technocratic, "throwaway" society to make room for women's rightful claims as individuals (partially constituted by liberalism). This means that the social compact cannot, in our time, be comprised of innocent do-gooders who sentimentalize the old ways. There can be no assent, without ambivalence, to a single scheme of things. We are all marked by the moral conflict of our age. "My body, myself" is a necessary corrective when communities overwhelm the individual and stifle the self. But that obsession with an abstract self, which is one defining feature of

---

[29]Ibid., pp. 41–42.

[30]As I write this, I feel uneasy: *Self-sacrifice* has become a dirty term to us precisely because our dominant surround is an atomistic one through which we must see in such terms a selfless self, a masochistic derangement. I fear that to write of self-abnegation in relation to this image may be to be presumptuously present-minded.

ultraliberalism, meshes all too perfectly with the market society. As more and more areas of social life are subjected to decisions made along the lines of a narrowly construed, liberal policy science, families and the remnants of traditional communities may serve as one key source of the preservation of social relations not reducible to instrumental terms. In the world of the social compact, human beings are ends in themselves, not means. No one is in a position to arbitrarily or capriciously assign value to the human life of another, for that value is a given; it is the rock-bottom starting point, the foundation of things.

Do any communities approximate this vision of the social compact? There are pieces of such communities in small-town and rural America, in working-class communities, or wherever people organize to preserve their way of life against the dissolving force of capitalist imperatives. Religious, radical, and some feminist communities aim explicitly at countering the atomism of this era. Harry Boyte, a populist, wrote:

> American history and tradition, like that of any nation, embodies contradictions between rapaciously individualist, democratic, and authoritarian elements. To reclaim the best in America's traditions and history is to rediscover the popular democratic heritage: our nation's civic idealism, our practices of mutual aid and self-help, our religious wellsprings of social justice.[31]

What political theorist Sheldon Wolin called rejectionism pervades our society—a form of rebellion that defies the terms of the wider system. We see such rejectionism, Wolin continued, in communities organized in the name of their common good against toxic waste, in rent-control movements, in environmentalism, and, I would add, in grass-roots aspects of the right-to-life movement, though we may disagree with some or all of the world view of antiabortion activists.[32] The social compact inspiring such movements is local, bounded, grass roots; it is a community, not a state, and its ethos is preserving, not acquiring. Such communities know they cannot change the society writ large. Instead, they are organized to defend and sustain what remains of a way of life not permeated by the forces of atomism, consumerism, and technological forms of control.

And families? One hesitates to use the term *traditional family,* but having spoken of a *modern traditional family,* I wish to convey the image of a set of human relations that, in their *raison d'être,* stand

[31]Harry Boyte, *The Backyard Revolution* (Philadelphia: Temple University Press, 1980).
[32]See Kristin Luker's most recent work for a discussion of the contrasting world views presented by pro- and antiabortion activists.

in opposition to the full sway of atomism. From the standpoint of the dominant ultraliberal discourse, such families are sites of the unfree and the suppressed. Yet, it is such a family that gave birth to generations of female activists, reformers, and social benefactors. And it is such a family that I am thinking about when I try to get a handle on what Stanley Hauerwas has called "the moral meaning of the family."

The ideal of the family is of an entity whose adult members have come together to create a mutual, ethical order; who acknowledge and accept the new identities that this coming together forges, making them social beings of a particular kind; and who commit themselves to responsibility for the future, either through rearing their own children or through other generative activities that link them to past and future beings. A collection of persons who happen to be under one roof at the same time does not make this family. Within the family of which I write, the animating ethos is to nourish humanity—not some vapid promise to fulfill an insatiably consuming self. This family is first and foremost an intergenerational institution, not first and foremost an intrapersonal association.

We seem to lack a descriptive vocabulary that aptly and richly conveys what we mean when we say *family* or *modern traditional family,* in order to distinguish this family, which exists in tension with the wider liberal surround in which it is situated, from families thoroughly suffused with contractualism and "nonbinding commitments" so that the members remain atomistic and "free." This latter family cannot transcend the point of contract. The intergenerational family must do so if it is to be true to its inner ethic and its moral purpose. For the ties of this family constitute us as historical beings. In Hauerwas's terms, "Set out in the world with no family, without a story of and for the self, we will simply be captured by the reigning ideologies of the day."[33] We do not choose our relatives—they are given—and as a result, Hauerwas continued, we know what it means to have a history.

But finally, we do require a language

> to help us articulate the experience of the family and the loyalty it represents.... Such a language must clearly denote our character as historical beings and how our moral lives are based in particular loyalties and relations. If we are to learn to care for others, we must first learn to care for those we find ourselves joined to by accident of birth.[34]

---

[33]Stanley Hauerwas, "The Moral Value of the Family," in *A Community of Character* (South Bend, Ind.: University of Notre Dame Press, 1981), p. 165.
[34]Ibid.

In a transformed traditional family, women are coequal partners and helpmeets as well as necessary and respected community members. To achieve this status, it is not necessary for each marriage partner to enjoy a precise parity of wage-earning power with the other. For this family is not a family defined by economic relations nor ground down in a Hobbesian struggle for power. If each person has a wide berth within a supportive communal surround for his or her activities, the marketplace *imprimatur* becomes less necessary and all-encompassing. One neither seeks nor takes advantage of those who are dependent on, or interdependent with, oneself. Dependency in the compact frame entails responsibility, not control.

As to how one might go about setting up such families, presuming that the vision I have sketched carries some resonance, that is a somewhat misplaced demand. One cannot gerrymander structures in a way that guarantees that Institution X or Y will pop up to perform Function Z. That is not the way in which institutions come into being: They are not designed by some rationalist artificer. The family that I have sketched will very likely unfold if the disintegrative pressures of the culture of productivity and consumption and the often sterile surround in which mothering currently takes place are eased or made more humane. We can trust to human beings to do the rest, for we are naturally social and bonding creatures.

None of this will convince the hard-nosed power realist or the committed atomist or the extreme liberal whose suspicions are raised by the mere suggestion of traditional—anything. And I have not yet addressed the social compact and abortion. Perhaps, I can undercut some disapproval as I complete my argument, but one point needs to be stated clearly: If one's view of society commits one to the image of a world dominated by force and infused by power relations that can be curbed only by counterforce, my social compact will look like the concoction of a starry-eyed optimist. I can only insist that this image does make contact with personal and political realities, as the current "gender gap" and women's reported understanding of political and social life indicate.[35] Moreover, I am open to this vision of mutual respect because I grew up in such a family and I have seen others struggling to create and to sustain such families. I am constantly struck by the uncommon, quiet heroism of ordinary people who trust themselves enough—and have sufficient hope—to bear and raise children under the strains that this society imposes.

---

[35]The "gender gap" shows that between the category "all women" and the category "all men," after one has controlled for age, education, class, and so on, an important distinction emerges on matters, primarily, of war and peace and social concern.

Family loyalty, devotion, constraint—all are unacceptable if one's model is atomism. Publicists for the market society are not threatened by liberationist arguments cast in the language of absolute choice and freedom. One recalls Aldous Huxley's prescient warnings in *Brave New World* that as political and economic freedom diminishes, sexual freedom may well tend to compensate. He concluded that a dictator would do well to encourage such freedom. To the extent that abortion advocates embrace this ideal of freedom, they immerse themselves in the infrastructure of consumerist values.

The compact order cannot readily support radical forms of individualism, that is, the self-identities of persons who position themselves wholly against the community. But ideally, this community would have sufficient elasticity so that it would not attempt to suppress individual expression and rebellion. More important, pressures and constraints would operate with similar force on men and women, though my hunch is that they would bear more heavily on women, who labor under a greater historical density and weight as communal beings. But none of this should be inflexible. One cannot and should not ignore the force of feminist protest. Nor can one undo altogether the self and the world that liberalism has wrought, even if one wanted (and I do not).

What are the implications for abortion? The social compact world cannot be an "easy" abortion society, though early-stage abortion would not be prohibited. Let me explain. Given that this image derives its moral identity from a noncontractual, nonatomistic ethos—one that repudiates instrumental rationality and technological fixes and that promises reconciliation (not domination), mutuality (not power politics)—the order must sustain the human being at each stage of the life cycle. Abortion-on-demand would represent an anomaly within this world, whereas in the atomized contract world, it would be an extension. In such a world, abortion would become what many supporters of liberalized abortion hoped all along it would be (though this did not turn out to be the case), a reluctantly agreed-to response to a desperate situation. If the compact community succors and forgives rather than punishing and condemning, it would have space for the woman who determined that an early stage abortion was her only possible course. She would not be ostracized or forced out of the community. But abortion-on-demand through the sixth month of pregnancy would present too sharp a moral disjuncture within an order that constitutes its members as communal rather than consuming. Its reigning symbols are those of mutuality and fructification, rather than that technologically engineered "equality" embodied in abortion-on-demand without qualification, the easy or ultraliberal stance.

The irony of the moment may well be that women, caught in the grip of the rationalist world view, wind up endorsing the image of freedom *from* nature that, historically, has invited the most insidious forms of domination—of women and of whole ways of life. It is a technocratic prejudice, not a liberating or democratic ideal, that we are somehow most "human" when we are in absolute control. This dictum, translated into the atomistic argument for abortion on demand, structures the human body through and through with the force of technocratic imperatives. The body, in microcosm, comes to mirror a controlling macro-order. As that order manipulates nature, the body controls human nature. What this controlling body-self fails to see is that she, too, is controlled by her own putative "power." With reference to the wider social body, she becomes self-policing; hence, that order can appear to sustain liberationist imperatives, can appear to be responding to radical demands.[36] But as long as these demands are to free the self from all the old shackles and to gain control over all areas of human existence, the social order is confirmed in its deepest structure. The covenant or compact frame puts pressure on this language of control by nourishing a vision of commonalities and attempting to realize some ideal of a shared human good. Abortion is not disallowed but it is "problematized," even as the language in which arguments for abortion are made must occupy the same linguistic terrain as other, partially countervailing tendencies. As a result, the easy, ultraliberal abortion arguments of the social contract frame are chastened even as the absolutist claims that give no weight to individual choice are called into question—though, clearly, the compact image does put heavy weight on the moral status of the fetus, as well as on that of the adult woman, and does insist that a social network be brought into play in making abortion decisions.

Some might argue that my social-compact ideal is too good to be true. But then, that is part of the point of an ideal of any sort: It sets up a standard toward which an individual or a whole people may strive. I am not persuaded by suggestions that we must wait for the full victory of a "socialist" or "feminist" morality before we can begin to think in more social and interconnected ways; that we cannot "transcend . . . the more individualist elements of feminist thinking" until we get the right historic conditions.[37] For to continue to act and to think, whether in matters of abortion or any other matter of

---

[36]I take the lead staked out by Michel Foucault in a number of texts, including *Discipline and Punish* (New York: Vintage Books, 1979), in making these observations.

[37]Petchesky, "Reproductive Freedom," pp. 669, 683.

deep importance and moral concern, wholly within the language of control, atomism, individualism, and so on, derails even the possibility that we might attain a more egalitarian future. One cannot sever men from any say whatever in the fate of their unborn children because we do not yet live in the new world, and then presume that men will get plugged in somehow as beings with some involvement in the future. Current presumptions widen a gulf between present and future until it becomes unbridgeable—unless one clings to an implicit teleological faith.[38] Indeed, we had best tend to many present danger signals if we mean to keep alive some alternative to atomism. It is to these alternatives that I now turn.

## CLEAR AND PRESENT DANGERS: MORAL AND POLITICAL

I shall be both mordant and brief. My intent is to alert us to those clear and present dangers imbedded in the technocratic, utilitarian faith that underlies ultraliberal abortion argumentation. This utilitarian ethic holds that nothing is of intrinsic value; hence, there are no intractable barriers to social engineering and experimentation. Neither the individuals nor the images of a social world are said to embody "good in themselves"; instead, good becomes a calculation of aggregate consequences. In our time the toting up of social "good" or "bad" is largely determined by cost-effectiveness and efficiency. Here are some examples.

First, the same ethic that undergirds those proabortion arguments that stress "wants" and measurements of the differential "value" of lives (presuming that one being can confer "value" on another) can also be used to justify claims that one can make all moral adjudications along cost–benefit lines. Some children's lives become more valuable, others more expendable. I shall have more to say on this subject when I mention eugenics, but I shall simply note here that under cover of such utilitarian formulae, one can readily envisage state-financed systems that mandate amniocentesis, genetic screen-

---

[38]Such a historical faith is evident in Petchesky, ibid., when she presumes that only at some future point, when we have become both a socialist and feminist society according to her specifications, may we consider what exceptions might pertain to a woman's absolute right to control her body. (Petchesky says that this right is not, at present, absolute, but she also claims that we have no morality to tell us what the exceptions might be, thus making it absolute by default.) She also attributes the failures of contemporary socialist societies to approach anything like a new, egalitarian community to the fact that the "socialist transformation" is not yet complete.

ing, subsequent compulsory abortion, and so on. One sign of hope is that many feminists who favor even the extreme liberal position on abortion also oppose such possible compulsions in the name of freedom.

Second, the technocratic world view buttresses the human arrogance that it may soon be possible for couples to aim for the perfect child. One could, in this image, abort all less-than-perfect models (as revealed through a panoply of tests). Should the one perfect child turn out, as all children must, to be less than perfect, it bodes ill for parent–child relations. More important, what is at stake here is our human capacity for risk taking, spontaneity, and welcoming. The new reproductive technologies, coupled with our throwaway ethos, buttress and reinforce our yearnings for absolute certainty and 100% control. In a less-than-perfect world, where deliberate choice and rational control ranged over only so much of human existence, and where contingency and the unexpected played themselves out in other areas, our demands for order and our hubris were bounded and chastened. That is less and less true. My concern is not just what will happen to families as this technocratic ethos spirals onward and upward, but the dire implications for democratic politics. Given human cravings for order and control, as well as the capacities of a technocratic world (at least, apparently) to satisfy these in ways that feed rather than sate the hunger, will our compulsion to control shift to the wider public sphere? Democracy is a chancy, unpredictable enterprise. Our patience with its ups and downs, its debates and compromises, indeed its very antiauthoritarianism, may wane as we become inured to more and more control—all in the name of freedom.

Third, more sophisticated control over reproduction, including foreknowledge of the sex of the fetus combined with the right to revolt, could lead to a future in which the natural balance of females to males will be undermined as more and more couples, in a society that remains male-dominated, choose male offspring. An article in *The Boston Globe* of July 20, 1982, reported the results of a nationwide poll done by the Princeton University Office of Population Research. Asked if they could choose the sex of their firstborn, what the sex would be, 45% of the respondents said male and 20% female. All the respondents were women.[39]

Fourth, one word: eugenics. This is a covert concern in much of the abortion debate, pro and con. We appear to be moving in this direction as more and more of the "imperfect" unborn and newborn are destroyed. The most dramatic example is the increased number

[39]Richard Cohen, "The Unequal Sexes," *Boston Globe* (20 June 1982), p. 17.

of cases in which Down's syndrome babies die lingering deaths when nourishment is withheld. A much celebrated "success" was signaled by the following *New York Times* headline: "Twin Found Defective in Womb Reported Destroyed in Operation." The case, the "first successful surgery of this kind in the country," risked the lives of twin fetuses in order to kill a defective one *while* it remained in the womb. Matter-of-factly, the *Times* reported, "The abnormal fetus was killed by withdrawing about half its blood through a hollow needle inserted in its heart, which then stopped beating."[40] This should make us queasy. Even if we refuse to extend our understanding of the community to include the developmentally disabled (as I do not), why should we assume that the targets of eugenics efforts— whether sporadic and localized or, at some later point, concerted and state-sponsored—will remain "only" the defective? How liberally will we begin to define *defect*?[41] Euthanasia bears a close relationship to the eugenics effort, for it aims to "rationalize" our approach to the old and dying, further severing images of the old from intergenerational ideals. The elderly, with the unborn or the disabled, get treated one way or another, depending on the "social costs" involved. To this, one must add the fears and concerns of blacks and other minorities in the matter of abortion and birth control policy. These fears have a base in historical practice and in the proposals "floated" from time-to-time concerning mandated abortion, sterilization, and so on.[42] One black writer has claimed that Planned Parenthood's policies have been those of upper-middle-class whites, who often express "a fetish about controlling the reproductive capacities of others, those who are poor and black."[43] The feminist argument for "reproductive freedom," construed as the absolute right to abort as well as freedom from coerced or enforced abortion or sterilization,

---

[40]Harold M. Schmeck, "Twin Found Defective in Womb Reported Destroyed in Operation," *New York Times* (18 June 1981), pp. 1, 19.

[41]The first targets of Nazi racial policy were the retarded, who were sterilized, aborted, and gassed. The mentally ill were among the first to be sent to their deaths.

[42]Erma Clarxy Craven, "Abortion, Poverty and Black Genocide," in Thomas W. Hilgren and Dennis J. Horan, eds., *Abortion and Social Justice* (New York: Sheed & Ward, 1972), reported that, in 1969 at a White House Conference on Hunger, a doctor with the National Institutes of Health recommended (1) mandatory abortion for any unmarried girl within the first three months of her pregnancy and (2) mandatory sterilization of any woman or girl giving birth out of wedlock for a second time. Alan Guttmacher, President of Planned Parenthood, apparently gave this proposal "his strong support," but it was quashed under the leadership of Fannie Lou Hamer (p. 231).

[43]Ibid.

does not seem reliable as a brake should our social ethos move further in the atomistic direction.

As this essay draws to a close, I am aware how powerless our words seem as we confront great social forces and tendencies. Nevertheless, if I am correct that our language of self-description and understanding and moral evaluation helps to shape those social forces and tendencies, it is important to bear witness, to articulate some possible *via media* between atomism and control, on the one hand, and the call for a return to some long-gone communal past, on the other. Rather than recalling that argument, I shall reflect, briefly, on what sort of people we are from the perspective of the position I have sketched.

More and more frequently, it seems, one finds the stated view that human suffering is bad and can never be a source of strength or a lesson in grace. It follows that families should not suffer, so retarded children must be allowed to die. The handicapped suffer—it would have been better had they not been allowed to live. Old people suffer, so we should find ways to kill them humanely. And there is "wrongful life." We feel sorry for those who should never have been born, so we must not force them to live. Or this imperative may be expressed as "the right to die": If one's birth was wrongful, that right is exercised by others in one's behalf. The possibilities in this direction are limited only by our capacity to conjure up yet another problem that can be solved by eliminating people or by not allowing them to be born.

Should a politics of technological control and an ethos of consequentionalism grow apace, as I fear they will, what might be the results for the family and the wider society? Minimally, there will be a rise in psychic numbing (some have already noted this), and an erosion of the bases of an ethics of stewardship, care, and trust, an ethic that respects the richness, the diversity, and the intrinsic value of forms of life and that sees the person as a caretaker, not primarily as an aggrandizer. We numb our moral sensibilities each time we acquiesce in a restriction of the concept of humanity, a restriction that *never* "enhances a respect for human life" but always threatens to erode that respect. Such restriction, Philip Abbott proclaimed, did not "enhance the rights of slaves, prisoners of war, criminals, traitors, women, children, Jews, blacks, heretics, workers, capitalists, Slavs, Gypsies."[44]

When we concurred, as a society, to a nearly full-scale redefinition that aimed to place fetal life altogether outside the bounds of

[44]Abbott, p. 145.

moral consideration, as a form of life having no weight in the scheme of things, we suffered a deep if subtle moral corruption. "The mystery of the silence of the unborn," wrote Daniel Berrigan. I think of others once hidden from view so that we were not required to see them. We seem more and more incapable of truly seeing what we are doing, and in acting unthinkingly, simply accepting the dominant terms of discourse of our age, we may one day slide over the precipice and tip the balance toward a society whose reigning symbols are violence, death, and expendability.

"Life is cheap in Casablanca," says Sidney Greenstreet to Humphrey Bogart.

Life is getting cheaper in the United States of America.

# Commentary to Chapter 3

## CAN SOCIAL COMPACTS EMANCIPATE US FROM SOCIAL CONTRACTS?

Elshtain is certainly not alone in wanting to avoid liberal solutions to the moral and political issues raised by the abortion dispute.[1] And in a society like ours, where political life and the economy are thought to be structured by liberal assumptions, liberal solutions to all policy issues need criticism. However, criticisms of liberalism have come from two different groups, both of which prefer "social compacts" to social contracts. These groups have different motivations for their criticisms, different visions of the alternative Good Life, and opposed strategies for achieving their goals. Which social compact vision motivates Elshtain's argument? And what guidance does either group's vision offer us in the abortion dispute?

Elshtain's paper does not provide obvious answers to these questions. The reason is that Elshtain's appeal to social compacts is an appeal to a "category of challenge" to excesses of social contract ideology and practice, rather than an appeal to the potential origins of a blueprint of an alternative structuring of the social order.[2] Whether

---

[1]Jean Bethke Elshtain, "Reflections on Abortion, Values and the Family," Chapter 3. Elshtain characterized the liberal solutions as "easy." However, the contrary is surely attested to by the resistence of white male legislators to the passage of the ERA, as well as by the virulent opposition to liberal solutions to the abortion issue. Conceptually, pure liberal solutions to any of the women's issues or to class and race issues are not only not easy, they are impossible. This is true because, as we shall see, liberalism cannot recognize as legitimate the "group rights" demanded by women, people of color, and the working class.

[2]Maurice Bloch and Jean H. Bloch discussed "nature" as a category of challenge in "Women and the Dialectics of Nature in Eighteenth-Century French Thought," in Carol MacCormack and Marilyn Strathern, eds., *Nature, Culture and Gender* (New York: Cambridge University Press, 1980).

---

SANDRA HARDING • Department of Philosophy, University of Delaware, Newark, Delaware 19711.

she makes a regressive or a progressive challenge is at least an open question.

I do not see how the social compact vision provides any more guidance on how to resolve the political and moral issues in the abortion dispute than it does on how to resolve any other social issues confronting us today. The notion of a social compact—even if "modernized"—is inextricably entangled with older ideological claims about the naturalness of kinship as the fundamental organizing principle of social life, and about the moral priority of community control of individuals. As Elshtain points out, we do not individually choose most of our relatives—our kin. However, as anthropologists note, neither are they given to us by biology. If reproduction is "natural," so, too, for our species is social and political life. Both exhibit the immense cultural variation possible for the species that remakes itself and its natural/social surround through historical processes. There is no such concrete entity as "the family" referred to in her title, let alone one called for by the "biologically human status of the fetus." Given the invariably sexist and often also racist and classist ideological burdens that social compact challenges carry, one is reasonably tempted to be skeptical of the emancipatory potential of Elshtain's argument.

## CONSERVATISM AND RADICALISM

Both conservatives and radicals today draw on long traditions of objection to liberalism's assumptions that humans are essentially possessive individuals with no necessary, noncontractual ties to other humans; that priority should be given to individuals' rights to—and choices for—life, liberty, property, and the pursuit of happiness; that the instrumentalism of social contract views of society is a worthy ideal; and that language, concepts, and methodologies both in social theory and in knowledge seeking must be value-neutral and morally distancing. In contrast, conservative and radical traditions conceptualize the community as a social compact—as morally, politically, and cognitively prior to the individual. They take this priority of community over individual to make positive contributions to morals, politics, and knowledge seeking: Both stress the positive role that emotions, collective social values, and responsibilities, perceptions, and the like—the "secondary properties" of the human part of nature—play in moral action, political organization, and knowledge seeking. Both stress duties and responsibilities to dependent others over rights of autonomous others, and collective projects and his-torically determined destinies over rational individual choice.

Overlooking the similarities in their conceptions of human na-ture and the social order, conservatives and radicals are often shocked to discover who their allies are when liberalism is the opponent. Politics may make strangers bedfellows; but cohabitation is not po-litical unity, and it often hides far more fundamental oppositions. Such is the case with conservatism and radicalism.

Conservatives think that the social aristocracy correctly mirrors the "natural aristocracy." They believe that human nature is essen-tially unchanging, and that either God or Mother Nature distributes natural talents and abilities in such a way as to fit individuals properly into the social hierarchies of the past and their remnants today. Consequently, they tend toward pessimism in the face of demands from the serfs for social change, and they adopt strategies that they hope will restore in the future what they perceive as the ideal societies of the past. The societies that they find ideal almost invariably are fundamentally structured by class, race, and sex hierarchies. In con-trast, radicals think that the social aristocracies distort the "natural democracy" of which humans are capable. They believe that human nature is extremely malleable in the hands of history, and that no social group has a corner on the talents and abilities necessary to participate as full equals in the social order. They tend toward op-timism in the face of demands from the oppressed for social change, and they adopt strategies that they hope will create in the future the social mirror of the natural democracy of which they believe our species is capable. Class hierarchy has been the leading target of radical criticism. Antiracism and antisexism movements similarly fo-cus on the social creation and maintenance of supposedly natural hierarchies. Which of these social-compact visions does Elshtain have in mind?

Quite apart from this question, Elshtain's essay also raises the issue of whether or not *any* social compact proposed so far offers unmitigated advantages to women today. When one examines crit-ically the knowledge claims, as well as the politics and the morals, concerning human reproduction and women's status—or the social relations between the sexes more generally—it becomes clear that neither social-compact tradition takes women to be as fully social creatures as men. In theory and practice, both appear to concep-tualize men and women more as two different species—say, humans and horses—than as full members of the same species. Finally, apart from these "women's issues," it is not clear to me that either the historical record or the theory of social compact societies, whether conservative or radical, offers any clear guidance to the appropriate ethical stance for us to take on "life-and-death" issues such as those raised by both sides in the contemporary abortion dispute.

My point here is not to defend social contract against social compact visions, for I agree with most of Elshtain's criticisms of social contract realities and concepts. Instead, I want to suggest why all of us, and especially women, should be equally critical of social compact theories. A major obstacle to either theory's becoming a theory for *human* emancipation is that neither contains the concepts that could make possible a critical perspective on social relations between the sexes.

## SOCIAL CONTRACTS

It is becoming increasingly evident that social contract theories have never, ever, anywhere, at any time, imagined women as a group as fully human—as fully social agents capable of making social contracts.[3] The reason appears to be primarily that social contract theories assume a rigid dichotomy between "the natural" and "the social" in which women's reproductive activities firmly mire women in the natural; in which the natural is seen as a threat to the cultural; and in which the history of culture is seen as a flawed but linear record of individual men's achievements in the public, social realm.

This problem is illuminated by attempts to reform social contract theory. Within social contract theory, inherently radical attempts to appeal to the goodness of the natural in order to reform the perceived excesses or degeneracies of the social have persistently been undercut and deradicalized by the reformers' refusal to recognize and/or act on the inherent logic of these arguments. If the natural is the ideal which we should pursue as a corrective in the social world, and if women are "closer to nature" than men, then women's natures and activities already stand as a model for men to emulate. The logic of this argument *within* social contract theory leads to the conclusion that it is uniquely women who can bring into balance the natural and the social. But it is this logical conclusion to their argument that the social contract reformers have been loath to recognize. They have consistently chosen to compromise—or sometimes to entirely abandon—the radical implications of their proposed reforms rather than

---

[3]Zillah Eisenstein, *The Radical Implications of Liberal Feminism* (New York: Longmans, 1979); Susan Moller Okin, *Women in Western Political Thought* (Princeton, N.J.: Princeton University Press, 1979).

having to admit women to the category of the fully human (let alone regarding women as models for men).[4]

This dilemma within liberalism reveals that it is not that social contract theories simply *happen*, through oversight, to exclude women and reproduction from the domains regarded as fully human. Nor, then, can social contract theories be revised to recognize women, too, as actual or potential moral, knowing, historical agents of culture. Such a revision would require the abandonment of the nature–culture dichotomy fundamental to the motivation for conceptualizing the social order as really or heuristically formed through social contracts. Thus, these theories must *begin* by assuming that only men *can* rise above the undifferentiated "merely natural" to unite as individuals to create culture, and that men *must* do this lest the distinctively "human" be overwhelmed and defeated by the forces of irrationality, passions, and bondage to natural social compacts. These latter forces are represented in liberal thinking both by the early history of the species and by the early history of men in their families of birth: Adult women thus represent the lurking presence of the "savage" and the childlike amidst the "civilized" and "tamed" social relations of adulthood.

Liberalism insists that individuals, not social groups, are the parties to social contracts. In contrast, feminism insists that neither men nor women really are capable of functioning as individuals. Both are members of sex classes in our kind of society, and it is an illusion beneficial only to the powerful to think otherwise. Everyone's rights, rational choices, psychological tendencies, and conceptions of the good are arrived at collectively, as members of sex classes as well as of hierarchically organized race, class, and cultural groups. From this perspective, social contracts are masculine, ruling-class protection rackets. They are conspiracies between ruling-class men to agree to give up some of their rights and powers to the state in return for the protection of their group interests *against other groups within their own societies.*

So, first of all, why do contemporary feminists buy into liberalism's social contract ideology? Why have feminists tried to force the state to protect women's rights to abortion, as well as to suffrage, to equal pay, to property rights, and to equal protection from such widespread phenomena as rape and wife battering? The answer is politically simple. American democracy was founded on social contract assumptions and remains more politically sensitive to appeals

[4]Bloch and Bloch. The eighteenth-century thinkers primarily discussed are Rousseau, La Mettrie, and Diderot.

and demands couched in liberal terms than to those couched in either conservative or radical social-compact terms. We are all forced to make our history in circumstances not of our choosing, as Marx pointed out. The abortion dispute is certainly not the only current political dispute in which the attempt to force our state to recognize everyone as fully human produces morally and conceptually inconsistent strategies. The availability of contraceptives and the right to private homosexual relations between consenting adults are defended by appeal to the liberal right to privacy in sexual relations. But the very same individuals and groups demand protection against battering husbands, marital rape, and sex with minors by arguing that there are limits to the sexual relations that the state can *justly* leave to be negotiated within the social compacts of the private sphere— "the personal is political." There is nothing very mysterious about why—in a society institutionally structured by racism, sexism, and classism, but espousing a liberal contract ideology—women and others conceptualized as less than fully human appeal to this contract ideology to gain formal status equal to that of the contractually favored groups. Nor have feminists been blind, as Elshtain implies, to either the general or the specific problems that women have with social contract assumptions and practices.[5]

In the second place, does not Elshtain herself, at least implicitly, appeal to the nature–culture dichotomy on which liberal theory is grounded? Does not Elshtain think that the excesses of liberalism, particularly evident in the feminists whom she criticizes, should be corrected by an understanding of the socially purifying function of the natural to be found in the "biologically human status of the fetus," "the family" as an anomaly "in the world of atomism and the social contract," women's "mission" to "protect vulnerable human existence," and the like?

## SOCIAL COMPACTS

Elshtain locates the historical origins of social compact visions in early Christian thought, and suggests that today

> There are pieces of such communities in small-town and rural America, in working-class communities, or wherever people organize to preserve their way of life against the dissolving forces of capitalist imperatives. Religious, radical, and some feminist communities aim explicitly to counter the atomism of this era.

-------------------------

[5]Eisenstein; Okin.

However, I understand the social compact ideal to be characteristic of traditional societies more generally—the "premodern," "preindustrial," and "primitive" societies that anthropologists and historians study—and also of the whole range of radical social-reform visions from Utopian socialism and Marxism to the various participatory-democracy visions emerging from our own recent New Left.

Historians and anthropologists point out that, in traditional societies, where kinship relations structure the economy, the government, and social relations more generally, "production" occurs in the realm of "reproduction"—in the family—whether the production is gathering and hunting, animal herding, agriculture, or craft industry. Here the separation between the public and the domestic, the social and the natural, is neither visible nor possible to create. Since women as a sex class are crucial to the reproduction of kinship but not to the reproduction of capital, women as a group tend to have higher status in traditional than in modern societies.[6] But what strategic advantage can we modern women and men find in this knowledge of an important cause of traditional cultures' social relations? As a social-structural possibility, social compacts based on kinship are gone forever for us modern and postmodern folks.

Furthermore, do social compact societies offer women and the rest of us unmitigated benefits over what we've got? Elshtain doesn't suggest that they do, but it is worth recollecting in more detail what social compact societies do permit. Finally, do social compact societies offer us guidance in ethical issues more generally, such as those raised by the abortion dispute? In both respects, I think not. After all, traditional social-compact cultures have produced untroubled acceptance of slavery, infanticide, human sacrifice, abandonment of the aged on ice floes, intimately conducted torture and mutilation of enemies, not to mention widow burning, enforced clitoridectomy and enfibulation, the cult of virginity, and other social expressions of the belief that women are "nothing": They are the collective property of the men who are the "compacting agents." And, of course, abortion itself has been practiced in every known society, often with general social approval. The point here is not that modern social-contract societies are more ethical or "humanitarian" than traditional

---

[6]Mary O'Brien pointed out that capital, unlike kinship, "breeds by itself." *The Politics of Reproduction* (Boston: Routledge and Kegan Paul, 1981). For the role of kinship and women in traditional societies, see Joan Kelly-Gadol, "The Social Relation of the Sexes: Methodological Implications of Women's History," *Signs* (1976), p. 4; Gayle Rubin, "The Traffic in Women: Notes on the 'Political Economy' of Sex," in Rayna R. Reiter, ed., *Toward an Anthropology of Women* (New York: Monthly Review Press, 1975).

societies; it is hard to understand what criterion would show such a claim, or its contrary, to be true. Rather, ethical norms and social practices are bold and creative attempts to deal with the particular realities of the social/natural surround as these are understood by those in a position to design and control cultures.

Nor have radical social-compact visions within modernism provided obvious blueprints for the future. The social compact vision to be found wherever "people organize to preserve their way of life against the dissolving forces of capitalist imperatives" is as often a conservative as a radical one, and pitifully few among the radical visions have even attempted to conceptualize how social relations between the sexes and the races structure social life.

Thus, although social compact visions do challenge social contract ones, I am more skeptical than Elshtain about the resources that social compact history and theory provide for emancipatory social projects today.

## CONCLUDING REMARKS

I suggest that Elshtain's concept of the *social compact* functions rhetorically as a category of challenge, and that her particular use of it is not obviously consistent with empirical fact or moral "progress." The term can reasonably be used to refer to an immense array of societies that share only the characteristic of not being social contract societies, and to refer to a wide variety of social visions created specifically as challenges to social contract assumptions. Like many of the latter, Elshtain's social compact challenge turns out to be grounded in the very nature–culture dichotomy central to social contract theory. Where the social contractors think that "nature" must be dominated by culture, Elshtain thinks that the excesses of liberal social contracts must be purified by a return to "natural" social compacts. Understanding women as essentially "a sex" is fundamental to this project. How an appeal to such an ideologically structured notion is supposed to help us to resolve in an emancipatory way the moral and political issues about abortion remains mysterious to me.

## CHAPTER 4

# A Family Perspective on Abortion

## THEODORA OOMS

### AUTOBIOGRAPHICAL STATEMENT

*Until quite recently, I had no doubts about which side of the abortion controversy I belonged to: I was a rather unreflective supporter of the prochoice movement. I began, however, to find that certain phrases of the prochoice movement grated on me, and that some of the arguments of the prolifers struck a resonant chord. I disliked the tactics of both sides and found that their strident certainty did not correspond to the way I believed most people, including myself, thought about the complex issue.*

*My prochoice sympathies grew naturally out of the values I learned from my family and from experiences as a child and a student in England. Both my parents were public health doctors and served as medical mission-aries in China, where I spent the first four years of my life. Their experiences in China, however, led to a loss of their once deep religious faith. I grew up as the eldest of three in an agnostic household guided by many Christian ideals. I remember always being aware of the problems of poverty, ill health, overpopulation, and the evils of war. My parents were both British socialists, and my father was an ardent pacifist. I went to a progressive boarding school where many of the faculty were left-leaning in their social and political views and many were Quakers. In college, I was active in socialist clubs and went on several peace marches. I don't ever remember discussions about abortion with family or friends, though we talked at length about the need*

The views expressed in this chapter are solely those of the author and do not reflect those of her institutional affiliations.

THEODORA OOMS • Director, Family Impact Seminar, Catholic University of America, Washington, D.C. 20064.

for the sexual revolution to be accompanied by responsible birth control use. I am confident that the pacifists I knew would have supported abortion, seeing no inconsistency in this position.

All of these factors led to my deep conviction that it was our duty both as a society and as individuals to attempt to remedy the evils of the world; and to my belief that the problems of poverty, ill health, and inequality could be remedied. Everyone, I thought, should be able to have as much control as possible over the circumstances and the direction of their lives: One important step toward this goal was controlling the size of one's family, and choosing whether and when to become a parent.

Later, in America, two close friends did have abortions for reasons that I did not question at the time. The main issue, for them and for me, was not the morality but the illegality of abortion: how to get a safe one. (The other issue was the absurdity of finding three doctors to certify that my friend was suicidal.) Luckily, I have never had to face an unwanted pregnancy myself, although when I was pregnant during the rubella epidemic, both my husband and I had no question about what we would do if I contracted rubella. I greeted the 1973 U.S. Supreme Court decision as one victory for good sense in the battle to overthrow a number of archaic and repressive laws concerned with sexuality. Although I was involved in several ways in the women's movement, abortion was not the central issue for me.

Ever since my undergraduate work in philosophy, politics, and economics, I have been interested in theoretical issues. However, my years of practice as a social worker and a family therapist have taught me to respect a diversity of situations and values, and to distrust any theory or policy that did not work in practice.

My work with families has profoundly changed the way in which I view the world. My professional growth parallels my own progress through the life cycle. When I was a young, unattached individual who was loosening my own family bonds, individual rights and freedom of choice seemed of utmost importance. Now that I am a wife, a mother of three, and a family therapist, I am more impressed by the value of connections, responsibilities, commitments, and context.

In particular, becoming involved with two families whose 16-year-olds became pregnant led to my interest in the family issues surrounding a teenage pregnancy. Directing a policy research study on the topic, I was disturbed to learn of the large numbers of teens getting abortions and the numbers of women of all ages who were clearly using abortion as a method of birth control. I realized that I no longer felt that abortion was an obvious or simple choice or indeed solely a woman's right. I knew that I needed to think through my position much more deeply.

Abortion is the most politically divisive of all the so-called family issues. Though a pregnant woman's decision either to abort or to give birth dramatically affects her family life, the family considerations that weigh in her decision are rarely mentioned in public debates and are seldom discussed in the volumes of writings on the subject. This chapter outlines what these family considerations are and argues that they should be given greater weight in both legal and ethical discussion.

## DEFINITION AND ASSUMPTIONS

*Family* has a wide range of meanings depending on the cultural and historical context, its descriptive or normative purpose, and the life cycle status of the user. If you ask a middle-aged American adult, "Who is in your family?", she or he usually replies, "My husband/wife and two sons," if married and a parent; but if single and not a parent, is likely to respond, "My mother, brother, and sister." But if the person comes, for example, from an Italian or Chinese background, the answer may be a long list that includes aunts, uncles, grandparents, and cousins. A Roman patriarch would have included everyone in his large household, including his servants. And Alex Haley would respond to this question by proudly showing the photograph of his last family reunion with over 200 family members.

For the purpose of this discussion, I shall use a quite restrictive meaning of *family*: those persons most closely related by blood, marriage, or adoption to the pregnant woman and the fetus, including her spouse or the expectant father, or, if she is an adolescent, her parents. Certainly, other family members can be very much affected by her pregnancy decision, but less directly so (for example, her siblings, children, grandparents, or the expectant father's own parents); and they will be given only minor attention here. The fetus, I would argue, needs to be regarded as a potential person and also as a potential family member. Thus, the fate and well-being of the fetus are of concern not only to the state but also to close relatives.

There is another kind of family unit that has an interest in the pregnant woman's decision, namely, a potential adoptive family, because if the pregnant woman decides to resolve an unwanted pregnancy by placing her baby for adoption, they will become parents. The existence in America of families waiting to adopt has, in my view, considerable influence on the moral aspects of the abortion issue and on the shape that appropriate public and private policy should take.

This use of the term *family* is relatively value-free because it does not imply any desired structure, roles, or functioning. However, I need to make my own biases on these topics clear, as they undoubtedly shape the argument that follows.

First, though I advocate that more attention be paid to family roles, rights, and relationships in the abortion issue (and many other issues), I am not guided by a romanticized ideal vision of family life. Families are a necessity. They are the crucible of the best and the worst in human nature, the source of our most positive and our most negative feelings and experiences. Many speak of the "essential" qualities of family life in our modern era as being the providing of love, loyalty, nurturance, and intimacy—a "haven in a harsh world." Yet in some families, many or all of these so-called essential elements are missing; and the harshness lies within the family, not outside it.

Second, I do believe that our society needs to shift from a patriarchal mode of family life to an egalitarian mode, particularly in the relationship between spouses. However, as a family therapist, I also believe that this democratization of families should not be carried too far. There is still a need—if families with children are to function at all—to retain some hierarchical boundaries between generations: Parents must still hold the gavel, and their votes must carry more weight within the family council.

I also approach this discussion with a particular set of assumptions about the nature of human behavior and society. These assumptions are derived from an ecologically based view that, in turn, draws on systems theory.[1] They have much in common with what others in this volume call *communitarian thinking*. The central assumptions of this ecological perspective are:

- An individual's needs, behavior, values, expectations and opportunities are the products of a continuous interplay between his or her biological makeup and personality and the systems within the immediate social environment, which, in turn, reflect or are influenced by external factors in the wider social environment. The primary social system for most people is their family.

[1]See, in particular, Urie Bronfenbrenner, *Ecology of Human Development* (Cambridge: Harvard University Press, 1979); Salvador Minuchin, *Families and Family Therapy* (Cambridge: Harvard University Press, 1975); Ludwig von Bertalanffy, *General Systems Theory: Foundations, Developments, Applications* (New York: George Braziller, 1968); Gordon Hearn, ed., *General Systems Approach: Contributions toward an Holistic Conception of Social Work* (New York: Council on Social Work Education, 1969).

- Within any one family system—whether it is within a household family or the extended kinship network—there are many aspects of family members' lives that are interdependent. A change in the situation, the behavior, or the feelings of one family member affects other members and produces a series of reactions that feed on one another. This series of reactions and counterreactions may dramatically shift the whole structure and functioning of the family, or it may be accommodated, with some minor adjustments.

- An ecological approach places great importance on the nature of relationships *between* social systems: the family and the workplace, social agency, school, and church. The quantity and the quality of the transactions between these systems are important if one is to understand the effects of one system on another. Professionals, agency staff, and bureaucrats are not neutral intervenors acting on individuals; they are parts of systems that interact with the family system.

- Families are the crucial building blocks of society. They perform certain critical functions—among them, rearing and educating the young and caring for dependents of all ages—that no other group or institution has been able to take over. Although the family has a curiously ambiguous place in democratic theory—as exemplified by the absence of any reference to the family in the U.S. Constitution—many have noted that families are perhaps the most important of a number of mediating structures that serve as a buffer between the individual and the state, and that they thus form a bulwark against authoritarianism.[2] (Most totalitarian regimes have sought to abolish or to seriously weaken family ties and integrity.)

A family perspective contrasts with the assumptions and the values of philosophical and scientific individualism. "Rational individualism," wrote political theorist Philip Abbott in his book *The Family on Trial,* "sees the world composed of self contained and autonomous units."[3] These atomistic individuals, John Locke said, enter into a voluntary contract with the state. This liberal tradition

[2]See Amitai Etzioni, *An Immodest Agenda: Rebuilding America before the Twenty First Century* (New York: McGraw-Hill, 1983), p. 99; Peter Berger and Richard Neuhaus, *To Empower People: The Role of Mediating Structures in Public Policy* (Washington: American Enterprise Institute, 1977).
[3]Philip Abbott, *The Family on Trial: Special Relationships in Modern Political Thought* (University Park: Pennsylvania State University Press, 1981), p. 5.

lies at the basis of American democracy, and it has dominated and permeated all aspects of our society. It holds that the liberty (autonomy) and the happiness of individuals are the supreme values and says very little about individuals' relationships with other persons or groups that may shape and qualify the nature of their autonomy and that may be a necessity for individual happiness or self-fulfillment. A family therapist, Salvador Minuchin, commented:

> Indeed it is difficult for anyone reared in Western culture to look beyond the individual. We are trained into both an ethical and an esthetic preference for individual self-determination. To think of the individual as a segment of a larger social and biological unit is distasteful at best.[4]

The current emphasis on what Etzioni termed "excessive individualism" leads to a society composed of "ego-centered" individuals and a deplorable weakening of community-based institutions and shared communal values. In Etzioni's view, the solution is not to retreat to a more Hobbesian societal model, where individual rights are totally subordinated to society and where the organized community is the source of all authority and legitimacy. Rather, he wrote, we need to seek to create an "open community," where there is a "wholesome relationship between community and member-individuals . . . based on a creative tension and a continuous search for balance, not domination of one by the other."[5] Both individuals and community are twin essential elements and need to have the same status, and to be kept in balance.

This essay attempts to counter what I claim to be an excessively individualistic view of the abortion issue. By focusing on family, I hope to provide one specific example of how to bring the interests of the individual and the community into better balance.

## THE LEGAL FRAMEWORK

The recent decade has seen a spate of expressed public concern about family matters, as well as a flurry of activity on all sides of the political spectrum.[6] This has been accompanied by an explosion of

[4]Salvador Minuchin and H. Charles Fishman, *Family Therapy Techniques* (Cambridge: Harvard University Press, 1981), p. 12.
[5]Etzioni, p. 20.
[6]For example, the three regional White House Conferences on Families, which were held in 1981; two American Family Forum meetings held in Washington, D.C. in 1980 and 1982; and the new House Select Committee on Children and Families established in February 1983, cosponsored by George Miller (D), Henry Hyde (R), and over 200 other members.

scholarship about the family among historians, psychologists, sociologists, legal scholars, and economists. The latest are the political theorists,[7] who are paying attention to what political philosophers wrote about the family in past centuries, and who are developing new contributions relating to the special nature of the family in a democratic society.[8]

Only a few philosophers, however, have even begun to grapple with the special claims that family members have upon one another and with the nature of family rights and responsibilities.[9] Not surprisingly, then, few discussions about the ethical issues in the abortion debate attempt to clarify the nature of family issues.

The U.S. Supreme Court decision that created the present framework for abortion policy did not directly address any family issues either. The *Roe* v. *Wade* (1973) opinion viewed the pregnant woman solely "in relation to the fetus within her and unrelated to husband, boyfriend, mother . . . she was conceived atomistically cut off from family structure."[10] Not until the *Danforth* decision in 1976 were the rights of the spouse and of the minor's parent considered, only to be dismissed.

Justice Blackmun wrote in the majority opinion in the *Danforth* case that "the decision whether to undergo or forgo an abortion may have profound effects on the future of any marriage, effects that are both physical and mental, and possibly deleterious."[11] But, he argued, we cannot give the husband the right to veto the woman's decision when the state itself lacks this right. The *Danforth* decision, however, left open the issue of whether parents or husbands should be *notified* of the pregnant woman's request for an abortion. Justices Stewart and Powell, in a concurring but separate opinion, suggested that parental notification, with some procedures for dispute resolution and mature minor exemption, would be constitutionally permissible. And Justice Stevens, dissenting in part, developed an extensive argument supporting parental consent.

---

[7]For an account of the recent multidisciplinary interest in the family, see Wesley Burr and Geoffrey Leigh, "Famology: A New Discipline," *Journal of Marriage and the Family,* August 1983.

[8]In addition to Abbott, see Jean Bethke Elshtain, ed., *The Family in Political Thought* (Amherst: Massachusetts University Press, 1982); and Susan Mueller Okin, *Women in Western Political Thought* (Princeton, N.J.: Princeton University Press, 1981).

[9]Stanley Hauerwas, "The Moral Meaning of the Family," *Commonweal* (August 1980), pp. 432–438.

[10]John T. Noonan, *Private Choice: Abortion in America in the Seventies* (New York: Free Press, 1979), p. 95.

[11]*Planned Parenthood of Central Missouri* v. *Danforth,* 428 U.S. 52 (1976) (Blackmun) C(9a).

The rights of married fathers have been defended on several grounds. One author based his argument on principles of sex discrimination, equal protection, and impairment of the husband's right of procreation.[12] The *Danforth* decision referred to a statement in the original Missouri brief for the Missouri District Court that "any major change in family status is a decision to be made jointly by the marriage partners," and pointed out that, in many states, joint consent requirements were necessary for the adoption of a child born in wedlock, for artificial insemination, and for sterilization. Thus, the challenged law stated, "Recognizing that the consent of both parties is generally necessary . . . to begin a family the legislature has determined that change in the family structure set in motion by mutual consent should be terminated only by mutual consent."[13]

Two U.S. Supreme Court decisions, *Stanley* v. *Illinois* (1972) and *Caban* v. *Mohammed* (1979), concerned the rights of putative fathers in adoption, and in most states today, notification must be given to the putative father of a mother's intent to relinquish her baby for adoption. It is difficult, then, to rationalize why the unmarried father should be consulted about adoption and should be expected to pay child support but should not be given any right to be consulted about aborting his potential child.

These twin issues of husband and parental consent and notification are very much alive. Several states have passed legislation requiring spousal and/or parental notification, and the U.S. Supreme Court reviewed a couple of such laws in the 1982–1983 session. In a 1981 U.S. Supreme Court decision on a Utah case, *H-L* v. *Matheson*, the court left open the possibility that a state parental notification law could be constructed that would be constitutional.[14]

The constitutional issue centers on the concept of family privacy. As Judy Areen, a family lawyer, pointed out:

> Prior to the recent moves to constitutionalize family law, family matters were normally left to the states. States in turn, generally followed a policy of staying out of family matters. There were of course some exceptions to this doctrine of family privacy. Among the more striking were the state laws regulating sexual activities and procreation. . . . The common law doctrine of family privacy became a constitutional standard in 1965. In *Griswold* v. *Connecticut,* Justice Douglas announced for the Court that there is a right of [family] privacy embodied in the penumbras

---

[12]Wesley D. H. Teo, "Abortion: The Husband's Constitutional Rights," *Ethics* 85, no. 4 (July 1975), pp. 337–342.

[13]*Danforth*. (Blackmun) C(8).

[14]*H-L* v. *Matheson*, 450 U.S. 398 (1981).

and emanations of the First, Third, Fourth, Fifth and Ninth Amendments to the Constitution.[15]

In the *Griswold* decision, and seven years later in *Eisenstadt* v. *Baird* (1972), the right to family privacy applied to what a married or an unmarried couple did in the privacy of their bedroom. However, in the latter decision, the right of family privacy became the right of the individual:

> If the right of privacy means anything, it is the right of the *individual*, married or single, to be free from unwarranted government intrusion into matters so fundamentally affecting a person as the decision whether to bear or beget a child.[16]

In these two contraceptive-related cases, the twin concepts of the individual and the family right to privacy were fused. However, as Areen succinctly wrote, "The stage was now set for the conflict the common law had long tried to avoid: a clash between the privacy claims of members of the same family.[17]

Thus, the *Roe* v. *Wade* decision in 1973 extended the right of privacy to include the abortion decision, but "this right is not unqualified and must be considered against important state interests in regulation." These interests were in preserving and protecting the health of the pregnant woman and a separate but distinct interest in protecting the potentiality of human life.[18] The abortion debate deals with the potential conflict between an existing person and a potential person who is totally dependent on her for life and sustenance. Injecting a family perspective into the debate sets up another conflict—between the interests and the constitutional privacy rights of existing persons who are related.

The *Roe* v. *Wade* decision failed to recognize another aspect of family factors involved in an abortion decision. Because the only legitimate state interests in permitting an abortion are the health of the mother, the several family considerations that may weigh heavily in a woman's mind as she struggles to make her decision (e.g., "I am not ready to be a parent"; "We do not have the resources to bring up another child"; "My family will suffer emotionally and economically") are not considered legitimate state interests, that is, legitimate

[15]Judy Areen, *Family Law, Teenage Pregnancy and Divorce Custody Disputes,* unpublished paper prepared for the Family Impact Seminar, Intervention in Family Conflict Project, July 1981.
[16]*Eisenstadt* v. *Baird*, 405 U.S. 438 (1972).
[17]Areen, *Family Law, Teenage Pregnancy.*
[18]*Roe* v. *Wade*, 410 U.S. 113, (Blackmun) VIII.

criteria for permitting abortion. Of course, in practice, the woman's health became broadly interpreted as including her mental and social health, which, in turn, included the stress that she (and her family) would experience if she bore a child.

## JUSTIFICATION FOR FAMILY INVOLVEMENT

*Why* should other family members be given any legal status or moral weight in the abortion dilemma? Two basic principles help guide us toward an answer. First, if it is agreed that the abortion decision is a moral decision—by which I mean that it is not a matter of purely personal choice—then, its effect on others must be considered. (If no other persons were affected, it would not be a moral issue.) Thus, said philosopher L. W. Sumner, in *Abortion and Moral Theory:*

> Moral issues arise when an agent's decision will affect the welfare of others. . . . Even if we leave the dependent person (child who may be born) out of the account, the addition of further individuals in a world of scarce resources cannot fail to affect the well being of at least some independent persons. . . . Thus the pregnant woman must not neglect its impact on others.[19]

Martha Brandt Bolton stated even more clearly how this principle applies to the abortion dilemma:

> It is clear that the decision to have, or not to have, an abortion does not affect the pregnant woman alone. It determines whether or not a new member will be brought into the woman's family, her living situation, and her community. Its outcome stands to affect a wide range of others, favorably or unfavorably; their welfare and interests are at stake.[20]

Moreover, she added, these interests and needs frequently conflict, thus creating the moral conflict between competing obligations.

Second is the basic principle of a political democracy: self-government, or at least representation. "The fundamental principle of a free society is that those who will be affected by the actions and decisions of others ought to have a voice in making those decisions."[21] In the case of abortion, this statement should be qualified

[19]L. W. Sumner, *Abortion and Moral Theory* (Princeton, N.J.: Princeton University Press, 1981), p. 211.
[20]Martha Brandt Bolton, "Responsible Women and Abortion Decisions," in Onora O'Neill and William Ruddick, eds., *Having Children: Philosophical and Legal Reflections on Parenthood* (New York: Oxford University Press, 1979), p. 47.
[21]Daniel Callahan, *Abortion, Law, Choice and Morality* (New York: Macmillan, 1970), p. 466.

to read "those *adults*" most closely affected. (Questions about how the fetus's rights and needs are to be represented and its inability to do so itself could also be discussed at length and, of course, underpin much of the prolife argument, namely, that society and its laws must protect the fetus by proxy.)

Before applying those two principles to my central thesis—that family considerations should be given more weight in the abortion dilemma—we need to ask several critical questions: What evidence do we have of the effects of the abortion decision on family members? Can these effects, as the woman perceives them, constitute legitimate reasons for choosing abortion? Who is best fitted to determine what these reasons are and their legitimacy? And finally, who speaks for the family: the pregnant woman, her physician, or the family members themselves?

## ABORTION DECISION'S IMPACT ON FAMILIES

On the first question, unfortunately we have very little systematic research to draw on, though a number of studies examine the impact of abortion on a woman's personality or psychosexual processes (or offer broad demographic statistics) without regard to her immediate social relationships.[22] There are, however, three published pieces of research that do examine the effects of abortion on a woman's close relationships. Mary K. Zimmerman and Kristin Luker conducted two separate research studies, interviewing 45 and 60 women, respectively, who had had abortions.[23] And Linda Bird Francke has published a very revealing anecdotal account of her interviews with a number of women who had had an abortion, a few couples, and some mothers of pregnant teenagers.[24] All three studies, however, concerned women who opted for abortion, and only Francke interviewed family members. We do not have any comparable studies of adult women who chose to carry the pregnancy to term, after considering and rejecting abortion. We do have a number of studies of teenage mothers, many of whose pregnancies were initially un-

[22]Mary K. Zimmerman, *Passage through Abortion: The Personal and Social Reality of Women's Experiences* (New York: Praeger, 1977), p. 26.
[23]Ibid.; Kristin Luker, *Taking Chances: Abortion and the Decision Not to Contracept* (Berkeley: University of California Press, 1975).
[24]Linda Bird Francke, *The Ambivalence of Abortion* (New York: Random House, 1978).

wanted, where abortion was at one point considered briefly as an option.[25]

To understand the various ways in which family members are affected by the abortion decision, we need to consider both the effects of remaining pregnant and having a child and of deciding to have an abortion.

Obviously, if a married woman decides against an abortion and gives birth, the effects of a new baby on her husband and their other children can range all the way from the very positive to the very negative. But what happens to the close relationships of a single (unmarried) adult woman who chooses to give birth? There is no recent research on this subject. Legally, however, the father of the baby is considered responsible for its financial support—even where, as in the recent New York *Serpico* case, he claims he was tricked into having unprotected sex.[26]

There has been considerable research recently on unmarried teenage mothers. We know that the lives of their parents and siblings, with whom most of them continue to live throughout the pregnancy and first year or two of parenting, are considerably changed. Few teens nowadays use pregnancy as an excuse to get married and leave the parental home. Instead, the parents provide financial support, housing, child care, and usually considerable psychological support. Sometimes, a grandmother may quit her job to care for the baby while the mother returns to school. Though on hearing of their daughter's pregnancy parents usually express a great deal of anger and disappointment, many families report that they feel closer together by the time the baby is born.[27]

Women who choose abortion do not usually do so without telling someone else. In the Zimmerman study 65% of the women had told their male partner or spouse when they first suspected that they were pregnant, and 95% by the time they had the abortion. No woman in Zimmerman's study underwent the abortion process alone. They all were accompanied by the husband, the boyfriend, or some other friend.[28] Not surprisingly, quite often the spouse or the boy-

[25]For example, Frank F. Furstenberg, *Unplanned Parenthood: The Social Consequences of Teenage Childbearing* (New York: Free Press, 1976), and a number of articles reprinted in Frank Furstenberg, Richard Lincoln, and Jane Mencken, eds., *Teenage Sexuality, Pregnancy and Childbearing* (Philadelphia: University of Pennsylvania Press, 1981).

[26]*Pamela, B.* v. *N.Y. Family Court*, 443 NYS2d. 343 (1981).

[27]Frank Furstenberg, "Implicating the Family: Teenage Parenthood and Kinship Involvement," in Theodora Ooms, ed., *Teenage Pregnancy in a Family Context: Implications for Policy* (Philadelphia: Temple University Press, 1981), pp. 131–164.

[28]Zimmerman, pp. 81, 113.

friend had a different view about abortion from that of the woman, which he may or may not have expressed.[29] But apart from the stress, anxiety, and possible conflict around the decision and the event itself, these few studies indicate that an abortion can have dramatic and long-term effects on the couple's relationship. In 55% of Zimmerman's cases, the women experienced a severe disruption in an important relationship, usually with the man.[30] Francke detailed some poignant stories of the deep hurt or rifts between married couples and between parents and teenage girls, though other women in the sample brushed the experience off quite casually. Francke also reported that several potential grandparents were deeply affected and hurt by the abortion and were grieved at the loss of a potential grandchild.[31]

One way of avoiding distress and anger is to keep the abortion a secret from the person whose reaction is feared (a husband or, more usually, a parent). The woman might then claim that an abortion would not affect her family relationships. Apart from the subtle and often destructive long-term effects of such deception, especially when the woman lives with a parent, this solution raises two other problems. First, the husband or boyfriend or parent who is tied biologically to the fetus has been deprived of the chance to express his or her views about being a parent or a grandparent, and to influence the decision. Sissela Bok reported on one study that claimed that, among those couples reporting, at least one parent did *not* want the child; in half of these cases, at least one parent *did* want the child.[32] Second, and more important, the pregnant woman or teenager may have made her decision to abort or to keep the baby based on misinformation, or wrong assumptions about how her parents or her spouse would react or be affected. This point is discussed below.

The second major question is: What kinds of family reasons can be considered legitimate grounds for an abortion? Beyond the studies quoted above, we have little research information on the reasons that women give for deciding on abortion. These, however, provide ample evidence that a woman rarely decides to have an abortion for reasons of her own physical health. In the Zimmerman study, financial inability to support a (or another) child was most frequently cited, followed by "the time was not right to have a baby" (or another

---

[29]Francke, pp. 161, 168.
[30]Zimmerman, pp. 189–190.
[31]Francke, pp. 211–223.
[32]Sissela Bok, *Ethical Problems of Abortion,* Hastings Center Studies, vol. 1, no. 1 (January 1974), p. 48.

baby right now)—a convenience factor.[33] In other words, in her judgment, she was either not ready to be a parent and to form a family, or the circumstances (such as being single) were not propitious, or her present family could not stand the stress, or the drain, of a new child on their financial or emotional resources.

The reasons range, as Bok noted, from those that most would recognize as compelling to those that most would think of as frivolous.[34] (Francke described several in both categories.) Consider the woman who learns from amniocentesis that she will bear a seriously defective child. In the view of many, this is a compelling reason for abortion: Such a child would put an intolerable stress on the family. Yet, many families are able to cope well with a retarded or handicapped child. In using family factors such as these, the pregnant woman is making a prediction about how she, and/or her family, will care for the baby: The difficulty is that some women make a very realistic assessment, whereas others may be unaware of their own or their families' coping abilities and resources, or of what unexpected joys or benefits may accrue. In judging the morality of her decision, how does one then decide which reasons are compelling and which are not? Or which women are good predictors and which are not? Can we develop guidelines, as Bok suggested, that might help such women make this decision? Given the diversity of family situations, circumstances, and values, how would this be possible?

## PARENT AND SPOUSE NOTIFICATION

This brief review of the family factors involved in an abortion decision leads to the third family question: How can the relevant family members' interests, concerns, and wishes best be ascertained? And when there are differences between the pregnant woman and her family, how can these disputes be resolved?

The first question seems simple: If a pregnant woman cites family factors (the reaction of her mother or her spouse, her lack of financial resources, and so on) as reasons for considering abortion, this belief should at least be checked out directly with the relevant family members. (There is no reason to believe that a strange physician or clinic counselor would know how her family would react.) In fact, this is what happens with the majority of adult pregnant women who do tell their spouses or male partners. However, Francke's interviews

[33]Zimmerman, p. 139.
[34]Bok, p. 45.

with a few of these men suggest that they do not always feel free to express their views, in part because they believe (interpreting the law accurately) that their views carry no legal weight, and that "It's basically her decision anyway." These unexpressed views can often fester, a fact that led Francke to wonder whether abortion counseling should not always involve the couple, presumably in order to draw the male partner's feelings into the open and to help the couple negotiate and talk through their differences.[35] It would be helpful to have more research on the male's feelings and experiences of an abortion dilemma and decision.

In the case of teenagers, we know that many who get abortions do not tell their parents. In fact, one of their major reasons for choosing abortion is fear of their parents' reaction.[36] This situation is regrettable, especially when the girl herself believes that abortion is an immoral act. Again, experience indicates that the great majority of parents, after initial shock and anger, end up being quite supportive, which suggests that teenagers should inform their parents despite their fears.[37]

To claim, as I do, that family members have an interest in the abortion decision is not to say that the family members' interests or views should carry *equal* weight with the pregnant woman's. I would agree with the *Danforth* decision that neither spouse nor parent should veto a woman's decision, but I do believe that they should have a chance to influence and to debate it with her. As Bok said:

> ... into her decision should go the awareness of the heavy price she will have to pay in the relationship with the father if she aborts their unborn child against his wishes. ... The father's reasons for wishing to continue the pregnancy should be given due weight, especially if he wants to share responsibility and care after birth.[38]

It is not clear whether Bok was talking here about the unmarried father as well, but one wonders how many unmarried pregnant women would be willing to go through the pregnancy and the birth in order to give up a baby that they definitely do not want to a father who *does* want the child and promises to care for it? The putative father, who has no legal relationship to the pregnant woman, is related to her through his blood tie with the fetus, through his potential fa-

[35]Francke, p. 151.
[36]Raye Hudson Rosen, "Help or Hindrance: Parental Impact on Pregnant Teenagers' Resolution Decision," *Family Relations* 30, no. 2 (April 1982), pp. 271–280.
[37]For a more lengthy discussion of the pros and cons of parental notification, see Theodora Ooms, "Family Involvement, Notification and Responsibility," in Ooms, ed., *Teenage Pregnancy*, Chapter 12.
[38]Bok, p. 48.

therhood. Does the father then have a moral right to ask her to go through the physical and emotional stress of pregnancy and childbirth so that he can raise his child? For me, this is a very difficult question.

Curiously, most discussions about informing the parent or the spouse assume that this process may curb the number of abortions because the legal issue of notification arises only when the pregnant woman has already requested an abortion and the informed family member *may* persuade her to change her mind. However, in my view, other family members should be informed at the point when the woman first has confirmation of her pregnancy. At this stage, she may still be quite ambivalent, and the views of her husband, boy-friend, or parents are more likely to carry weight in her decision. To the best of my knowledge, none of the current legal notification laws or proposals suggest this approach.

Many who find the argument quite persuasive up to this point will insist that family members should be informed on a voluntary basis only: The pregnant woman should be encouraged to talk her decision over with her husband or parent. Mandatory notification conjures up specters of spouse or child abuse and violates notions of patient confidentiality. The fear is that the angry parent or husband would become excessively violent and might exert undue pressure on the pregnant woman. Although this may occasionally happen, I believe it is a mistake to design our laws based on worst-case examples that apply only to the very few. The onus should be on the pregnant woman to cite evidence why this notification could result in her being seriously abused (or why notification does not apply because the pregnancy is the result of rape or a very casual encounter).

Conflict, argument, anger, and violence are, however regretta-bly, an integral part of family life in America. And it has never been the state's role to protect family members from disagreements with each other. Gradually, however, we have adopted some fairly broad standards and have set up better—but far from perfect—procedures and services for state intervention when an adult or a child needs to be protected from serious violence or abuse. These standards and procedures should be applied to the situation of the pregnant woman.

An additional point that relates to family integrity and autonomy was made by Justice Stevens in a partial dissent to the *Danforth* decision. In his view, the state's "interest in having parents involved in the decision making process was quite independent of any estimate of the impact of parental consent on the total number of abortions.[39] In other words, if one believes that family members need to take

[39]*Danforth* (Stevens partial dissent).

some part in the decision, one must also respect the outcome of that process of family decision making. Thus, as some will surely choose abortion, the family perspective that I have thus far outlined requires that abortion should remain legal (at least, within certain parameters). Few prochoice activists, however, would accept this compromise.

## THE OPTION OF ADOPTION

If the baby is unwanted by the biological parents, an alternative to abortion is giving the unwanted baby up for adoption. The evidence at the moment is that pregnant women, especially teenagers, do not consider adoption a viable alternative to either abortion or keeping the baby. Teenagers say, "After I have carried my baby for nine months inside me, I couldn't give it *away*," as if this would be an act of rejection. But there is some evidence that agencies that develop special programs to present adoption as a real option for pregnant teenagers (such as asking families who have adopted to join in discussions with pregnant teens) have some success in helping girls to decide that the way to show their love for their baby is to give it parents who are longing for a child and are able to care for it.

Adoption statistics are virtually nonexistent in this country. We have no records of the number of legal or illegal adoptions each year, or of the number of parents wanting to adopt. The general impression is that there are large numbers of couples waiting to adopt babies, including black families. Thus, the supply of adoptive homes is ample (at least, for young, healthy babies). This fact places the abortion decision in a different moral context. If an unwanted pregnancy could result in a happy adoption, how can the pregnant woman decide that abortion is the right decision? Do we have a moral right to expect a woman to undergo the risks and stress of pregnancy and birth and then place her baby for adoption, thereby avoiding the tragic choice of killing her fetus?

I am inclined to say that we do, but this points again to the need to change agency practices and the general climate and opinion about the adoption option.

## PROLIFE AND PROCHOICE VIEWS OF THE FAMILY

The debate between prolife and prochoice is usually expressed in individual rights language as a conflict between the autonomy of the individual woman and the right to life of the individual fetus.

Both positions are, in Daniel Callahan's terms, "one value solutions
. . . arguing that the problem is not one of balancing a variety of
values but of defending and promoting one transcendent value."[40]
In their debates, the nod to family concerns is a token one.

Though the prochoice proponents do not rest their central arguments on any explicit family considerations, they sometimes point
out the undesirability of a child's being "unwanted": This could be
described as a family argument, as they are asserting that being wanted
is a critical ingredient in family functioning. This argument does not,
in my view and in the view of others, hold up under close scrutiny.[41]

Prochoicers, I think, take it for granted that many women want
to have abortions for "family reasons," not just on the grounds of
their own physical and mental health or convenience; but they do
not talk very much about what these family factors are. In fact, much
prochoice language emphasizing a woman's "control over her own
body" and her "reproductive rights" suggests that a pregnant woman
is primarily concerned with her own needs. But many women, especially those who are married and have children, may be thinking
more of their obligations toward the other people who are dependent
on them. Even an unmarried woman may not be acting selfishly—
she may long to have a child—but may consider it unfair to bring a
child up in a single-parent family. The prochoicers might garner
stronger support if they sounded less selfish and expressed their
arguments, where appropriate, more in terms of family responsibility.

Carol Gilligan, a psychologist, carefully listened to how women
described their feelings, their dilemmas, and their moral conflict
concerning the abortion decision.[42] She found that they emphasized
care, responsibilities, and relationships and used terms such as "selfish" or "self-sacrificing." These women's moral concepts do not jibe
with the current framework and language of the abortion debate,
which in Gilligan's view is threaded through with men's moral conceptions about rights, justice, and fairness. Her book provides con-

---

[40]Callahan, p. 1.

[41]See especially Callahan, p. 455, and Juliet Cheetham, *Unwanted Pregnancy and
Counselling* (London: Routledge, Kegan Paul, 1977), where she noted: ". . . this
is a complicated and muddled world where unplanned pregnancies may be wanted,
where wanted children may emerge from unwanted pregnancies, where the offspring of wanted pregnancies may be rejected, where infatuation with infants grows
cold and where children may be wanted solely to meet their parents' pathological
needs" (p. 3).

[42]Carol Gilligan, *In a Different Voice: Psychological Theory and Women's Development*
(Cambridge: Harvard University Press, 1982).

siderable evidence that women's moral thinking is different from men's, and that women's moral problems arise from conflicting responsibilities rather than from competing rights.

Two prochoice writers and philosophers, Daniel Callahan and Sissela Bok, have argued cogently for the rights of fathers and parents of teenagers to have some part in the abortion decision[43]; however, the prochoice movement has been adamantly opposed to any *legal* requirement that would give a voice to the spouse, boyfriend, or minor's parents. Physicians or counselors may encourage the pregnant woman to tell the "significant other," but on a voluntary basis only. And existing counseling manuals give very little guidance on *how* to counsel the couple, and on what to do if the pregnant woman and her partner or pregnant daughter and parent disagree over the decision.

It seems ironic, as prolife advocate Bernard Nathanson pointed out, that the feminists who have pushed so hard to have men included in the birth process and in child care should deny males the right to be involved in the abortion decision.[44] Although feminists are correct in insisting that the consequences of sex have to date been borne almost exclusively by women, campaigning for free access to clinics that offer only female methods of birth control and for women's autonomy over the abortion decision would seem to encourage the very male disengagement and irresponsibility that they deplore.[45] (Bok, Callahan, Manier, and Lui have made this same point.[46])

The core of the prolife position on abortion is, likewise, based on individual rights: this time, the paramount right of the fetus. However, in various conservative and prolife writings, attention is paid to the family issue; certainly, in the political rhetoric and jargon, *prolife* and *profamily* have recently become almost synonymous.

Prolifers are curiously silent, however, about whether any family reasons might be considered weighty—even if not overriding—indications for abortion. Their writings are imbued with a romantic and totally positive view of the value of children and motherhood; it seems difficult for them to empathize with women with large families who are living in overwhelming conditions of poverty and stress, and who have negative experiences as parents. Luker suggested that those involved in the prolife movement have not had much personal

[43]Callahan, p. 466; Bok, p. 48.
[44]Bernard Nathanson, *Aborting America* (New York: Doubleday, 1979), pp. 256–257.
[45]Nathanson, p. 257.
[46]Edward Manier and William Lui, eds., *Abortion: New Directions for Policy Studies*. (University of Notre Dame Press, 1977), p. 174.

experience with families living in extreme poverty.[47] (We learn from several sources,[48] however, that only a very small percentage of abortions are a result of a request from the "overburdened tired mother.") Luker also learned that a good number of prolife activists have had direct experience with handicap—but this makes them more, not less, determined to protect the life of handicapped fetuses.

Prolifers are strong advocates for the rights of the other family members to be part of the decision-making process. Recent "pro-family" legislation, such as the Family Protection Act, and conferences such as the American Family Forum include in their incoherent list of profamily actions both parental and spouse consent for and notification of abortion and, in the case of minors, contraceptives. John Noonan cited several U.S. Supreme Court decisions conferring a number of other rights on unmarried fathers and then said, "It could reasonably be argued that, if biology conferred rights, a father had as much interest in the unborn child of eight weeks as in an infant of eight months."[49] Nathanson emphasized that, because the man is equally involved in the sex act, he should be held accountable for its result, although "since abortion is legal, the father should probably not have an absolute veto, but he absolutely must not be excluded. Notification of the abortion plan should be a minimum requirement." He believes there are no arguments at all for forbidding notification of a minor's parents. "Thus," he concluded, "has the Court unravelled the family."[50]

The prolifers' support of family rights, it seems, is a contingent one. A major underlying assumption of their arguments for at least notifying the husband or the parent of a teenager is that doing so would result in a smaller number of abortions. We have no evidence to prove whether this prediction is valid. If husbands, boyfriends, or parents were notified of the *fact of the pregnancy* at an earlier stage, there could be more or at least as many abortions as now.[51] (In the case of teens, a mother is frequently more realistic than her pregnant daughter about the effect of giving birth on her daughter's life and is likely to urge her daughter, however reluctantly, to abort. Too

[47]Kristin Luker, *Abortion and the Politics of Motherhood* (Berkeley: University of California, 1984). Also see Chapter 2 in this volume.
[48]Including Mary Ann Lamanna, "Science and Its Uses: the Abortion Debate and Social Research," in James T. Burchaell, ed., *Abortion Parley* (New York: Andrew and McMeel, 1980), pp. 99–158.
[49]Noonan, p. 91.
[50]Nathanson, pp. 256–257.
[51]See Ooms, *Teenage Pregnancy,* p. 384.

often, however, mothers are informed by their daughters when it is too late to get a safe abortion.)

Do conservatives, when they argue for family involvement, genuinely respect the family members' rights to make a decision, even if their involvement results in more abortion? Do they really respect *family* privacy, or only when the resulting decision agrees with prolife morality on abortion? If the latter is true, as I suspect, then in this important sense, they are *not* profamily.

Underlying the prolife position is a set of deeply held values about sexual morality and family life. The prolife banner symbolizes their dislike and disapproval of the behavior and the attitudes that are associated with (and, in their minds, caused or at least encouraged by) liberal abortion laws: Premarital and extramarital sex, for example. In addition, conservatives in general tend to value the traditional sex-role divisions within the family and to hold up patriarchal structures as the ideal[52]; abortion threatens this ideal by giving greater control to women over their lives, and by making it easier for women to enter the marketplace and to function at home on more egalitarian terms.

Thus, the abortion controversy, which on first examination appears to be a conflict between two individualistic philosophies, is also, after all, a conflict between two different ideals of family life. The prochoice position, to the extent that it leans on feminist ideology, stakes out a claim to a vision of a more egalitarian, less burdensome, and more "free" form of family life—one that Jean Bethke Elshtain fears could become "family deconstruction,"[53] and the prolife position clings to the traditional patriarchal model. In these extreme versions, both ideals of the family seem irrelevant to modern times, to the real-life, varied experiences of today's families.

## THE SPECIAL NATURE OF FAMILY RELATIONSHIPS

The prolife assertion that abortion is antifamily may reflect something important about the special nature of family relationships that the prochoice advocates have ignored. I believe that prolifers strongly resist the idea of *choice* and impermanence in family affairs in part because they realize that it is the involuntary nature of family

[52]For an elaborate New Right argument based on a curious view of economic history, see George Gilder, *Wealth and Poverty* (New York: Basic Books, 1981), Chapter 6, pp. 68–74.
[53]Jean Bethke Elshtain, "Family Reconstruction," *Commonweal* (August 1980), pp. 430–431.

relationships and the permanence of family commitments that distinguish families from other groups and associations. This feeling has not been well articulated by their writers, with the exception of Stanley Hauerwas:

> We tend to forget that the family has traditionally not been rooted in contract but in biology . . . the great strength of the family has everywhere been consanguineal rather than conjugal. And here not affection, but duty, obligation, honor, mutual aid, and protection have been the key elements.[54]

Judith Jarvis Thomson, in her well-known philosophical defense of the prochoice position, was surely mistaken about family relationships when she said, "Surely we do not have any special responsibility for a person unless we have assumed it explicitly or implicitly"; she added that parents "do not simply by virtue of their biological relationship to the child who comes into existence have a special responsibility for it. They may wish to assume responsibility for it or they may not wish to."[55] She was talking about their relationship to the fetus, but the statement can also be applied, on her premises, to a newborn.

The Christian marriage service statement "for richer for poorer, in sickness and in health" is what family relationships are, at their core, all about. Of course, good families require more than this: Affection, love, and what Urie Bronfenbrenner has called "an irrational, intense, enduring commitment." When these qualities exist, children are more likely to thrive, and other family members flourish also. But even in less-than-ideal circumstances, we do not choose to give our family members away. Of course, sometimes we fail: There are child and spouse abusers, too many "throwaway" and "runaway" children whose parents do, in essence, give them away, and parents who petition the courts to take over the guardianship of their "incorrigible" child. But we think of these situations as failures, not as the result of the exercise of "free choice."

The rapid rise in divorce, however, has begun to change our notions of the special nature of family relationships, and we seem to be moving closer to the social contract theory of family, at least with regard to the marriage relationship.[56] In marriage, we are now saying, if the other person does not "fit" our needs, we can choose to "give him/her back," to "undo" the family tie. This, of course, is just what

---

[54]Hauerwas, p. 434.
[55]Judith Jarvis Thomson, "A Defence of Abortion," in *Philosophy and Public Affairs*, 1, no. 1 (Fall 1971), (Princeton, N.J.: Princeton University Press, 1971).
[56]Abbott, p. 293, who critiques this trend.

we do when we choose abortion: When having a child does not "fit" with our plans, or the child will not be perfect, we proceed to "undo" the family tie. (Because divorce is also a fundamental threat to these traditional notions of family, it seems strange that we do not find the prolifers campaigning against divorce as intensely as against abortion. The reason is possibly that in divorce it is harder to establish an innocent, vulnerable party whom the prolife, "profamily" movement can defend.)

It may indeed be that we have come too far and are in danger of losing and forgetting the distinctive "special" aspects of family relationships.

Although the conservatives' analysis has usefully drawn attention to some real problems in the present trends in our society, their diagnosis of the origins of these problems is wrong, and their prescriptions for cure are unrealistic and backward-looking. We need to find a way of redressing the balance and realizing that, if we want to have the benefits of family life (caring, intimacy, love, guidance), we need to commit ourselves more strongly to relationships and accept circumstances, such as unwanted pregnancy, that we might not freely "choose." We need, as Elshtain said, to find a way of "reconstructing" the family[57] that encompasses greater equality within the marriage, individual autonomy, and control over the size and economic circumstances of one's family, without sacrificing commitment, obligation, responsibility, and acceptance that are the essence of family relationships.

## TOWARD A FAMILY-CENTERED ABORTION POLICY

My development of a family perspective as applied to the abortion issue leads me to three immediate conclusions.

First, certain family members have a right to be involved, through notification, in the decision about a woman's pregnancy. But involvement does not mean a veto. The pregnant woman must, for ethical and practical reasons, take the final responsibility for making the decision. No one can or should force her to have an abortion or to be a parent, and no one can or should force her to take care of herself during her pregnancy.

Second, the effects of the abortion decision on the family are legitimate moral criteria and may thus constitute sufficient justification, in a particular case, for an abortion.

[57]Elshtain, 1980.

Third, the existence in the United States today of a supply of
✓ adoptive families that are eager to give homes to babies profoundly
influences the context of moral decision making about abortion.

Abortion is always a tragic choice. But although I believe that
taking away life from a potential person and family member is a
moral wrongdoing, it may sometimes be the least bad alternative.

In America today, where some, though not abundant, resources
are available to assist women during pregnancy and child rearing,
and where adoption is available for all healthy babies, few circumstances would make abortion the least bad alternative. However, in
our pluralistic society, where there is so much confusion, uncertainty,
and disagreement about which circumstances are justified, it is unwise
to attempt to codify into law in which precise circumstances abortion
would be justified. Thus, I believe that the present law permitting
abortion—within certain parameters—should stand, with some
minor though important modifications that I will specify.

If these changes were made, some, and probably many, abortions
would continue to take place that I personally feel are wrong and
not justifiable. However, government at all levels, together with
voluntary agencies and the public, can put more energy and resources
into trying to prevent unwanted pregnancies and should encourage
and support women and their families to consider the alternatives.
Several of the moderate prolife individuals and organizations have
made this point repeatedly and eloquently.[58] And yet, although few
prochoice advocates or supporters are at ease with the present rates
of abortion, the numbers of teenage abortions, and the rates of repeated abortions, the prochoice movement has not on the whole
responded to this challenge or joined in constructive discussion and
debate about how these goals should best be accomplished.

I will briefly discuss four components of such an effort that
follow from this family perspective.

## MODIFICATION OF THE EXISTING LEGAL FRAMEWORK

The present constitutional framework for permitting abortion
should be modified so that:

- The rights and interests of the pregnant woman's family (narrowly defined) are considered legitimate interests for state

[58]For example, see Marjory Mecklenburg, *An Examination of Life Supportive Policies
in the Public and Voluntary Sectors,* a statement by the then president of American
Citizens Concerned for Life, Inc., before the Subcommittee on Constitutional
Amendments, Senate Committee on the Judiciary, 19 June 1975.

protection in addition to the present state concern about the health of the mother and the potential life of the fetus.

- The physician, or designate, should be responsible for informing the appropriate family members of the confirmation of pregnancy and should offer them and the pregnant woman counselors trained to assist them in making decisions about the pregnancy, and in any disputes that might arise between family members within the framework of protecting the woman's right to make the decision.

- If the pregnant woman claims that such notification would result in serious harm to her, and/or if she claims that her fetus was a result of rape or a casual encounter, then she should be asked to designate an (adult) representative from her extended family, friends, or community to serve as a surrogate for the parent/partner/spouse.[59]

These suggestions would result in a law that would be a flexible and sensitive instrument: Is this a contradiction in terms? Would such a legal framework be practical? Could it be implemented? Not being a lawyer, I am on shaky ground here. But I am impressed with a recent example of the implementation of a Massachusetts notification and consent law for minors that was a result of the *Bellotti and Baird* U.S. Supreme Court decision of 1980. The court decision called forth voluntary legal and community resources that successfully facilitated prompt recourse to a court hearing in an informal and nonburdensome way for pregnant minors who did not want to inform their parents and claimed mature minor status.[60] I believe my suggestion of a surrogate parent from her community who knows the woman would be both easier to implement and more constructive than recourse to a strange judge.

The requirement of providing trained counselors is much more difficult to implement, but it might be approached by the next suggestion.

## TRAINING OF PREGNANCY COUNSELORS

A national council, or several councils, should be established (with joint public and private funding) to study the current status of pregnancy counseling and to recommend guidelines for training

---

[59]See Ooms, "Family Involvement," p. 388.
[60]Patricia Donovan, "Your Parents or the Judge: Massachusetts' New Abortion Consent Law," *Family Planning Perspectives* 13, no. 5 (September–October 1981), pp. 224–227.

counselors to work in all facilities that provide medically adminis-tered pregnancy testing. Ideally, the members of this council should represent all major religious denominations and all views on abortion. The guidelines could spell out the ethical issues that follow from a variety of basic religious beliefs or value systems. They should in-clude information about what other options and financial and service resources are available.

The lack of skills and the bias of the counseling currently offered by abortion clinics and the nonexistence of counseling in many for-profit clinics have been criticized by prolife groups and others, and these criticisms deserve study.[61]

More serious, in my view, is the timing: Most counseling comes too late, after the woman has basically made up her mind. Imple-menting this suggestion would be an expensive, ambitious, and com-plex task. It might also be difficult to get prolife groups to work cooperatively with those who believe that abortion is sometimes permissible.

## ADOPTION AS AN ALTERNATIVE

Agencies, clinics, and private offices that offer pregnancy testing and counseling should be made aware of adoption procedures and services, and in particular of the many new efforts currently being developed to present adoption as a morally viable alternative to teenagers. The National Committee for Adoption and other groups could be very helpful in developing and disseminating this kind of information.[62] Their efforts should not concentrate only on pregnant teens, however: Adult women, many of whom now resort to abor-tion, should also be informed about adoption.

## PREVENTION OF UNWANTED PREGNANCY

Many more efforts and resources need to be directed toward preventing "unwanted" pregnancy, and these should emphasize strongly that men are equally responsible for prevention. In the past few years, community-based agencies, including a number of youth-serv-ing agencies, have been developing (largely with the support of pri-vate funding) community awareness, sex education, and family-plan-

---

[61]Juliet Cheetham, "Alternatives to Termination—Making the Decision," *British Journal of Family Planning* 8 (1982), pp. 101–104; Mecklenburg, 1975.

[62]The National Committee for Adoption in Washington, D.C., provides information and advocacy on adoption through a variety of reports, a newsletter, conferences, and other activities.

ning activities, which should be continued and encouraged. (Unfortunately, the politicization of sex education, and of the invaluable family-planning programs, has placed federal and state funding of these efforts in jeopardy.)

Some of these efforts are attempting to involve teenage males. But society as a whole, the media, and the structure and direction of funding for contraceptive research and family-planning services continue to assume that women should bear the responsibility for pregnancy prevention.

If we are to recognize the limited rights of the male partner in abortion decisions, then it is even more important to insist that he also bear equal responsibility for preventing unwanted pregnancy.[63] The difficulty of implementing this goal should not be underestimated.

Neither mediation nor compromise is possible on the abortion issue as long as we accept the terms of the debate as defined by the polar positions of prolife and prochoice: as being between two mutually exclusive individual rights and two radically differing ideals of family life. However, the great, and largely inactive, majority appear to be in broad general agreement. Numerous polls, as Lamanna pointed out, demonstrate that most people do want to protect and respect fetal life yet also agree that abortion should sometimes be permissible. It would be a pity if efforts were now to concentrate on attempts to define—and then codify—what these permissible circumstances should be. This approach would surely lead to a no-win situation. Instead, the search, the discussion, and the debate should focus on the processes and procedures that would best balance and reconcile the competing interests of individuals, families, and the community as well as encouraging more responsible moral decision making and a choice of alternatives so that abortion becomes truly a last resort.[64]

[63]I am grateful to my colleague Susan Brown for this point.
[64]The development of my ideas in this essay owes a great deal to the discussions in our two project meetings. I especially want to thank Mary Segers, for drawing my attention to several relevant articles, and Mary Mahowald, for her initial helpful critique.

# Commentary to Chapter 4

## MARY B. MAHOWALD

That *prolife* and *prochoice* labels are much too simplistic to accommodate the subtleties of a carefully reasoned argument on abortion is abundantly clear in Theodora Ooms's approach to the issue. Her focus on the family, with its critique of individualistic elements on both sides of the debate, represents a sane and realistic alternative to the extreme positions. Moreover, her proposal of the family as mediator between individual and social values may be viewed as both radical and conservative in its implications. It is conservative of the root value of the family itself, by which individuals throughout time have sought to develop their unique identities; it is radical in that it challenges that variety of individualism which our culture recommends.

Although agreeing with Ooms's criticisms of individualism, I think her critique has not gone far enough. In fact, a more subtle form of individualism may underlie an emphasis on family values. Further, there is a basic inconsistency between Ooms's advocacy of "squeal" legislation (such as the Akron ordinance, ruled unconstitutional by the U.S. Supreme Court) and support for the right of a pregnant woman to choose abortion.[1] That right also seems compromised by Ooms's suggestion that the wishes of the putative father or the possible adoptive couple might determine the outcome of abortion decisions. Before developing any of these points at greater length, however, I would like to consider the basic category of Ooms's proposals: The family unit.

---

[1]Cf. *City of Akron* v. *Akron Center for Reproductive Health, Inc.*, No. 81–746, as cited in *The United States Law Week*, Supreme Court Proceedings 51 (4768), Bureau of National Affairs, Inc., Washington, June 14, 1983. What has been popularly labeled *squeal legislation* by the media is the requirement that minors seeking abortion first obtain parental or judicial consent for abortions. Ooms, however, advocates parental notification rather than consent.

---

MARY B. MAHOWALD ● School of Medicine, Case Western Reserve University, Cleveland, Ohio 44106.

## THE FAMILY

At the outset, Ooms defines the family as "those persons most closely related by blood, marriage, or adoption to the pregnant woman and the fetus." She then specifies the persons about whom she is concerned: the pregnant woman's "spouse or the expectant father or, if she is an adolescent, her parents." Ooms's use of the disjunctive *or* here (between references to the expectant father and the adolescent's parents) may mean that she intends only one or the other side of the disjunction to be recognized as family. In other words, whom one counts as family members depends on whether the pregnant woman is an adolescent or not. Yet, the individuals on both sides of the disjunction may be relevant to adolescents as well as to adults considering the option of abortion. For example, responsibilities to an elderly parent may be a significant factor for a pregnant adult; and the responsibility *to* (as well as *of*) the expectant father may be relevant to a pregnant teenager. Possibly, Ooms is less concerned about adults who seek abortions than about adolescents, about whom she has written elsewhere.[2] However, only about one third of those who have abortions are younger than 19 years old.[3] Among the remaining two thirds are some adults for whom marriage and family are irrelevant considerations because their primary support systems are not based on blood, marriage, or adoption. There are also adults, both married and unmarried, for whom other children figure more prominently in abortion decisions than do their male partners.[4]

In some cases, the spectrum of those who count as a family unit is so narrow that it comprises only the pregnant woman and her fetus, for example, where a pregnancy is the result of a casual encounter between single, independent adults. Unless the fetus is construed as an actual rather than a potential person, it hardly seems appropriate to view "family considerations" as relevant in such a situation. A similar problem arises with regard to possible adoptive parents, as actual beings surely have a stronger claim to moral standing than do merely possible beings of the same species. Moreover, even when the pregnant woman is married, her husband may not be

---

[2]Theodora Ooms, ed., *Teenage Pregnancy in a Family Context* (Philadelphia: Temple University Press, 1981).

[3]Cf. Centers for Disease Control, *Abortion Surveillance, 1978,* issued November 1980 by U.S. Department of Health and Human Services. These figures are applicable only in the United States for the year reported.

[4]According to the above government report, the following are the pertinent figures for those who had abortions in 1978: 26.4% were married, 73.6% were unmarried, and 43.4% already had children.

responsible for the pregnancy. When she is thus a member of two couples, it is unclear which "family" concerns are paramount if there is conflict. Responsibilities to close friends or to one's profession may also take precedence over a duty to those related by blood. Consider a lifelong friend dependent on a pregnant woman for emotional or material support; or consider professional commitments that deeply affect the lives of others, as in medicine or the ministry. Surely, such nonfamilial ties are also pertinent to abortion decisions.

Because the families affected by pregnancies (whether defined by blood, by adoption, or by marriage) are often multiple and overlapping, we cannot neatly draw concentric circles illustrating a priority of familial responsibilities from the innermost circle outward. True, there are at the center a pregnant woman and her fetus, but the possible family configurations that proceed from that center are so numerous that "family emphasis" is utterly vague beyond the center. Whatever the configuration, however, one factor is pertinent: These concerns play a part in the morality of abortion decisions. So also do the social configurations that arise from other-than-familial reasons: friendships, religious or political commitments, and so on. Unfortunately, Ooms's emphasis on the family ignores these other ties, with which family interests may conflict.

## AN EXTENDED INDIVIDUALISM

Ooms deserves credit for pointing out the antifamily elements in the popular prolife view of abortion, as well as the inegalitarian or sexist interpretation of family roles that that view assumes. However, her critique does not recognize that an emphasis on a traditional or nuclear family may be a not-too-subtly disguised individualism in its own right. Instead of looking out exclusively for the interests of the pregnant woman *or* the fetus, as do many on either side of the abortion issue, this extended form of individualism entails looking out exclusively for a single family unit, that is, a man, a woman, and their children. Because one family's wealth or welfare may be obtained at the price of another's, all sorts of chauvinistic behaviors may be justified in the name of such family individualism. If the fetus counts as a family member, then abortion is never permissible on the basis of the pregnant woman's wishes alone, or on the basis of social costs, for example, in cases of severe fetal defect. If the fetus does not count as a family member, the abortion of a healthy, viable fetus is permissible even for trivial reasons, such as the convenience of a family member. In either case, family interests would overrule social responsibility to the fetus as a separable, valuable individual, whether person or not.

It seems to me that an excessive emphasis on the family, especially in its biological caste, tends to limit the autonomy of individual women deciding for or against abortion. Typically, young women are socialized into thinking that they are primarily, even exclusively, responsible for the fate of the fetus, as well as for any future child. Where their own immaturity, economic instability, or a serious fetal defect makes it impossible for them to care for a future child, their range of options is obviously restricted by these factors. A family support system *may* increase the options available to the pregnant woman, but reliance on that system places her in a position of dependence on family members. If our social structure and our socialization process were such that pregnancy was generally acknowledged as a contribution and a burden to be shared even beyond the family community, her options would then be broadened; clearly, she would not be as alone and limited in her decision as individualistic or even family considerations suggest.

My own view is that all moral decisions are social, but they are not always familial. Especially when the pregnant person is a minor, dependence on family has sometimes exerted considerable pressure to choose a course in conflict with her own moral conviction. I am thinking, for example, of a case in which the parents of a seriously ill young woman threatened to cut off necessary support if she were to continue her pregnancy. Eventually, the woman acquiesced to her family's wishes, but such acquiescence is hardly interpretable as a free decision. As Ooms points out, then, a profamily position is not necessarily prolife. However, neither position is necessarily moral because "family," like "life," is often, but not always, a *good* to be promoted. Neither, in other words, is an absolute value.

Ooms's critique of the individualism expressed on both sides of the abortion debate would be strengthened, I believe, by a fuller treatment of what such individualism entails, and why it is wrong. The philosopher Josiah Royce once explained a distinction between individualism and individuality that is apropos. Individuality, as he described it, refers to the unique core of someone's personality, the congruence of characteristics that makes the individual distinctive and unrepeatable. In contrast, individualism entails an attempt to extend and enrich that core of uniqueness by pursuing the goal of a "separate, happy self."[5] Unfortunately and ironically, this ideal of individuality is unrealizable because ongoing social interactions are

[5]See Josiah Royce, *The Religious Aspect of Philosophy* (Boston: Houghton Mifflin, 1885), p. 201.

essential to the fulfillment of individuals as such. Their individuality will ultimately be stifled rather than developed through purely individualistic pursuits. Thus, the genuine community that is essential to the full flowering of individuality is at odds with individualism.

Applied to the abortion issue, an exclusive emphasis on the right to life of the fetus or on the right to choose of the pregnant woman ignores the social fabric with which both are inextricably interwoven. To treat the pregnant woman as an isolated individual, standing alone in her decision, is insulting in that it strips her of the very context that is integral to her identity. It may be less insulting to define her identity in the limited context of her family. The reality to address, however, is that the pregnant woman stands at the center of multiple social relationships, some of which may be deeper than familial. The fulfillment of her individuality is intimately linked with all such relationships, as well as with her fetus. Her morality is similarly linked with those relationships.

## ADVOCACY OF MANDATORY NOTIFICATION

Josiah Royce might also enlighten us regarding the "squeal legislation" that Ooms defends. Communication is obviously essential to community, according to Royce, but it is necessarily a communication that comes from the heart or the spirit, rather than from legal notice or mandate. It is also essentially respective of the different language capacities of individuals, that is, their ability to interpret one another.[6] Where such communication occurs, families already know of the pregnancies of their daughters (or their partners), and where legislation is necessary to provide that information, the revelation is surely not equivalent to communication. As for Ooms's expectation that parents who initially react angrily to news of their daughters' pregnancies will later rally in support, there is to my knowledge no documentation to that effect, and there is substantial reason for thinking otherwise. On the basis of studies concerning the quality of parent–adolescent interactions and the motivations for pregnancies, it seems at least as likely that greater divisiveness between parents and pregnant adolescents may occur—especially after the critical period of decision making regarding the abortion has passed.[7]

[6]Cf. Josiah Royce, *The Problem of Christianity*, ed. John E. Smith (Chicago: University of Chicago Press, 1968).
[7]Cf. Susan Phipps-Yonas, "Teenage Pregnancy and Motherhood: A Review of the Literature," *American Journal of Orthopsychiatry* 50, no. 3 (July 1980), pp. 403–431.

The best argument in support of mandatory notification concerning pregnancy and abortion decisions distinguishes between those
dependent on and those independent of others for their support.
Perhaps because abortion is a medical procedure, like others for
which parents are responsible concerning their children, parental
consent as well as the pregnant daughter's consent ought to be required. But this reasoning clearly is in conflict with the privacy argument of *Roe* v. *Wade*.[8] Because Ooms supports that legislation, I
see few grounds for approval of the requirement to inform families
of pregnancies and requests for abortion. Consistency would demand
that minors be permitted to make unilateral decisions regarding abortion only to the extent that they are permitted to make such decisions
for other procedures. If parents are imputed to be responsible for
these decisions—morally, legally, economically—then they have a
justifiable claim to be informed about abortion, but their claim is
based on justice rather than on family interest.

## THE ROLE OF PUTATIVE FATHERS OR ADOPTIVE PARENTS

One last problem concerns Ooms's suggestion that a putative
father may have the right to determine whether a pregnant woman
will continue an unwanted pregnancy. Her suggestion is based on
his blood tie (*sic*) to the fetus as well as on his intention of raising
the child that the woman wishes to abort. But this recommendation
is inconsistent with Ooms's rejection of the inegalitarian or sexist
aspects of the patriarchal family model. If equality or justice is to be
respected, the woman alone has already contributed part of herself
over a considerable period of time in the interests of the fetus,
whereas the putative father or a possible adoptive parent merely
hopes or plans to spend part of his or her future in the fetus's behalf.
To put it crudely, the principle of "equal pay for equal work" may
be at stake.

However, *asking* is not equivalent to *requiring*. Thus, although
it seems wrong to coerce a woman to undergo the risk and pain of
childbirth, it may not be wrong to *ask* her to do so for the sake of
another (including the fetus). An important proviso to the legitimacy
of such asking is that the woman be truly free to decline the request.

[8]Cf. 410 *United States Reports* 113, decided January 22, 1973: "This right of privacy
. . . is broad enough to encompass a woman's decision whether or not to terminate
her pregnancy."

The distinction relevant here is between legality and morality, or between an ethic of obligation and an ethic of virtue. If Ooms were to deal with such a distinction regarding the role of putative fathers and adoptive parents (whether couples or not), her puzzlement about the weight of their views might be reduced. To be consistent with her support for the pregnant woman's legal right to choose abortion, she might then clearly reject their right to determine a different outcome. It would not be inconsistent to maintain at the same time that the pregnant woman ought to consider the willingness of others to care for the fetus she is carrying—especially where the pregnancy is relatively risk-free. To the extent that the woman honors such a wish for the sake of others' interests (those of the putative father or the adoptive parent, for example), she would be acting virtuously or supererogatorily.

The legality–morality distinction is a useful one for summarizing points of agreement and disagreement between Theodora Ooms and me. Although we concur that the law ought to allow individuals to make their own decisions regarding abortion, I disagree that the law should coercively inform family members about pregnancies or abortion decisions. In the area of morality, however, I agree that the individual should take full account of the impact of abortion decisions on her family, but I also maintain that broader social considerations provide a vantage point from which family interests themselves must at times be assessed and challenged. In other words, on the basis of an essentially social and egalitarian framework—the one that I have attempted to elaborate in my own contribution to this volume—the family perspective on abortion is useful but ultimately inadequate.

## CHAPTER 5

# Children, Personhood, and a Pluralistic Society

## VIRGINIA ABERNETHY

### Autobiographical Statement

*In the Dickensian tradition, I was born. Not only was I a firstborn, but I was to remain an only child. My early years were spent in Havana, Cuba. My first schooling was at a British day and boarding school in Buenos Aires, Argentina, where my father was an executive with ESSO. The headmistress was later decorated by the queen for her work in educating British youth who had been sent abroad to avoid the London blitz. I walked to school past a forbidding estate, guarded by a steel fence and fierce Airedales, that was said to be a Nazi spy headquarters. Our beautiful German maid (who took me to hear the violins at a Viennese tearoom when we were supposed to be in the park) married a lieutenant from the* Graf Spee, *scuttled outside Montevideo harbor.*

*At school, we learned in English in the morning and had similar subjects taught in Spanish during the afternoon. Math twice a day, but the schema for long division differed with the culture. Occasional lunches at school were punctuated by criticism of my table manners: "Americans don't even know which fork is theirs."*

*Patriotic observances at school featured "God Save the King," "There'll Always Be an England," and the Argentine national anthem. As the world learned during the Falkland Islands invasion, the Argentine war flag carries a sun, but the civil flag is two plain stripes of sky blue with white*

VIRGINIA ABERNETHY • Department of Psychiatry, Vanderbilt University School of Medicine, Nashville, Tennessee 37232.

*between. Las Malvinas have long aroused irredentist fervor in Argentina, and I learned about them in second-grade history (afternoon curriculum).*

*As an American in Argentina, I learned that we were all* Americanos, *and that I was a* Norteamericana. *There is no patriotism like that of an expatriate. By age 5, I knew by heart four verses of the "Star-Spangled Banner," but my only chance to sing it was at the annual Fourth of July picnic at the American School featuring hotdogs, mustard, and speeches by the American and British ambassadors.*

*We returned to the United States near the end of World War II. Instead of Germans, English, Argentines, North Americans, and Yugoslavs uneasily tuned to their short-wave radios, we were at home now with Americans, who would, of course, be like us. My fine patriotism survived only a few repetitions of the Pledge of Allegiance, although I still like to sing the "Star-Spangled Banner" at the beginning of each Nashville Symphony Orchestra performance.*

*In New York, I learned that I did not speak like the average cab driver, nor did I aspire to that, so I cultivated my parents' border-states speech: "Oh Maryland, My Maryland," and "Carry Me Back . . . ."*

*Was I a Democrat or a Republican? As a self-defined southerner in suburban New York, I was happily different as a Democrat. But that position became intolerable when our history lesson moved beyond Reconstruction and I learned how, in 1932, "they stole our party." I was forced then to become a Republican (ESSO reclaiming its own); lately, I would like to vote Libertarian but have resisted the symbolic gesture.*

*This history may explain why I admit of no truth except the fine truth of pluralism. I have seen too much fervor, too much genuine sincerity and heroism, and, above all, too much certainty attached to entirely opposite ideas and causes.*

*Science suits me well. In science, our hypotheses are tentative and testable. A scientific hypothesis is, by definition, in jeopardy. If a hypothesis is not in jeopardy—that is, falsifiable by the results of an appropriate test—it does not meet the minimum criteria for science. Beyond that, it is a good hypothesis if it appears to provide a parsimonious explanation for a great body of data. All this means that my views can be changed by data, or by new questions that illuminate the significance of new data sets. My thinking is also modifiable by appeals to any value that I already hold. Show me how my value is relevant to a particular idea or action, and you can influence me.*

*I am not easily swayed by, or even much existentially interested in, appeals to values that others see as important or ultimate. Your absolute value is not mine. Values are personal and cultural. Values are not absolute.*

*It follows that there is rather little in the way of ultimate goodness, although in a society of shrinking resources it may yet suit us to pretend otherwise. But the latter, cynic's view has been anticipated. Dostoevsky saw it well, and Marx articulated its application: "Religion is the opiate of the masses."*[1]

Attitudes toward children or child rearing are often extrapolated to abortion. My discussion focuses on abortion primarily but is not confined to it, as the essence of the current controversy over abortion is missed by not addressing the larger philosophical issue. The broader aspects of the debate cannot, responsibly, be ignored because attitudes toward the child and child-rearing data presented here strongly validate the reasonableness of a particular political and philosophical position, a pluralist position. Pluralism protected by separation of Church and State is constitutionally affirmed by the First Amendment (the establishment clause). Yet, this political heritage is at stake when the abortion debate is cast as a prochoice–prolife dichotomy. Choice in the matter of religiously based beliefs is constitutionally guaranteed and should not have to be debated.

While accommodation to divergent moral values within a heterogeneous society is addressed in the concluding section of this essay, the initial focus is on inferences about attitudes toward children and child rearing that can be drawn from cross-cultural, anthropological, sociological, and historical data. Two dimensions appear salient: Why children are wanted, either by their parents or the society at large; and how and when personhood is attributed to individuals. The questions themselves, of course, imply a willingness to be guided by data rather than by "moral insights" that would *a priori* define as wrong (or untutored and barbaric) any attitude that does not conform to a particular set of beliefs.

## THE VALUE OF CHILDREN

Cross-culturally, there appear to be at least five categories within which a desire for children can be understood. Briefly, children may have affective value, they may function as status markers for parents, and they may make economic contributions to the family. They may also have a *future* value in enhancing their parents' financial or emo-

---

[1] For a contemporary treatment, see D. Callahan, "Minimalist Ethics," *Hastings Center Report*, vol. 11, no. 5 (1981), pp. 19–25.

tional security. For the family and society, children are a primary source of recruits, contributing to survival and future vitality.

The notion that children are intrinsically *lovable* and *affectively rewarding* is widely held cross-culturally.[2,3,4] However, this positive view is not unalloyed in either the Western tradition or elsewhere. Historically, medieval European society appears to have had little awareness of the specialness of childhood, and interest in children seems to have depended on the extent to which they could participate in adult life. Seventeenth-century New England Puritans departed even from this essentially neutral attitude toward childhood: Their theology taught the concept of original sin as "the innate depravity of the human being at birth," with the consequent and immediate imperative that less sinful ways should, by any means, be instilled in children.[5] Finally, there is evidence of a growing ambivalence about the emotional rewards of being a parent in contemporary culture. William Kessen observed, "No longer can we smile comfortably at Faraday's quip, 'What good is a newborn child?' In many young minds, the question has become serious."[6]

Both clinical and research studies reveal something of the mechanisms that underlie modern parents', and especially mothers', discomfort with their role. It appears that women who lack a strong support network of friends and relatives, who have moved often, and who do not carry a mental image of good mothering derived from their own childhood experience are more likely than others to feel frustrated and trapped by the parental role. Such women comment that they need regular relief from their children to keep them refreshed or, more seriously, to keep them from sinking into depression.[7] Child abuse, a tragic symptom of disregard for children, has also been attributed to the absence of a mental image of good moth-

[2]Virginia Abernethy, *Population Pressure and Cultural Adjustment* (New York: Human Sciences Press, 1979).

[3]Virginia Abernethy, "American Marriage in Cross-Cultural Perspective," in H. Grunebaum and J. Chirst, eds., *Contemporary Marriage: Structure, Dynamics, and Therapy* (Boston: Little, Brown, 1976), pp. 33–51.

[4]E. Waldman, A. S. Grossman, H. Haygle, and B. L. Johnson, "Working Mothers in the 1970's: A Look at the Statistics," *Monthly Labor Review* (October 1979), pp. 39–49.

[5]L. F. Newman, *The Cult of Childrearing: Eighteenth and Twentieth Centuries* (Boston: Annual Meeting, American Association for the Advancement of Science, 18 February 1976), pp. 1–2.

[6]William Kessen, "Ambiguous Commitment," *Science* 193 (23 July 1976), p. 310.

[7]Virginia Abernethy, "Social Network and Response to the Maternal Role," *International Journal of Sociology of the Family* 3, no. 1 (1973), pp. 86–92.

ering, combined with a dearth of attention to the mother's own immediate emotional needs.[8]

The effect of the first child on the conjugal relationship also needs to be factored into the definition of attitudes toward children. Intimacy and affection between spouses is a highly valued objective in modern marriage, but recent studies tend to conclude with increasing consistency that parenthood is negatively related to this state of man–woman bliss. Family-life-cycle literature consistently shows high initial satisfaction in marriage followed by a decreased satisfaction that coincides with the advent of children. This dissatisfaction is most pronounced during the preschool years. There appears to be a gradual resurgence of satisfaction in the "empty-nest" phase of the marriage, with fluctuations in marital well-being more visible for wives than for husbands. Case studies also suggest that parenthood threatens communication, intimacy, and mutuality in marriage; that husbands sometimes anticipate parenthood with ambivalence; and that immature wives regress into pathological states under the stress of motherhood. These findings are consistent with survey data in which childless couples report higher marital satisfaction than do parents.

There is enormous variability not only in the belief that children are emotionally rewarding to parents individually and within the marriage, but also in the *weight* that societies attach to such ties. In many non-Western societies, a relatively strong mother–child affective bond is acknowledged, but children are regarded as the father's property, so that the mother may not have prior claim in case of divorce or her husband's death. Even if there is a nursing infant at the time of marital dissolution, the cultural definition of the marriage contract may require that the mother relinquish the child to the father's family as soon as it is no longer suckling. There have been similar understandings in the United States: The idea that the mother's presumably more intense affective relationship with the child gives her a prior claim to custody after divorce gained no legal recognition until around 1921. The traditional emphasis was on conjunction of the father's obligation to support his children with his rights to their presence, obedience, and services.[9]

In other contexts, dismissal of the importance of affective relationships continues despite the basically child-oriented goals of

[8]H. P. Coppolillo, *A Conceptual Model for Some Abusing Parents* (Nashville: Vanderbilt Medical School, Department of Psychiatry), manuscript, 1974.
[9]A. P. Derdeyn, "Child Custody Contests in Historical Perspective," *American Journal of Psychiatry* 133, no. 12 (1976), pp. 1369–1376.

American society. Adoption practice suggests that "there is still considerable judicial unwillingness to break completely with the concept that parents have something closely akin to a legal property right in their children."[10,11] For example, in *Moreland* v. *Craft* (1971), the court returned a child to his biological mother even though she had signed a written surrender for adoption when the child was 3 months old and he had lived with the presumptive adoptive family from that time until he was 4. This judicial insensitivity to the child's attachment needs is not unique; it makes an indelible statement about our valuation of children.[12]

In summary, the positive affective valence of children is widely, but not universally, acknowledged. Moreover, the importance accorded to affection, compared with other principles or standards applied to children, varies to such a degree that the view of children as property not infrequently outweighs considerations of their emotional well-being and their reciprocated loving relationships.

In both personal and highly ritualized ways, children also serve as achieved *status markers* for parents. In the United States, the status and the sense of competency associated with parenthood appear to be more prominent in sectors that have few other sources of self-esteem. For example, it has been noted that motherhood marks the transition to adult status in some lower-class subcultures. Similarly, fatherhood has been cited as a major source of self-esteem among lower-class men.[13] A New Orleans study of black women who could not afford medical care showed that one of the best predictors of discontinuing contraceptive use was revealing the fact of use to a husband or a boyfriend, who would object.[14] If some men who expect to make little or no contribution to a child's support are intolerant of women's attempts to limit pregnancy, it suggests that they see public evidence of potency as a major testimonial to manhood, and that this evidence is one dimension of the value of children.

Data have also been adduced to show that, in preindustrial societies lacking organized political machinery, power depends on the

[10]A. P. Derdeyn, *Child Abuse and Neglect: The Rights of Parents and the Needs of Their Children* (Charlottesville: University of Virginia School of Medicine,), manuscript, 1976.
[11]A. P. Derdeyn and W. J. Waddlington III, "The Rights of Parents versus the Best Interests of Their Children," *Journal of Child Psychiatry* 16, no. 2 (1977), p. 238.
[12]Ibid.
[13]Lee Rainwater, *And the Poor Get Children* (Chicago: Quandrangle Books, 1960).
[14]D. McCalister and V. Thiessen, "Prediction of the Adoption and Continued Use of Contraception," *American Journal of Public Health* 60 (1970), pp. 1372–1381.

size and the cohesiveness of kinship groups. Therefore, power ultimately derives from control of the reproductive function. Menarche, marriage, parenthood, and other biological or behavioral markers assume vital social significance in this context, and individuals gain status through successfully negotiating these life-cycle events.[15] Thus, it is congruent with the cross-cultural evidence to suggest that children are often wanted because of their positive effects on their parents' social standing within the local community.

The *economic contribution* that children make appears to be another factor influencing the norms of community family-size norms and the value of births. Even at young ages, children do substantial work in agrarian economies, and their usefulness continues through the early stages of industrialization. In the mid-1700s, Adam Smith, visiting the American colonies, saw families of up to 20 children and observed, "Labour is there so well rewarded that . . . each child, before it can leave the parents' house, is computed to be worth a hundred pounds clear gain to them."[16] Richard Easterlin, who recently studied a 100-year span of U.S. family-size and population-density data, has concluded that the more open land there is, the greater is the expected value of children and the higher is the fertility rate.[17]

Fertility in Ireland shows a similar response to economic opportunity. It rose dramatically in the same century that saw the introduction and the spread of potato culture. However, the cycle that began with higher productivity and higher fertility eventually became a treadmill; it was necessary to drudge over marginal land in order to support the newly enlarged population. In this diminished environment, individuals reduced their expectations for prosperity, and fertility began a decline that became precipitous by the time of the 1840s potato famine.[18,19] It is difficult to observe this sequence without concluding that children became first more valued and then less valued, according to their marginal economic effect on families. Sim-

---

[15]Karen E. Paige and Jeffrey M. Paige, *The Politics of Reproductive Ritual* (Berkeley: University of California Press, 1981).

[16]Quoted in Waldman, 1979, p. 42.

[17]Richard Easterlin, "Does Human Fertility Adjust to the Environment?" *American Economic Review* 61, no. 2 (1971), pp. 399–407.

[18]K. H. Connell, *The population of Ireland 1750–1845* (Oxford, England: Clarendon Press, 1968).

[19]M. Drake, "Marriage and Population Growth in Ireland, 1740–1845," *Economic History Review, 2nd Series* 16 (1963–1964), pp. 303–305.

ilar cycles have been observed in other European and non-European societies.[20,21]

In mature industrialized societies, children have few or no opportunities to contribute to the family economically and, in fact, have a negative financial impact. Costs include outright monetary expenditures, as well as the opportunity cost of a mother's lost earnings. In 1978, nearly 48% of mothers in two-parent families with children between the ages of 3 and 5 were in the labor force, but the proportion dropped to just under 38% if there were children under 3. Thus, it appears that many women do choose between childbearing and paid work. The President's Commission on Population Growth and the American Future (1977) estimated that the direct cost of a child to a family with a median annual income of $18,750 was in the neighborhood of $64,200; but when "the earnings foregone by the mother were included, the estimated costs of raising children skyrocketed"[22]: Small wonder, one journal commented, "the ambiguity of commitment Americans have to children."[23]

The data invite speculation that as long as a society remains agrarian or preindustrial and children contribute economically, the material dimension takes precedence over consideration of the emotional value of children. Significantly, the 1930 U.S. Census first revealed an *urban* residence for more than half of the native-born, white American population, and this demographic shift coincided with a new legal recognition that a mother's greater emotional investment gave her a strong claim to her children in the case of divorce. As long as our society was predominantly rural and children had economic value, the emotional basis for such claims carried little weight; with a shift to predominantly urban residence, where children become an economic liability, the mother's presumptively greater emotional commitment to her children gained new legitimacy as the basis for custody awards. Currently, a closer balance between the rights and duties of mothers and fathers seems to be in the making.[24]

In many societies, the value of children resides less in the present than in the *future*. In much of the developing world, children provide economic security for aged parents. On the other hand, the dominant cultures of some industrialized societies explicitly reject the notion of children becoming an economic asset for their parents. In these

[20]Abernethy, *Population Pressure.*
[21]M. Drake, *Population and Society in Norway 1735–1865* (New York: Cambridge University Press, 1969).
[22]Waldman, 1979, p. 42.
[23]Kessen, p. 310.
[24]Abernethy, *American Marriage.*

societies, the old person who becomes financially dependent on an adult son or daughter may feel stigmatized and inadequate. Although the covert wish that children will function as old-age security no doubt exists at some level, it is an illegitimate expectation in northern European culture and can be articulated only in jest. Consider the cockney renegade in *My Fair Lady*: "I'm getting married in the morning . . . I'll be supported by my children . . . and never have to work again."

The refusal of economic contributions from adult children should not be equated with an absence of other demands on children. The demands unmistakably exist, but they are attuned to psychological, rather than material, goods. Insofar as children are valued as objects of affection, they are expected to return love and care as they mature. Mother's Day and Father's Day are institutionalized opportunities for children to express love and gratitude. A consistent and culturally legitimate expectation is that adult children should stay in touch with their aging parents and provide emotional security for them.

However, many perceptive parents are troubled by the recognition that their demands for closeness to their children may be self-defeating. Indeed, the isolation of old people, as well as the present demand for even those nursing homes where conditions are terrible, suggests that parents are not receiving the anticipated dividends in emotional security. This outcome is particularly ironic insofar as the neglected parents are the very generation that invested heavily in their children and set themselves the goal of doing materially better for their children than their parents had done for them.

Given these conditions, some of today's adolescents and young married couples can hardly fail to conclude that one benefit supposedly accruing to parenthood is evanescent: The much publicized failure of communication between generations and the unwillingness and inability of geographically and socially mobile families to care for an old person must, inevitably, shake the belief that children are rewarding in the long run.[25,26]

Finally, societies that do not have effective means of *recruiting* new members lose vitality and die out. Reproduction is the only reliable recruitment mechanism over time, as groups such as the Shakers discovered too late when they tried to rely on converts. Because societies invest in children as recruits, centralized nation-states have sometimes officially adopted pronatalist policies in reaction to individual behavior of a distinctly antifamilial cast. The

[25] Ibid.
[26] Kessen, p. 310.

Roman Empire provides one example of a complex society in which growing scarcity apparently motivated individuals to restrict their family size at the same time that an official pronatalist policy was embodied in legislation.

Growing scarcity in Rome can be inferred from a doubling of the population in the 150 years beginning with the Augustinian period (30 B.C.); from the political turmoil that by Hadrian's time (A.D. 117–138) was inspiring frequent, publicly supported circuses to distract a restive populace; and from the later, rapid turnover of officially installed emperors: 27 emperors in the last 50 years of the second century. At the same time, there was an acceleration of the trend toward small family size and antifamilial attitudes, which were apparent in the patrician class as early as the Augustinian period. While individuals were avoiding the responsibilities of parenthood, the government strained to encourage large families, especially in the aristocracy:

> Legislation intended to raise the family's prestige included imposition of civil disabilities on the unmarried and childless as well as incentives for family formation. For instance, the unmarried were forbidden to inherit property; fathers were given preferential treatment in the allocation of public offices; and matrons were awarded the right to wear distinctive costume. . . . In addition, family allowances were given for children, and abrogating a traditional paternal right, infanticide was made a capital offense.[27]

However, the pronatalist legislation fell short of its desired effect because the public apparently saw its interests as being best served by restricting fertility:

> . . . as economic conditions in Rome deteriorated, it appears that prostitution and other non-familial outlets for sexuality increased, that coitus interruptus (the only known contraceptive method) was more widely practiced, that the average age of marriage rose to 18 for women and 26 for men, and that both abortion and infanticide became increasingly frequent in all social classes.[28]

It is not always so clear that government policy is intentionally pronatalist. For example, French law forbade contraception other than coitus interruptus and rhythm until the 1960s, but the underlying rationale may equally have been religious or pronatalist. In either case, French women obviously found means (through abstinence, contraception, and abortion) to limit reproduction, because small family size has been the statistical norm in France since the

[27] Abernethy, *Population Pressure.*
[28] Ibid.

1850s. On the other hand, when in the early 1970s four Eastern European governments with authoritarian regimes attempted to curtail the widespread use of abortion, the pronatalist intent was clear: "The change in policy derived not from medical, moral or juridical concerns but from fears that a precipitous decline in births would lead to too small a labor force."[29]

Other reasons for positively valuing children conceivably exist. I do not claim that the possibilities for why children are wanted are exhausted by the notions that children (1) are lovable; (2) reinforce a parent's self-image or social worth; (3) produce more than they consume; (4) are a source of comfort and security for elderly parents; or (5) contribute to a society's continuity and vitality. This list is limited to reasons characterized by some material or emotional benefit that is thought to attach to the child or to be conferred by the child.

In each of these value categories, the benefit may, or may not, be present. Therefore, children may, or may not, be wanted. This view is distinct from any intuitive position, such as that a child is good because it is good, or that it is good because it is willed by a divine or other nonhuman force.


## PERSONHOOD

When, in the development proceeding from the fertilization of a human egg by a human sperm, does a life gain entitlement to the range of rights that a community affords? Answers have varied by place and time, as have societies' evaluations of children, and the two domains are very probably linked. Rights issues have deep political significance, however, and merit separate attention.

The right-to-life position, as is well known, claims that entitlement to full rights and protection begins at the moment of conception. However, a widespread and contrary opinion holds that there are essential differences among forms of human life, and that limits on rights are associated with these differences.

The view that human life is not morally unitary is denoted by various linguistic usages. The term *human life* is often used to refer to that stage of development where the organism would for the first time become entitled to such rights and legal protection as a community affords. However, *human life* also has a biological, species

---

[29]*Planned Parenthood–World Population Washington Memo* (New York: Alan Guttmacher Institute, 27 February 1976).

referent (human life as opposed to dog, cat, or monkey life, for example), so it can fail to convey the intended meaning, or the meaning becomes a matter for debate.

*Person* more clearly captures the intuition that human life is not morally unitary, and that a certain specialness adheres to some but not to all stages in human development. Except when quoting an informant whose intention to restrict the meaning of *human life* is clear, *person* is used here to denote the particular forms of human life that are entitled to whatever rights a community affords.

Two approaches to defining *person* stand out: a philosophical definition in the tradition expanded by Tristram Engelhardt and others, and the cross-cultural social anthropologist's approach. There is broad common ground between these. Both could agree with the biologically derived insight that *developmental individuality* is a necessary (although still a gravely insufficient) condition for personhood.

Clifford Grobstein suggested some commonsense criteria for assessing developmental individuality and concluded that the eight-cell fertilized egg does not attain this standard. Specifically, research with fertilized nonhuman mammal eggs shows that cells in the "packet" of up to eight cells multiplied by mitosis

> are not yet tightly adherent, nor do they seem to be significantly interdependent developmentally. To all intents and purposes they behave as individual cells rather than as cell-parts of a multicellular individual. Second, in conformity with this interpretation, each cell, if isolated from the others, can form a complete embryo. Third, again in conformity, if two four-celled stages are fused, they form a single embryo whose cells give rise to a mosaic adult.[30]

Thus, an eight-cell fertilized egg meets not even the most concrete, biological criteria for the individuality that seems a *sine qua non* for personhood. The shortfall for any stage of fetal life is still greater from the sociological and philosophical perspectives.[31]

Postulating that the distinguishing characteristic of humanity is its ideal of a moral community, philosopher Tristram Englehardt defined persons as "the moral agents of the universe":

> One is . . . interested in the concept of person due to its role in ethical theory. Thus, . . . one will be interested in identifying those entities that are self-conscious, rational, and self-determining, because they will, as well, be the moral agents of the universe. They will be the entities

---

[30]C. Grobstein, "The Moral Uses of 'Spare' Embryos," *The Hastings Center Report* 12, no. 3 (1982), pp. 5–6.

[31]Virginia Abernethy, A. C. Wentz and C. H. Garner, *Human in Vitro Fertilization: A Response to Tiefel* (Nashville: Vanderbilt Medical School, Departments of Psychiatry and Obstetrics-Gynecology), manuscript, 1982.

who are responsible for their actions and who are bearers of both rights and duties.[32]

He continued, "Not all humans will be persons in this sense. Nor will appeals to potentiality secure persons the standing of actual persons. If X is potentially Y, it follows that X is not Y."

Infants, because they "are not moral agents," are among those who are not persons in the strict sense:

> If by person one will mean a self-conscious, rational and self-deter-mining entity, it is reasonable to hold that, though normal adult humans are such beings, infants are not. Or if one regards the issue from the moral point of view, infants are not moral agents, though normal adults usually are.[33]

However, Engelhardt suggested that extending to other humans, such as infants and young children, the rights legitimately reserved for persons *in the strict sense* is an option continually available to any society. For example, he said, "We currently accord humans the status of persons at birth and remove that status at brain death." The option of extending personhood may be exercised in order to promote social interests such as parental care for children and "concern and sympathy for the weak":

> Our treatment of instances of human life that are not also persons must be explained in terms of general practices established to secure important goods and interests, including the development of kindly parental attitudes to children, concern and sympathy for the weak, and protection in ambiguous circumstances for persons in the strict sense. This practice of imputing personhood thus depends upon the moral geography of a particular community... In addition to the strict sense of person as a bearer of rights and duties, we will often have good moral grounds for creating other senses, which confer upon instances of human life certain of the rights of persons strictly, though none of the duties, due to the absense of moral agency... Where precisely one draws the compass of such social senses of person will depend upon utilitarian and other consequentialist considerations.[34]

Thus, philosophical reasoning on personhood in the strict sense becomes the base on which societies are seen to embroider their own meanings, emphases, and expansions. Extension of personhood to the infant at birth should be understood in this framework. Such an extension is an arbitrary decision, so there is no *logical* reason for

---

[32]H. T. Engelhardt, Jr., "Viability and the Use of the Fetus," in W. B. Bondeson, H. T. Engelhardt, Jr., S. F. Spicker, and Daniel Winship, eds., *Abortions and the Status of the Fetus* (Dordeicht, Holland: D. Riedel Publishing Co., 1983).
[33]Ibid.
[34]Ibid.

expanding or not expanding the meaning to an even earlier stage in development, or for withholding personhood or not until some later time.[35-38] Nonetheless, Engelhardt suggested that there are compelling pragmatic and rational reasons for using birth to define the early limit of when "personal human life" may begin.

Coming to similar conclusions, the sociological analysis of personhood begins with the premise that sociality has a biological basis:

> The social dimension is not a human creation, constituted by choice for the convenience of individuals, nor is it merely an aggregate of individuals. Sociality is a natural, inalienable state of affairs. We are social by nature, not by choice.[39]

Moreover, *rights*, by definition, make sense only in a social context: A claim of rights implies the existence of some other being who has a complementary duty to yield a good or to perform a service:

> A convivial order is the condition for the possibility of a rights claim. Assertions of rights *by me* are claims for recognition within the moral commons. Acknowledgment of rights claims *on me* are recognition that others are also members of that commons.[40]

To the extent that persons are physically able to exercise choice about assuming duties or obligations to others, it follows that all rights are conveyed and may be withheld by societal processes. *Personhood* denotes a multitude of rights and is therefore conditional on a social definition.[41]

If these sociological premises and the conclusions that flow from them are correct, one would expect to find variation cross-culturally and over time in the forms of humanity that are granted personhood by their respective societies. A few examples from Western and non-Western cultures illustrate the point.

According to W. A. Silverman, early Jewish law (especially the Pharisaic Code) proscribed infanticide but excluded infants younger than 1 month from this legal protection. Again, early Roman law

[35]H. T. Engelhardt, Jr., "The Ontology of Abortion," *Ethics* 84, no. 3 (1974), pp. 217–234.

[36]H. T. Engelhardt, Jr., "Ethical Issues in Aiding the Death of Young Children," in Marvin Kohl, ed., *Beneficent Euthanasia* (Buffalo, N.Y.: Prometheus Books, 1975), pp. 180–192.

[37]H. T. Engelhardt, Jr., *Old Problems, New Technologies, and Changing Values: The Challenge of Biomedicine* (Washington: Georgetown University), manuscript, 1982.

[38]Engelhardt, "Viability."

[39]L. R. Churchill and J. J. Simon, "Abortion and the Rhetoric of Individual Rights," *The Hastings Center Report* 12, no. 1 (1982), p. 11.

[40]Ibid.

[41]Abernethy et al., *Human in Vitro Fertilization*.

proscribed hastening the death of a relative but excluded the killing of a child by its father from the general prohibition. Similarly,

> Early Christian leaders thundered against infanticide as a heathen practice: they insisted that all human life be held inviolable (although the exact fetal age at which ensoulment and thus "true humanness" was considered to take place was a matter of shifting doctrine). However, the proscriptive attitude of the early Christian emperors was not universally held. Constantine never explicitly forbade infanticide and later emperors did nothing to abolish exposure of infants or the sale of children as slaves.[42]

Moreover, Silverman said, one early Christian code explicitly commanded the father "to destroy deformed children." By "the Middle Ages," he pointed out, "infanticide was punishable by law, exposure was not." Eighteenth- and nineteenth-century Europe also tacitly condoned the abandonment of infants to orphanages, where up to 90% died in the first two years; moreover, mothers essentially known to have murdered their infants were never prosecuted, although several countries had laws against taking infants into the parental bed because accidentally rolling over was so frequently offered as an explanation for a baby's suffocation.[43] As recently as a decade ago in the United States, federal funding for family-planning programs in impoverished areas was sought as a means of reducing the number of unwanted births ending in infant neglect or more overt forms of infanticide. Inferences about the causes of infant death appear to have had merit, because nonwhite infant mortality in nine Maryland counties dropped at least 25% between 1969–1970 and 1972–1973; this change coincided with the introduction of family-planning programs but no other general improvement in area living conditions.

Behaviors in non-Western countries also illustrate a variety of social definitions of when a human infant is a person. For example, the first birthday marks the introduction of a Japanese baby to family friends because, although he or she has until then been "alive," he or she was not yet a "human life." That is, the baby is accepted into the community only after "a year in which it has been doing well."[44] At the end of the life cycle, some Australian Aborigine communities appear to withdraw personhood from an ailing relative by withholding water and care and beginning to sing, in the patient's presence, clan songs mourning loss. In most reported cases, the patients appear

---

[42]W. A. Silverman, "Mismatched Attitudes about Neonatal Death," *The Hastings Center Report* 11, no. 6 (1981), pp. 12–16.

[43]W. L. Langer, "Checks on Population Growth: 1750–1850," *Scientific American* 226 (1922), pp. 92–99.

[44]Atsuko Toko Fish, personal communication, 10 May 1982.

to acquiesce in this redefinition of their status and do not attempt to reach water.[45]

Thus, the philosophical and sociological views of personhood converge on the social community as the effective unit that confers the status of "person" on any human individual. The philosophical tradition defines *moral agency* as the capacity that humans must have in order to be persons in the strict sense, but it adds that societies may extend the compass of personhood in order to promote particular goals or objectives. The sociological tradition begins with the intrinsically *social nature* of humanity and notes that, logically, a claim to "rights" makes sense only in the social context because such a claim implies that "duties are incumbent on others." Thus, only the community can grant the legitimacy of rights; the social group controls what duties and obligations it will assume. Because the status of person connotes entitlement to a bundle of rights, the community grants or withdraws personhood. This decision is obviously not formal in the usual sense, or lightly taken, but is the outcome of particular historical traditions and environmental pressures.

## SEPARATION OF CHURCH AND STATE

Data demonstrating the temporal and geographic variability in (1) attitudes toward children and child rearing and (2) the social attribution of "personhood" suggest that it is difficult to support as right (in the absolute, moral sense of *right*) any particular set of criteria in these domains. Even within the Western, Christian-Judaic tradition, there is insufficient consensus on which to base any conclusion except that societies control the expansion or the contraction of the compass of personal (contrasting with the more inclusive category of biological) human life.

Thus, any claim that human life is morally unitary and that entitlement to rights should begin from the moment of conception is based on a moral insight that has a minimal relation either to historical tradition or to demonstrable reality. It is insupportable either by ordinary observation or by the most rigorous scientific methodology. It is, simply, a moral insight: an apprehension of truth that springs full-blown. It is not subject to analysis or proof. These characteristics place it in the realm of belief.

Now, it has never appeared that the right to believe in this way

[45]H. D. Eastwell, "Voodoo Death and the Mechanism for Dispatch of the Dying in East Arnhem, Australia," *American Anthropologist* 84 (1982), pp. 5–18.

is in dispute. On the contrary, the privilege of any individual or group to believe that the human conceptus is morally indistinguishable from later, rational stages of human life, or to act on that belief by personally foregoing abortion or even contraceptive use, is acknowledged. The so-called abortion debate is joined only when adherents to the view that human life is morally unitary attempt to control the behavior of others; specifically, when it is asserted that a conceptus is entitled to the protection accorded to persons, and when important claims (the necessary complement of rights) are made on fully vested members of the society without their consent.

In the "abortion debate," adherents of the right-to-life movement are attempting to force the behavioral consequences of their beliefs on others. The debate exists because a moral insight apparent to just a portion of the citizenry has been infused into the political process and is being proposed as the law of the land.

The debate, one finds, is not just about when biological human life acquires the rights associated with personhood. The debate is about whether this nation shall depart from its constitutionally designed heritage of separation of Church and State. The principle of separation will be violated if the beliefs of one sector of the population become law.

Such a law would surely be deemed unconstitutional. Legal scholar Lawrence Tribe has written about the abortion controversy that "the question [turns on] a decision as to what characteristics should be regarded as defining a human being"; he stated that this decision "entails not an inference or demonstration from generally shared premises, whether factual or moral, but a statement of religious faith upon which people will invariably differ widely." Tribe then noted that preventing a union of government and religion is "the 'first and most immediate purpose' [of] the establishment clause" of the U.S. Constitution, adding that the absence of a demonstrable secular purpose in a law makes "excessive entanglement" of Church and State a "definitional certainty." For example, its "religious motivation" resulted in the invalidation of a 1968 Arkansas law that forbade teaching evolution.[46]

Tribe went on to elaborate his perception of a threat to the establishment clause "whenever the views of organized religious groups have come to play a pervasive role in an entire subject's legislative consideration for reasons intrinsic to the subject matter as then understood." Tribe later modified this strong rejection of the "value

---

[46]Laurence H. Tribe, "Forward: Toward a Model of Roles in the Due Process of Life and Law," *Harvard Law Review* 87, no. 1 (1973), pp. 21–23.

TABLE 1. Percentages of Women's Responses to Questions on
Morality and Legality of Abortion

|                              |     | Abortion is wrong | | |
|------------------------------|-----|-----------|-----|-----|
|                              |     | Yes       | No  |     |
| Abortion should be legal     | Yes | 23[a]     | 44  | 67  |
|                              | No  | 33        | 0   | 33  |
|                              |     | 56        | 44  | 100 |

[a]This table shows that 23% of women think that abortion is wrong, but that it should remain a legal option.

of allowing religious groups freely to express their conviction in the political process,"[47] but he continued to see

> the argument for preferring majority rule over the woman's choice in matters of reproduction as thin to the vanishing point. Among other things, that argument at least suggests, though it does not logically compel, the conclusion that majority rule should prevail over the woman's choice even when her preference is for life and the majority's is for death. It bears recalling that the original case in the series of which *Roe* v. *Wade* is a part was *Skinner* v. *Oklahoma* (1942) where the Court affirmed the value of reproductive autonomy over a majoritian decision in favor of sterilization.[48]

In closing, I return briefly to fresh and interesting data. A Yankelovich, Skelly, and White poll[49] shows that 56% of the women polled believed that abortion is morally wrong, but *two thirds thought it should be legal* (Table 1). The critical subset was those women who thought that abortion is wrong but that it should nonetheless remain a matter of personal choice.

By subtraction (100% − 56%), 44% disagreed that abortion is wrong. If it can be assumed that these women favored the continued legality of abortion, this leaves 23% (67% − 44% = 23%) who thought that abortion is wrong but would not force their views on others through law. The distinction is congruent with the principle, the separation of Church and State. Theirs is a constitutionally sound position that commands respect.

In summary, the continuity of the developmental process, both before and after birth, defies scientific resolution of questions about

---

[47]Laurence H. Tribe, *American Constitutional Law* (Mineola, N.Y.: Foundation Press, 1978), p. 928.
[48]Ibid.
[49]Edward Cromer, "Study on Abortion Shows Women's Ambivalent Beliefs," *The Tennessean*, Nashville (30 April 1982), p. 50.

when a human fetus or child acquires the status of person. It is not surprising that answers, as revealed cross-culturally in attitudes toward children and child rearing, are extraordinarily variable. As there is no demonstrable basis for a decision, certainty about the moral rightness of any particular answer bespeaks beliefs. It is precisely against such an infusion of religiosity into government that the First Amendment to the U.S. Constitution guards.

The political imposition of a nonconsensually held morality is one of the most serious violations that a freely constituted society can suffer. The right-to-life position, insofar as it aims at coercing a large and unconsenting sector of the nation by curtailing individual choice on an essentially private issue, is an attack on the secular and pluralist tenets of government. Restated by Tribe, "The 'first and most immediate purpose' of the establishment clause was to prevent 'a union of government and religion [that] tends to destroy government and to degrade religion.'"[50]

---

[50]Tribe, "Forward: Toward a Model of Roles," p. 22.

# Commentary to Chapter 5

Professor Abernethy's discussion is full of disquieting implications that she either does not see or chooses to ignore, or that do not trouble her. Her position is either inadequate or filled with foreboding moral and political implications, or a combination of the two. Although my comments are prompted by her essay, they are more broadly applicable to certain powerful tendencies in contemporary American society. These trends would transform our understanding of moral and social life by *redescribing* social beliefs, institutions, and practices in narrowly medical, functionalist, econometric, or sociobiological language that strips us of our capacity to make moral evaluations.

The broad theoretical perspective that underlies Abernethy's discussion is best described as narrowly functionalist. She views social institutions and practices, including parenting and the family, through a lens that dictates the assessment of those institutions and practices from an externally imposed standard. She reasons from the existence of a practice that it serves a function—for example, infanticide—and hence cannot be questioned or condemned but only analyzed "logically," with matter-of-fact acquiescence in what "is." She suggests that we cannot quarrel with, or make judgments about, various social practices concerning the treatment of children because we must be "guided by data." But being guided by data is not the value-free, scientifically neutral enterprise that Abernethy suggests. Any explanatory framework, including functionalism, secretes a set of valuations, establishing those positions that are automatically defended and those that are eschewed or challenged.

A problem with Abernethy's approach is not that she has embraced a particular theoretical framework, but that she is unaware of how it undergirds her own evaluations, creating a value slope that

JEAN BETHKE ELSHTAIN ● Department of Political Science, University of Massachusetts, Amherst, Massachusetts 01003.

admits of certain possibilities in the creation and the maintenance of human society even as it denies or negates the validity or "good" of other possibilities. The scientific data that she turns to for support are not bluntly self-evident, as she believes, but require interpretation. It is her perspective, not some simple fact-of-the-matter, that dictates her insouciance when confronted with incidents of infanticide or, less dramatically, widespread abortion on demand. She feels no compunction in arguing for her own theoretical framework, however, because, being "scientific," she sees it as being above the fray. Other points of view are "intuitive" or emotional or value-laden and must be repudiated by the hard-nosed fact follower.

This will not do. Take the following example, drawn from the history of political thought, to illustrate the terrible dilemma in which Abernethy unwittingly places herself. Aristotle, in his masterwork *The Politics,* discussed the distinction between household and *polis* with compelling teleological certainty. His argument bears implications for how we think about public and private life to this day. But Aristotle, like Abernethy, wound up being complacent with reference to the social arrangements of his time, including slavery. He went beyond acceptance to buttress quite explicitly what "is" by seeing it as functional, hence necessary, hence required: If an institution or practice exists, it is because, somehow, it is meant to exist. Aristotle was guided by the data. Those data showed, empirically, the existence of slavery as a social institution. The mere fact of its existence as a widespread social phenomenon justified it as functionally required, as bearing some good.

If one accepts a hard or maximal version of empirical consequentialism (a theory whose crudity distances it from Aristotle's teleological sophistication, though both may be said to buttress what exists), it becomes impossible to challenge or to argue against *any* social practice, including slavery, the degradation of women, and the mercy killing of "defectives" (I think of the Nazi *Gnadentod,* or euthanasia program). The point is not that Abernethy, if pressed, would endorse all empirically evident social practices—including, say, rape—as good, but that she has no basis from which to challenge such practices, given her wholesale embrace of an amoralist functionalist framework—in the name of science.

The central marker of Abernethy's substantive case is argument from "value theory." Importing language drawn from neoclassical market economics (an econometric discourse) into the discussion of abortion, Abernethy makes her own case concerning children and their "value," as if one were talking about some market product. Children, like automobiles or investment property, may be more or less valued, depending largely on the material conditions that pertain in any given era at a particular point in time. (Although Abernethy also uses the language of value to treat the emotional links between parents and children, material imperatives, for her, take precedence.) A kind of cost–benefit calculus is present in her discussion. But this sort of accounting in relation to the question at hand conveys an image of irrationality if people, despite the "cost," have children. It does so because a whole range of human goods, ideals, thoughts, and emotions fall through the grid of econometric reasoning.

Think about the formulation "affective value of children" for a moment. Why is this language so far off? It doesn't get to the heart of the matter, to parent–child bonds, because it conjures up the notion that children may have *attributed* to them the value of being lovable and cuddly, and hence, it may be *affectively rewarding* to have them around. The calculation going on here distances us from the intensity and the intimacy of family life and ties and the unique claims a child makes for care and love. This language leaves us bereft of a moral anchor. Within the terms of "affective value," children are on a par, say, with household pets, which are also lovable and "affectively rewarding." But surely this won't do: It misses the deeper roots of our ties to our children. Rather than being of intrinsic value, as Kantian ends-in-themselves, Abernethy's children are valued for extrinsic reasons—only if they somehow contribute to their parents' happiness or to their economic status or well-being. There are particular dangers in this kind of argumentation.

For example, Mary Anne Warren,[1] an analytic philosopher, in the course of making a strong proabortion argument, admitted that her position justifies infanticide, to which she personally does not object. But she recognized that most people, "emotionally," would consider it a form of murder. The only argument that she could come up with against infanticide, given her prior theoretical commitments, was a kind of watered-down utilitarian calculation: People would be "deprived of a great deal of pleasure" if the infant were destroyed, about on the level of having one's stereo and Beatles' albums stolen. To locate the value of children not in themselves, as concrete and irreplaceable beings, but in the fact that they may, or may not, make parents feel good, cuts off the moral foundation of society at the roots.

Having said this, I want to indicate that I do not disagree with

---

[1]Mary Anne Warren, "On the Moral and Legal Status of Abortion," in Marshell Cohen, Thomas Nagel, and Thomas Scanlon, eds., *The Rights and Wrongs of Abortion* (Princeton: Princeton University Press, 1980), p. 136.

Abernethy's historical evidence that children played a more direct productive role in household and domestic economies in preindustrial epochs or as partial bread winners in the early and quite hideous stages of industrialization—hideous in their impact on most human beings, but especially on the many young, poor, exploited, and oppressed. But Abernethy can no more argue against the earlier economic roles that children played, emerging stunted, exhausted, and often destroyed, than she can argue for some other alternative, for the issue, to her, revolves around an externally applied standard of "value." If one views matters through an economic lens it becomes, as I suggested above, irrational or "dysfunctional" to have children when they are of little or no economic value. This language distorts human relations and motivations. It washes out the possibility that human beings might choose, as familial beings, to play a *heroic* role, to devote themselves to others, to be the authors of a story of people who take on responsibilities and carry them through. Instructive in this regard is Sennett and Cobb's *The Hidden Injuries of Class* or Robert Coles's rich volumes on *Children of Crisis.*[2]

Stanley Hauerwas has argued that it is a sad state of affairs when parents are encouraged to think of themselves as managers turning out a product to which they, or others, may attribute value.[3] There is an image of market imperatives gone wild. I find it unimaginable that anyone would conceive of bearing and raising a child on such terms. Very different is the sense that I, as a parent, or potentially a parent, am a culturally defined being, sharing a particular world and, as a sign of hope and commitment to that world, I have a child who will become a part of it through the moral education that I have to offer.

The implicit Malthusianism running through Abernethy's discussion emerges in the casual way in which she attributes value to children or withdraws it, depending on the circumstances. Particularly instructive in this regard is her treatment of infanticide. Finding no serious moral values involved, she simply indicates that there is greater "tolerance" of infanticide under conditions of extreme scarcity. But surely this fact tells us something dreadful: That human beings may be driven to extreme acts under circumstances that strip them of their humanity. Maria W. Piers, in her book *Infanticide: Past and Present,* argued, "Massive infanticide has . . . always occurred in connection with famines and hopelessness."[4] In other words, human

[2]Robert Coles, *Children of Crisis*, 5 vols., (Boston: Little, Brown, 1967–1977).
[3]Stanley Hauerwas, *A Community of Character* (South Bend, Ind.: University of Notre Dame Press, 1981).
[4]Maria W. Piers, *Infanticide: Past and Present* (New York: Norton, 1978), p. 39.

beings are capable of blunting their moral sensibilities under extreme stress. But just as we condemn the Nazi extermination camps as a deformation of human possibility, a horrific working out of some of the most evil possibilities of human nature, so we must condemn those circumstances that drive individuals to the destruction of the helpless and the vulnerable. Yet, for Abernethy, this becomes just another form of population control.

That infanticide is as old as human history or has sometimes been widely practiced does not, *pace* Abernethy, indicate a presumptive force in its favor, should we find it empirically evident. Although infanticide may be evident as a practice, it is a practice that has always required atonement or justification.[5] It is not a practice on which to base a moral code that makes life itself, or the ideal of a way of life, possible. Rather, the abandonment of that practice is universally taken as one sign of moral advance; moreover, it has been shown that if the situational catalysts, particularly dire economic exigency, are eased or removed, the more natural human instinct is not to abandon infants but to care for them. Abernethy has no way of discussing these issues through terms of moral discourse because she separates rigidly her hard-headed calculations of "value" and individual "want" from an "intuitive position, such as that a child is good because it is good." The entire moral community is threatened should this consequentionalism deepen and become more widespread, as Abernethy's treatment of the "person" and "personhood" demonstrates clearly.

Abernethy's understanding of the person or personhood is narrowly abstract and legalistic. Interestingly, she takes recourse to what she condemns in her discussion of the value of children and the position of right-to-life spokesmen and spokeswomen, namely, a moral "intuition" that only the term *person* can capture. Yet, she veers away from this usage almost immediately to discuss personhood as something we "attribute to" others if we are "guided by data," the sacrosanct facts and nothing but the facts again. For Abernethy, it turns out, personhood must be earned; a life must "gain entitlement to the range of rights." We—we dominant members of society—can withhold or admit others into our status and some particular forms

[5]Urban C. Lehner, "Japanese Ceremonies Show Private Doubts over Use of Abortion," *Wall Street Journal* 6 January 1983, p. 11, discussed the rituals of atonement that women in Japan by the thousands go through for their aborted fetuses. He quoted a licensed abortionist as saying such ritual is "a way of saying sorry to the fetus." Despite the official legitimation, even encouragement of abortion, many feel the need to do penance. This seems to suggest a depth of feeling that no amount of legalistic, medicalized distancing can, or does, negate.

of "human life" may not qualify. Quoting Tristram Engelhardt's definition of persons as "those entities that are self-conscious, rational,
and self-determining," Abernethy fails to *see* the dangers inherent in
such a formulation. Widespread infanticide and euthanasia are two
such morbid possibilities, both readily justifiable, given Abernethy's
insistence that the "extension" of personhood "is an arbitrary decision, so there is no *logical* reason for expanding or not expanding
the meaning."

I am arguing, remember, not that Abernethy favors either infanticide or euthanasia but rather that there is nothing in her own
position to prevent such abuses. Indeed, she argues forcefully that
conferring personhood or "imputing" should be an arbitrary decision
on the part of already-established "persons." She says clearly that
even the "extension of personhood" to the newborn infant is "arbitrary" and is not required by logic. But whose logic? What logic?
There is no logic as such; rather, there are many forms of thinking
that bear the stamp of human reason. Abernethy seems to believe
that there is only one clear-headed way of going about things—her
own utilitarian, functionalist, scientific way—and that all other points
of view are fuzzy or intuitive or attempts to impose arbitrary moral
standards. Yet, she calls her own standards arbitrary, for she accepts,
apparently, nearly any coolly thought-out rationale for withholding
personhood from infants, the seriously handicapped, the infirm, and
a host of others who would fail to meet her test of personhood, if
that is what society "chooses." Abernethy might respond that I have
put her on a slippery slope here. But as a political theorist, I am
deeply aware of the horrible abuses, up to and including eugenics
and even genocide, invited by arbitrary denials of personhood. Her
perspective squeezes out the moral and the conceptual space within
which one might begin to consider these matters.

Finally, Abernethy trivializes the abortion debate by her presentation of the prolife people as a group of religious fanatics determined to force "the behavioral consequences of their beliefs on
others." This is a gross oversimplification, as the work of Kristin
Luker and others has shown. Mary Ann Lamanna's essay also demonstrates that the vast majority of the American population, not
simply one sector, oppose abortion on demand and the view that
refuses to give any moral status to the fetus. Abernethy might reply
that whatever their moral beliefs, most people oppose legal restrictions on abortion. But even this assertion is open to dispute. More
important for my purpose is the fact that Abernethy's treatment of
the abortion issue would preclude by fiat the intrusion of *any* "religiously based beliefs" into our public morality. This is terribly ironic,

of course, when one considers the opening words of the preamble to the constitution: "We hold these truths to be self-evident," and those self-evident truths flow, in a direct line, from religiously based notions of natural or higher law. The very principle that Abernethy cherishes—our commitment to particular understandings of the free human personality—is based on a set of rock-bottom, foundational views of the human being that have their roots in our Judeo-Christian heritage. Her argument would also preclude the efforts of a Martin Luther King, Jr., to base a movement for racial equality on religious beliefs concerning the brotherhood and sisterhood of humankind. To strip our social life and our political discourse of religiously based beliefs would be to deprive us of our history and our present.

Abernethy's use of the establishment clause is most peculiar. That clause prohibits Congress from establishing an official religion, but it says nothing about the use or abuse of religiously based beliefs. From "Thou shalt not kill" to the abortion debate, such beliefs have been central to our public life. To claim, contrary to any serious constitutional law arguments with which I am familiar, a prohibition *against* any and all religiously based beliefs as constitutive of American public life in the establishment clause is to see what is not—and *should not* be—there.

CHAPTER 6

# More Trouble than They're Worth?

## Children and Abortion

### MARY MEEHAN

## AUTOBIOGRAPHICAL STATEMENT

*My opposition to abortion and other forms of killing comes partly from my experience of growing up in a large family, where each new child was greeted with joy and love. There is so much diversity in our family that I resist the tendency to deal with persons in the mass, as statistics, with the assumption that they are very much alike and that all are expendable.*

*The experience of living on a farm, from the time I was 9 until I was 18, also influenced my outlook. I cared for many young animals and observed the care that their mothers gave them. Protecting the young thus seems to me a very natural thing—an instinct that we share with other beings. Living on a farm gave me lessons in the wonder and beauty of life. I saw more than one calf struggle up on its wobbly legs just after birth and watched puppies play before they could even see.*

*It also showed me the ugliness of wounds and death. I was shocked to find that a sow with a protein deficiency had eaten her piglets; to see my horse with his chest torn open, apparently by another horse in sheer meanness; to watch buzzards eat dead animals; to hear that a friend's father had been badly gored by a bull. Life and death on a farm are very real, not much like the movies or television. Perhaps this is why John Hersey's* Hiroshima, *which I read while on the farm, had great impact on me.*

*Studying history and reading a daily newspaper also influenced me. They suggested to me that the Dark Ages are always at hand, that the*

MARY MEEHAN ● Free-lance writer, 23 2nd Street, N.E., Washington, D.C. 20002.

*tides of violence always threaten, and that tragic mistakes are often made by good and well-intentioned people.*

*I was strongly opposed to the war in Vietnam and worked full time in Eugene McCarthy's antiwar presidential campaign of 1968. In the early 1970s, I was increasingly puzzled and disturbed by the tendency of the political Left to favor legalized abortion. How could people who were so troubled by the violence and killing in Vietnam so easily accept the violence and killing of abortion? I did not understand this; nor did I understand why abortion was a centerpiece of the women's movement, which I sympathized with in many other respects.*

*Thinking that perhaps others on the Left knew something that I did not know, I watched and waited, read about the issue, looked for enlightenment. None of the standard arguments of the prochoice position satisfied me; and some, such as those of Garrett Hardin, appalled me. Information on fetal development and on the brutal techniques of abortion increased my opposition.*

*A friend from peace politics invited me to join him on the January 1978 March for Life in Washington. I found that the marchers were not the angry fanatics suggested by the liberal press, but nice and friendly people deeply committed to an ideal. I have been marching with them ever since. I am a member of Feminists for Life and of the peace–prolife group called Prolifers for Survival.*

*A free-lance writer, I have written for publications such as* America, Inquiry, The Progressive, *and the* Washington Post. *I write in opposition to abortion, infanticide, the death penalty, and war.*

For most of my life, and especially for my last 16 years as a political activist and writer, I have been concerned with problems of violence and killing. Growing up in the bloody twentieth century and learning about the violent history of humankind have convinced me that the central problem of politics is how to keep people from killing one another. Explaining and protecting the right to life seem to me the most important tasks of political theory and political practice.

Although I am not a pacifist, I believe that each person's right to life is bounded only by another's right to self-defense. The right of defense is implied by, or a part of, the right to life. If there were no right of defense, there would be no way to stop the bullies who have no respect for anyone's life. Even in dealing with a bully or an aggressor, however, one is bound to spare his life if that can be done while protecting one's own. The theory of just war, when it is as carefully applied as I believe it should be, is in harmony with this principle. So is opposition to the death penalty; self-defense does not justify killing a prisoner.

Abortion, it seems to me, involves primarily the taking of human life. It is a violent act, one that usually involves dismemberment of the human embryo or fetus. The violent nature of abortion is often overlooked in philosophical discussions that are detached from reality. It should not be overlooked. Just as we cannot adequately discuss modern warfare without considering the effects of napalm and nuclear bombs, we cannot deal fully with abortion without considering its methods. But the violence of abortion, though important, is secondary to the fact that it ends a human life. If abortion involved "only" the severance of one limb, and if the victim always survived, it would still be a serious moral problem, but it would not have such terrible finality.

In writing about children and abortion, therefore, I deal first with the right to life. This discussion is followed by a discussion of parents' obligations toward the new human life that they cause to exist and then by an outline of how I believe the law should deal with abortion. I suggest, however, that law can be only a part of the solution, and that our society must learn to welcome and value children. A consideration of the positive values of children is followed by responses to widespread objections to children (which are also rationales for abortion): that they are too expensive; that many are unwanted; that rearing them takes too much time and trouble; that some are handicapped; that some are conceived through rape; and that they add to an overpopulation problem. Finally, I suggest practical ways in which persons on all sides of the abortion issue, while continuing their philosophical and political debate, can cooperate.

## THE RIGHTS QUESTION

Wherever we come from—whether from God or from chance—the very fact of existence gives each of us a claim to continued existence. That claim or right is as nearly absolute as human rights can be. It is more than a property right, for although we might say that each of us "owns" or "has" our own existence, we can also say that each of us "is" our existence. The right to continued existence is a precondition of all other rights. Without it the others are all in danger. Technically speaking, the rights to free speech and assembly exist in some totalitarian countries. But persons who exercise those rights are likely to find themselves before a firing squad in Iran or decapitated by a roadside in El Salvador, so that their claims to free speech and assembly seem rather academic. Without the right to life, human society is reduced to a kind of warfare in which force decides every major issue. In the words of Thomas Hobbes, life is "solitary, poor, nasty, brutish, and short."[1]

In discussing the right to life, especially with respect to abortion, some insist that we must weigh it against "competing rights" or "competing values." They do not recognize the overriding value of life in a practical sense. Without life, one has no other rights; one simply does not exist and thus has no chance to debate "competing rights" or anything else. The phrase "live to fight another day" has application here. If our right to free speech or a free press is taken away, but our right to life is respected, we may be able to reestablish our freedom. This is one reason that the effort to abolish the death penalty in totalitarian countries is so important.

## RELIGIOUS VIEWS, SECULAR VIEWS

The right to life may be most firmly grounded for those who believe that there is a God of goodness and that humans are made in God's image. Pope John Paul II stated it this way: "Human life is precious because it is the gift of a God whose love is infinite, and when God gives life, it is forever." John Paul said that "every child is a unique and unrepeatable gift of God."[2] The same thought is expressed in the Book of Isaiah, when Zion complains, "The Lord has forsaken me; my Lord has forgotten me." And the Lord responds:

> Can a mother forget her infant,
>   be without tenderness for the child
>     of her womb?
> Even should she forget,
>   I will never forget you.
> See, upon the palms of my hands
>   I have written your name . . .[3]

Certainly, this view of the worth of each human is different from the one now dominant in our culture: that each of us results from

[1] Thomas Hobbes, *Leviathan* (Oxford, England: Basil Blackwell, 1946), p. 82.
[2] Pope John Paul II, Homily at Mass in Washington, D.C., 7 October 1979, published in *New York Times* (8 October 1979), p. B-6.
[3] Isaiah 49:14–16 (New American Bible).

accident and evolution and that each is easily replaced. One woman who had an abortion later told an interviewer, "I had no feelings about the baby. . . . I had no emotional attachment to it. Hell, you can make one of those things every month."[4]

Yet, the absence of religious belief does not remove all support from the notion of human rights. Dostoyevsky's character was wrong when he suggested that, if God does not exist, then "everything is lawful."[5] Other people still exist, and their very existence imposes obligations on us, just as our existence imposes obligations on them. The first obligation is a negative one that, if observed, would end most violence. It is the rule not to harm one another. If this rule is not self-evident, it is close to being so. In the form of the Golden Rule, it is found in most ethical systems. It is expressed in the lofty language of our Declaration of Independence, which speaks of the rights to liberty and to the pursuit of happiness but—first of all— the right to life. It is also expressed in the wisdom of the streets: "Your right to swing your fist ends where my nose begins."

Bernard Nathanson, speaking of the ancient rule of "Do unto others as you would have them do unto you," wrote that

> unless this principle is cherished by a society and widely honored by its individual members, the end result is anarchy and the violent dissolution of the society. This is why life is always an overriding value in the great ethical systems of world history. . . . Looked at this way, the 'sanctity of life' is not a theological but a secular concept, which should be perfectly acceptable to my fellow atheists.[6]

## POTENTIAL OR ACTUAL?

Medical and scientific textbooks affirm that the life of each human begins at fertilization (conception). Those who deny this elementary fact, or who say that it cannot be known, ignore a wealth of scientific evidence, including the recent experience with the *in vitro* fertilization of the "test-tube babies." Some of their statements appear to be guided by sociopolitical goals rather than scientific interests. As Senator John East remarked during hearings on this question;

[4]Quoted in Linda Bird Francke, *The Ambivalence of Abortion* (New York: Random House, 1978), p. 105.
[5]Fyodor Dostoyevsky, *The Brothers Karamazov*, trans. Constance Garnett (New York: Modern Library, 1937), p. 629.
[6]Bernard N. Nathanson and Richard N. Ostling, *Aborting America* (Garden City, N.Y.: Doubleday, 1979), p. 227.

> It strikes me that there is a tendency here simply to deny the obvious.
> It is like saying the earth is not round, it is flat, because one is uncom-
> fortable with the result that comes from acknowledging it is round.[7]

Some say that the unborn should not have the protection of legal personhood because they are only "potentially human" or "potentially rational."[8] Yet, the unborn are actually human; scientifically, there is no question about this. At the earliest stages of life, they are only potentially rational, and some people believe that it is permissible to take their lives before their brains have developed enough to make them rational. But if this becomes the criterion, what does it say about children and adults who are severely retarded? Have we the right to declare them less than human? If we start grading people's worth by their intelligence quotient, there will be no end to the injustice visited on those who do not score very high.

Some arguments for abortion are based on the tiny size of, say, an 8-week-old fetus. She can be held in the palm of one's hand. Does this somehow make her less valuable, less human? Those of us who are small in stature have problems with that concept. And there is a special unfairness in penalizing the unborn for not having size or abilities that, if left alone, they will surely develop. It is almost like saying, "In another few months, you will grow to the point where we cannot kill you because you will be too much like us. Therefore, we will end your lives now; we will get you before the cut-off date; for a limited period, we will have open season on the unborn." A developmental approach to abortion, with a slight twist, can even be used against adults. Thus, Germain Grisez, imagining a situation in which an embryo could speak in his own defense, said that "he might contend that the life of an adult is of less worth than his. After all, the adult has less time left to live, and all that he has gained in actualization he has lost in possibility." The embryo, said Grisez, could argue that "my life is far better than yours, for my life is a

---

[7]Senator John P. East in U.S. Congress, Senate, Committee on the Judiciary, Subcommittee on Separation of Powers, *The Human Life Bill: Hearings on S. 158,* 2 vols., 97th Cong., 1st sess., 20 May 1981, vol. 1, p. 114. See pp. 14–16 of this volume for many quotations from medical textbooks on the beginning of human life. See pp. 48–61 for an example of a doctor who claimed that he could find no scientific evidence on when human life begins.

It seems ironic that many individuals and groups who are relentlessly scientific in other areas (who oppose, for example, the teaching of "creationism" in public schools) have decided to ignore or to deny scientific fact on fertilization. They practice a selective agnosticism that undermines their approach to other issues.
[8]Some adults have mornings when they feel only "potentially human" and "potentially rational," at least until their first cups of coffee.

process of development and ever increasing vitality, while yours is a process of deterioration."[9]

Grisez's conjecture also suggests one of the major problems of the abortion debate, which is that the unborn cannot speak or act for themselves. A pamphlet of one prolife group includes this quiz:

> Under current U.S. law, which is not a person?
> a) A Supreme Court judge
> b) A corporation
> c) An unborn child
> Hint: Who can hire the fewest lawyers?[10]

Rights are of the greatest importance to the unborn because rights are all that they have. They have no clothes, no money, no property, no power. They cannot speak or organize to defend themselves. If their right to life is not recognized and protected, then they are completely vulnerable to power and violence and death.

I believe that the unborn do have a right to life. They are members of our species; they are our smallest brothers and sisters. Every unborn child is, to borrow Willa Cather's phrase, "one of ours."[11]

## PARENTAL OBLIGATION

Doris Gordon, Coordinator of Libertarians for Life, has developed the concept of parental obligation in a way that bears directly on the rights of the unborn:

> Unborn children don't cause women to become pregnant but parents cause their children to be in the womb, and as a result, they need parental care. As a general principle, if we are the cause of another's need for care, as when we cause an accident, we acquire an obligation to that person as a result. . . . We have no right to kill in order to terminate any obligation.[12]

Gordon said that

> unborn children are, in a sense, "captives" of their parents. Parents have no right to harm them, for there is no right to cause another to be

---

[9]Germain G. Grisez, *Abortion: The Myths, the Realities, and the Arguments* (New York: Corpus Books, 1970), p. 305. Grisez added, "I do not suggest that the embryo's argument would be sound." But he said that it "would be no more fallacious than ours, if we measure his worth by his degree of development."

[10]"Equal Rights: Or How Society Protects Almost Each and Every Person" (Minneapolis: Soul, n.d.), p. 12.

[11]This is the title of Cather's novel about a Midwestern farm boy in World War I.

[12]Doris Gordon, letter to the editor, *Life Report* (published by Maryland Right to Life), April 1979, p. 7.

utterly dependent, to be in harm's way, and then negligently or intentionally fail to prevent the harm from befalling that person.

She added

> All children, born or unborn, are human beings with the general, human
> right to be free from aggression. They also have a special right to be
> given support and protection by their parents.

Further:

> All children, born and unborn, also have the right of self-defense and
> so the right to be defended by third parties. The law should not deny
> any child these rights, nor grant a special privilege to do so.[13]

I believe that lawmakers have a positive obligation to protect
the unborn from assault, as they do to protect other humans from
assault. One can argue that government has an even greater obligation
to protect the weak and helpless. Certainly, this is the tradition of
our common and statutory law with respect to children, the retarded,
and the insane. It is also the tradition of the political Left—a tradition
undermined by the Left's support of abortion today. But some within
the Left, represented by groups such as Feminists for Life and Prolifers for Survival, are saying quite clearly that the Left betrays its
defense of the vulnerable when it supports abortion.[14]

## WHERE I STAND

All of this leads me to believe that abortion should be outlawed
except in those rare cases where the mother's life is at stake. Thomas
Aquinas wrote that "it is natural to everything to keep itself in being,

---

[13]Doris Gordon, *Abortion Is Aggression: Libertarianism Is Pro-Life,* an unpublished
paper, n.d. Libertarians for Life, which Gordon heads, is a group of Libertarian
Party members who oppose abortion.

[14]This and similar points are developed at greater length in Daniel Berrigan, "The
Dying and the Unborn" (interview), *Reflections* (Fall 1979), pp. 1–2; Daphne de
Jong, "The Feminist Sell-out," in *Pro-Life Feminism* (Milwaukee: Feminists for Life
of America, 1980), pp. 3–6; Jesse L. Jackson, *How Shall We Regard Life?* 8 pp.,
n.p., n.d.; Juli Loesch, "Pro-Life, Pro-Peace," *Sign* (September 1981), pp. 11–14;
Mary Meehan, "The Other Right-to-Lifers," *Commonweal* (18 January 1980) pp.
13–16, Mary Meehan, "Abortion: The Left Has Betrayed the Sanctity of Life,"
*The Progressive* (September 1980), pp. 32–34; William Raspberry, "A Liberal against
Abortion," *Washington Post* (23 January 1980), p. A-23.

as far as possible."[15] Whether he knew this from others' experience or from his own, I do not know, but anyone whose life has been seriously endangered understands what he meant. Yet, even in self-defense, one has an obligation to spare the other's life if possible. For this reason, when self-defense is offered in court as an excuse for killing, the law requires evidence that the use of deadly force was justified. Likewise, the "unity" constitutional amendment supported by many in the prolife movement would provide that

> No unborn person shall be deprived of life by any person: Provided, however, that nothing in this article shall prohibit a law allowing justification to be shown for only those medical procedures required to prevent the death of either the pregnant woman or her unborn offspring, as long as such law requires every reasonable effort be made to preserve the life of each.[16]

This proposed amendment is close to the actual laws of many states before the 1973 U.S. Supreme Court decisions legalizing abortion.

Although I support it, I am under no illusion that it can be passed or ratified in the near future. A statutory approach, such as that of the various "human life bills" introduced by Senator Jesse Helms and others, is the only approach that has any chance of success soon.[17] But no amendment or bill by itself can end abortion. In the 11 years since the 1973 Supreme Court decisions, the practice has become deeply embedded in our law, our culture, and even our economy. Many years of dialogue, education, and action will be needed to restore legal protection to unborn children. A major part of that effort must be devoted to persuading our society to welcome children again, to look on each child not as a burden but as a sign of hope.

---

[15]Thomas Aquinas, *Summa Theologica,* Part 2-2, Question 64, Art. 7. Self-defense is usually understood as defense against an unjust aggressor. Some ethicists say that it does not apply in the case of abortion because the unborn cannot intend injustice and because their growth is a natural process that does not constitute aggression. I am still troubled by this problem, but I feel that the "unity" amendment noted below may be the best solution.

[16]"NRLC Board Reaches Historic Consensus on HLA Wording," *National Right to Life News* (13 October 1981), pp. 1, 8. The reference to the medical procedures required to prevent the death of the unborn apparently means induced labor or Caesarean section.

[17]The Helms bills in the 97th Congress were S. 158, S. 1741, S. 2148, and an amendment to the debt ceiling bill. See U.S. Congress, Senate, 97th Cong., 2d sess., *Congressional Record,* 18 August 1982, p. S 10736, for the text of the amendment to the debt ceiling bill. It was tabled by a 47–46 vote after several unsuccessful efforts to end a filibuster against it. Ibid., 15 September 1982, p. S 11575.

## THE VALUE OF CHILDREN

Most adults, if left to themselves, seem to like children. We like them because they are human, small, curious, often joyous, sometimes incredibly funny. We value them especially for their innocence and for the hope they represent for the future. Someone who grew up in a community where there were many Jewish survivors of Nazi Germany remarked that "our parents looked upon us as living proof that Hitler lost."[18] And the chief nurse of a public-hospital emergency room—one that handles victims of car accidents, drug overdoses, knifings, and shootings—once said that "when a baby is born here, it creates an emotional boost like no tomorrow. You see so much of life going out that it's an extreme pleasure to see a life coming in."[19]

Children are a fresh start, a chance to make up for the accumulated mistakes of humanity, a chance to do it right this time. They also offer the possibility of doing things we have never done before. This view was expressed by Rep. Henry Hyde when he said that abortion proponents

> suffer from a failure of imagination. . . . Do they ever think of the secrets that are undiscovered, the diseases that are uncured, the frontiers that are uncrossed, the music and the poetry that are unwritten? Do they ever think that maybe they have destroyed somebody who might have solved some of the great problems—space, time, disease?[20]

Some object to this line of reasoning, saying that it could be used to promote everyone's having as many children as possible. I suppose that it could, but it need not be. Hyde was speaking of humans already in existence, so that a better analogy would be soldiers killed in war. We often wonder what they might have accomplished had they not died so young.

It seems ironic that a conservative like Hyde says this, whereas many people on the Left—traditionally the place of optimism—have become prophets of gloom and doom. *They* are the ones who say, "But look, the child might be handicapped; poverty might be too

[18]Quoted in Blaine Harden, "Whatever Happens, Doc, I Love You," *Washington Post Magazine* (21 February 1982), p. 16.

[19]Lucille Frank, quoted in Sandra R. Gregg, "D.C. General: Emergency's Chief Nurse," *Washington Post* (16 July 1981), p. D.C. 1.

[20]Henry Hyde, "A Congressman's Thoughts on the Pro-Life Movement," *Georgetown University Right to Life Journal* (Spring 1980), p. 10. The article was taken from a speech that Rep. Hyde delivered at Georgetown in October 1979.

much for her to overcome; she might suffer from being unwanted; and besides, the bomb will get us all anyway." This is not to deny the reality of hard cases, which are considered in some detail below. But it is to suggest that the Left suffers from an excess of pessimism. It comes very close to turning against the future.

## The Price-Tag Approach

The traditional and hopeful approach to children suggests that people should not have them merely for self-fulfillment or as a substitute for personal immortality. Nor should we view children as consumer products that, when "defective," may be "recalled." Nor should we put price tags on them. Yet, children are priced rather carefully these days. In 1982, *Time* magazine reported a government estimate that "raising a child born in 1982 to the age of 18 will cost from $85,000 to $134,000 in an urban community." Then, as though speaking about a new car, *Time* added that "there are many additional options" and gave estimates on child care, college education, and other items.[21] In a story bound to frighten most parents below the Rockefeller income level, the *Washington Post* later reported an estimate that rearing a boy born in 1980 through age 22, with college education, will cost $226,000. The estimate for rearing a girl was even higher: $247,000.[22]

The price-tag approach to children is part of the strange ambivalence that surrounds the abortion issue. Some people seem to assume that an unborn child has no right to life but that, if her parents allow her to be born, she then has a right to an extremely comfortable existence, fashion jeans, her own television and stereo, video games, a car as soon as she is old enough to drive, and a college education. The average number of children per family has declined, but an only child today may consume more than several children did 30 years ago.

Even so, if we take the highest child-rearing estimates at face value, it is easy to calculate a little further and conclude that the very expensive child will go on to become a very productive worker—

---

[21]"The New Baby Boom," *Time* (22 February 1982), p. 58.

[22]Spencer Rich, "Bringing Up Baby Costs $200,000+, New Book Says," *Washington Post* (8 July 1982), p. A-11. Lawrence Olson, author of the book in question, indicated that the costs of transportation and recreation are higher on the average for girls than for boys.

and may, in fact, "earn back" his or her cost in about 10 years.[23]
Perhaps, though, we should not pay too much attention to calculations like these. They lead to embarrassing questions about how
much each one of us costs—not only the direct cost to our parents,
but the larger economic cost of our lifetime consumption. In a "Peanuts" cartoon strip, one of the children says that Snoopy "is more
trouble than he's worth." And Charlie Brown responds, "Most of us
are."[24]


## WANTED OR UNWANTED?

Prochoice advocates often say that, if a child is not wanted by
her parents, she is bound to be unloved, unhappy, and possibly
abused. Better that she never be born, they say, than face a life of
unhappiness.[25]

There are many problems with the concept of "wanted children"
versus "unwanted children." Not least is the implicit determinism:
We are asked to believe that a child unwanted before birth will
necessarily be unwanted after birth and that the condition of un-
wantedness will blight the child throughout life. Many parents who
were despondent, or at least ambivalent, about pregnancy love and
cherish the child after birth. Others who do not want their child after
birth and show this by abuse or neglect did want the child before
birth, but in effect "unwant" her after. Neglect and abuse can indeed
blight a child's entire life, but this is the fault of the parents, not of
the child's existence. Whether the parents do not want the child
before or after birth, or both, they have the option of releasing her
for adoption. Many adoption agencies are eager for more children
to place, and Mother Teresa has issued a standing invitation to parents:

---

[23]But children do not have rights to fashion jeans, television, a car, or even a college
education. Many would be better off without some of those items. It is, for
example, a biased assumption of college-educated and middle-class people that a
college education is needed for a complete life. Some highly intelligent people
are miserable in school but happy and productive outside it. Others are "successful"
in school but seem to learn little from it.

[24]Charles M. Schulz, "Peanuts," *Washington Post* (30 October 1980).

[25]Curiously, some Christians use this argument. I remember only one instance in
the Scriptures in which Christ said, "It were better for that man if he had not
been born." He was not speaking of a leper, a cripple or some "unwanted" person,
but of Judas Iscariot, who was about to betray him and to commit suicide. Matthew
26:24 and Mark 14:21.

If any of you don't want the child, I want it. Give me that child because that child is the greatest gift of God. To the family, to the nation, to the whole world. Our sisters are in many places here in the United States. Just bring the child to them.[26]

Other problems with the wanted-unwanted dichotomy are psychological and political. Sidney Callahan has suggested that it is "destructive of family life for parents even to think in these categories of wanted and unwanted children. By using the words you set up parents with too much power, including psychological power, over their children." She made a point that many other feminists have missed when she said that, often, through history, "a woman's position was precarious and rested on being wanted by some man. The unwanted woman could be cast off when she was no longer a desirable object."[27]

When Graciela Olivarez dissented from a 1972 presidential commission's recommendation of abortion on request, she viewed the wanted-unwanted distinction from the position of minorities:

Many of us have experienced the sting of being "unwanted" by certain segments of our society. Blacks were "wanted" when they could be kept in slavery. When that ceased, blacks became "unwanted"—in white suburbia, in white schools, in employment. Mexican-American (Chicano) farm laborers were "wanted" when they could be exploited by agri-business. Chicanos who fight for their consitutional rights are "unwanted" people. . . . Those with power in our society cannot be allowed to "want" and "unwant" people at will. . . . I believe that, in a society that permits the life of even one individual (born or unborn) to be dependent on whether that life is "wanted" or not, all its citizens stand in danger.[28]

## CHILDBEARING AND CHILD-REARING RESPONSIBILITIES

Feminists often say that women should have a right to abortion on request because all of the burden of bearing children falls on women and because most of the burden of rearing them falls on women. The first point is undeniably true, the second often so (al-

---

[26]Mother Teresa Bojaxhiu, transcript of filmed speech to the 1982 National Right to Life Convention. The film was shown in Cherry Hill, N.J., 17 July 1982; the transcript was supplied by the convention press staff.

[27]Sidney Callahan, "Talk of 'Wanted Child' Makes for Doll Objects," *National Catholic Reporter* (3 December 1971), p. 7.

[28]Graciela (Grace) Olivarez, separate statement in U.S. Commission on Population Growth and the American Future, *Population and the American Future* (Washington: US Government Printing Office, 1972), pp. 161, 163.

though it need not be). But many feminists overlook the point that abortion is a men's solution. This is especially the case when children are conceived outside marriage. So much stress is placed on the social and financial difficulties of women in this situation that we tend to overlook the problems of the men who are involved. Abortion is a much simpler solution for them because they do not have to undergo it. They merely have to encourage their female partners. Sometimes, they must pay for it, but $150–$200 for an abortion is far cheaper than paying child support for 18 years.

As Juli Loesch said, "In the bad old days, if an unmarried woman got pregnant, the father-of-the-child was expected to accept some degree of accountability." She added, "Now the responsible thing is to put up the cash for an abortion ('No hard feelings, OK?'); and if the man actually goes to the clinic with the woman—if he holds her hand—why, he's a prince."[29] This is the easy way out, the cheap way out. Prolife feminists believe it is no coincidence that the Playboy Foundation has put a great deal of money into groups supporting legalized abortion.[30] The Playboy dream of carefree, no-fault sex has been realized at last. For men.

In a thoughtful letter published in the newspaper of a prolife–peace group, one man remarked that

> too many men have sex for entertainment, sex for experience, sex for status, sex out of boredom, sex to make you feel like "a hell of a man." If a man has sex and abandons the woman, and the woman abandons her child, who's the real abortionist?[31]

The irresponsibility of men is a major cause of abortion, and I doubt we can come close to solving the problem until more men recognize this.

On the question of child rearing, I have doubts about the practice of placing very young children in day-care centers for extended periods. It would be good to see more genuine sharing, to see more "househusbands" who take time off from careers to be with their young children and to do the housework while their wives take a

---

[29] Juli Loesch, "Our Bodies, Their Lives," in *Pro-Life Feminism*, p. 11.

[30] The Playboy Foundation, a division of Playboy Enterprises, has given financial support to the ACLU Campaign for Choice, Abortion Rights Mobilization, Catholics for a Free Choice, the National Abortion Federation, the National Abortion Rights Action League, the Religious Coalition for Abortion Rights, and other proabortion groups. See "The Playboy Foundation" brochure, various years; *Playboy* (May 1977), pp. 194–195; and Ann Marie Lipinski, "Playboy's Strange Playmates," *Chicago Tribune* (30 March 1980), Sec. 12, pp. 1, 4.

[31] "Male Attitudes," a letter from an unnamed man in *P.S.* (Prolifers for Survival newspaper), December 1980, p. 7.

turn at work outside the home. The development of "cottage industries," whether involving crafts or computers or real estate, is another possibility for parents who must work but want to spend time with their young children. There is nothing sacred about commuting or the eight-hour day; in fact, they are responsible for much of the stress and unhappiness of modern life.

The women's movement should end its condescension toward women who choose to stay home full time and care for young children. The movement hails men who do this but largely scorns stay-at-home women. Why the difference? Such women often have an awesome combination of skills: They are cooks, carpenters, nurses, gardeners, psychologists, tutors, seamstresses, occasionally farm managers, and often highly skilled craftswomen. Many develop careers in the "real world" after their children are in school (sometimes feeling, however, that the corporate world is less real than the other). What is wrong with this? Why all the pressure for parents to prove themselves supermen or superwomen in business or professions before spending time with their children?

## THE HANDICAPPED

Selective abortion of the handicapped unborn has been promoted—and accepted by many—partly because of a belief that handicapped people cost more than they are worth. Thus, in 1979, three government workers published in a major health journal a report on the economic benefits of screening and selective abortion in cases of neural-tube defects such as spina bifida. They concluded that society would save a great deal of money by avoiding the costs of medical care and special education and the lost productivity of people with such problems. Their discussion of "benefit-cost ratio" and "net lifetime economic cost" sounded like a Pentagon study.[32] Significantly, the government went from defending the right to life, to allowing abortion, to paying for many abortions, and finally to pointedly suggesting that some of us are more economic trouble than we are worth. Anyone who does not find this progression disturbing should take another look at the deplorable record of governments in the twentieth century.

[32]Peter M. Layde et al., "Maternal Serum Alpha-fetoprotein Screening: A Cost-Benefit Analysis," *American Journal of Public Health* 69 (June 1979), pp. 566–573. Two of the three writers were medical doctors.

Down's syndrome children are major targets of amniocentesis screening, in which a pregnant woman's amniotic fluid is tested to see whether the fetus is "defective." (Again, the comparison with consumer products is striking.) Most Down's children are retarded, and many have heart defects and other physical ailments. They require special care and training, but most of them can lead happy lives—possibly happier than most, because of their special innocence. After attending a conference on Down's syndrome children some years ago, *Commentary* editor Norman Podhoretz reported his conversation with a noted scientist who said "he saw no reason why anyone who accepted abortion should balk at infanticide, particularly when the infant in question was known to be defective." Podhoretz responded that certainly Down's children are defective, "but so are many other kinds of people. Some are blind, some are deaf, some are halt, some are lame, and some have missing limbs; some are given to madness and some are the prey of disease." If Down's children "can be put to death," he asked, "why not these, and if these, why not anyone who fails of absolute perfection?"[33]

Significant portions of the legal profession and of society at large are moving beyond abortion to "passive infanticide" for Down's syndrome children and others with serious handicaps. Handicapped newborns have been denied treatment in many American hospitals, despite state laws forbidding child neglect and child abuse, discrimination against the handicapped, and homicide. Here are a few examples:

- In 1973, two pediatricians at the Yale-New Haven Hospital (New Haven, Connecticut) reported that, over a 2½-year period, 43 handicapped babies had died after treatment was withheld or withdrawn. The handicaps included Down's syndrome, spina bifida, and heart-lung problems. The doctors indicated that, although some of the babies would have died in any case, others would not.[34]
- In 1977, the parents of Phillip Becker, an 11-year-old Californian with Down's syndrome, refused consent for the heart surgery that their son needed. Without the surgery, doctors said, Phillip would suffer unnecessarily and probably die at an early age. California courts upheld the parents, and the

---

[33]Norman Podhoretz, "Beyond ZPG," *Commentary* (May 1972), pp. 6, 8.
[34]Raymond S. Duff and A. G. M. Campbell, "Moral and Ethical Dilemmas in the Special-Care Nursery," *New England Journal of Medicine* 289 (25 October 1973), pp. 890–894.

U.S. Supreme Court refused to hear an appeal on Phillip's behalf.[35]

- In 1981, Jeff and Scott Mueller, Siamese twins joined at the waist and missing a leg, were born in Lakeview Medical Center, Danville, Illinois. Nurses later indicated that a doctor, at the request of the twins' parents, ordered that the boys be given no food or water. The state intervened, saved the twins' lives, and charged the doctor and the parents with attempted murder. The prosecutor said that he could understand the parents' pain, "but you also have to feel sorry for the children, hearing the nurses' statements: how they cried in pain because they were hungry; how the cries dwindled down to whimpers." A judge dismissed the charges against the doctor and the parents.[36]

- In 1982, a Down's syndrome baby was born in Bloomington Hospital, Bloomington, Indiana. "Infant Doe" had no connection between his esophagus and his stomach and thus could not eat normally. His parents decided against surgery to correct the problem and also decided against intravenous feeding. Infant Doe died after six days without food or water—and after the Indiana Supreme Court had followed lower courts in refusing to order the treatment requested by the child's court-appointed guardian and by a county prosecutor. A coroner reported that the baby died of "natural causes," and the county prosecutor decided against criminal charges.[37]

In the outcry following the "Bloomington baby" case, the Reagan administration notified 6,800 U.S. hospitals that the Rehabilitation Act of 1973 forbids discrimination against the handicapped

---

[35]Jim Mann, "U.S. Supreme Court Refuses to Order Heart Operation for Retarded Boy, 13," *Los Angeles Times* (1 April 1980), part 1, p. 21. Later, a California judge awarded custody of Phillip to another couple, and the heart surgery was performed successfully despite years of delay. "Retarded Youth Gets Surgery after Dispute," *Washington Post* (1 October 1983), p. A-4.

[36]Joyce Wadler, "Siamese Twins' Parents Charged," *Washington Post* (12 June 1981), pp. A-1, A-9; Joyce Wadler, "Criminal Counts Dropped in Siamese Twins Case," *Washington Post* (18 July 1981), p. A-12. Although doctors had said that the twins could not be separated, they were, in fact, separated by surgery in July 1981, and both survived. "Siamese Twins Listed in Good Condition," *Washington Post* (24 July 1982), p. A-2.

[37]*Herald-Telephone* (Bloomington, Ind.), 15 April through 20 April 1982; Stephen Chapman, "From Abortion to Infanticide," *Chicago Tribune* (22 April 1982), sec. 1, p 24.

by recipients of federal funds and warned them that withholding medical treatment from the handicapped could lead to a "termination of federal assistance."[38] The American Hospital Association suggested that the administration's action was "simplistic" and complained that it could lead to "an adversarial relationship between hospitals and parents."[39]

In responding to arguments for abortion of the handicapped, Henry Hyde once asked, "Do you have to pass a physical examination with perfect marks in order to be admitted to the human family? Is that what we want to do?"[40] Good questions, to which one might add: What are the practices of selective abortion and infanticide doing to the hearts and minds of handicapped children and adults? Do they now suspect that everyone wishes they had never been born? More depressing than a handicap must be the thought that one is regarded as an unfortunate "mistake" who lives at the sufferance of others.

In *Pre-meditated Man,* Richard Restak tells the story of a retarded boy whose mother went through amniocentesis because she feared that the next child too, might be retarded. When the mother came home from the testing, her retarded son was hiding in a closet. For several days afterward, "he had trouble sleeping because of nightmares that someone was trying to hurt him."[41] One participant in the 1982 Feminists for Life conference walked with a noticeable limp. In a "group sharing" session during the meeting, she revealed that a major reason she joined the prolife movement was that "I was

---

[38]U.S. Department of Health and Human Services, "Notice to Health Care Providers," by Betty Lou Dotson (Washington: U.S. Department of Health and Human Services, 18 May 1982), pp. 1, 2; *HHS News* (Washington: U.S. Department of Health and Human Services, 18 May 1982), p. 1.

[39]Quoted in Cristine Russell and Charles R. Babcock, "Hospitals Warned on Handicapped Babies," *Washington Post* (19 May 1982), p. A-21. Medical groups opposed the administration's later actions in court in 1983–1984.

[40]U.S. Congress, House, Rep. Henry Hyde speaking on *Conference Report on Labor-HEW Appropriations,* H.R. 12929, 95th Cong., 2d sess., 12 October 1978, *Congressional Record* 124 pt. 27, p. 36391.

[41]Richard M. Restak, *Pre-meditated Man: Bioethics and the Control of Future Human Life* (New York: Viking, 1975), p. 87. This kind of reaction is not limited to handicapped children. Dr. Edward Sheridan, a psychiatrist who teaches at Georgetown University, told a recent interviewer: "I have had children who suffer from night terrors and who fear to fall asleep because they overheard their parents discussing an abortion they had or planned to have. These children fear they may be gotten rid of the next time they make their parents angry." "The Psychological Effects of Abortion: An Interview with Dr. Edward J. Sheridan," *Georgetown University Right to Life Journal* (Fall 1981), p. 1.

born with spina bifida."[42] A bright, helpful, contributing member of the conference, she had slipped into the world years before the amniocentesis–selective-abortion package was available.

## RAPE AND ABORTION

Is abortion justified when a woman has been made pregnant by a rapist? This question is hard to deal with for three reasons. First, the woman did not consent to intercourse and thus lacks the usual parental obligation toward the child. Second, it is unjust for her to have to bear the discomfort and expense of a pregnancy that was literally forced on her. Third, as Mildred Jefferson has written, to some people rape is "an unpardonable sin which taints sinner and victims alike. The child is never thought of as an entity deserving of consideration—only a blot to be removed."[43]

On the other hand, the child has done no wrong and should not be punished for the father's crime. Rape is no longer punished by execution of the rapist (a change for the better), but now, the child is executed instead. What does this say about our sense of justice? Certainly, it is unjust that a woman must carry to term a child conceived through rape. Yet, it is a far greater injustice to kill the child. Injustice cannot be avoided in this situation; the best that can be done is to keep it to a minimum. The first injustice, which lasts for nine months of a life, can be relived both financially and psychologically. But the second injustice ends a life, and there is no remedy for that.

As one woman said, "The answer to rape is not abortion, it's stopping rape."[44] There is no reason for us to accept a situation in

[42]The writer's notes on Feminists for Life Conference, Milwaukee, Wis., 4 June 1982. Many prolife activists, including Senator Jesse Helms, have handicapped children. Helms and his wife, who already had "birth children," adopted a child with cerebral palsy and saw him through a series of operations. By 1981, the boy was a college senior; he said that "Mom and Dad always stressed that whatever your talents, just do the best and you'll make it." *Time* (14 September 1981), p. 30.

[43]Mildred F. Jefferson, "Rape and Incest Emotional Issues," *International Life Times* (14 March 1980), p. 13. In some cases, a woman may not know whether a pregnancy was caused by voluntary intercourse with someone just before the rape or by the rapist. I assume in this argument that she does know it was caused by the rapist.

[44]Valerie Evans, quoted in Mary Claire Blakeman, "New Generation of Right to Lifers," *Los Angeles Times* (16 September 1980), pt. 2, p. 5.

which women are at risk for rape throughout their lives. I realize
that this stance adds another item to a long and wearying list of things
that should be done to make a safer and more civilized world. Members of the prolife movement are beginning to feel somewhat like
Sisyphus as he pushed his rock up the hill. It is hard going in any
case; but at every pause, someone asks us, "But what about the
handicapped? What about the hungry? What about rape victims?"
And we say, "We must do more to help the handicapped and their
parents"; and, "There is enough food, but we need better distribution"; and, "We just have to stop rape." We also say, "Abortion
seems like a shortcut to solving these problems, but it does not really
solve them. It does not end hunger or rape. These problems are not
the children's fault; we should not blame the children or punish them
for the failure or crimes of others."

## OVERPOPULATION?

With many U.S. schools closing because of declining birth rates,
and with the social security system in trouble for the same reason,
we no longer hear dire warnings about overpopulation in the United
States. But the population control movement still views the Third
World as one huge "hard case" that needs the quick fix of abortion.
Foundations and government agencies have poured millions of dol-
lars into the distribution of abortifacients in poor nations, on the
assumption that curbing their birth rates would improve their economies. Some population-control enthusiasts have taught abortion
techniques and encouraged their use against explicit laws of the nations involved.[45]
    But the Malthusian assumptions on which these programs are
based have not been subjected to much critical analysis by the popular
media, which have done so much in the last 25 years to frighten
people about the "population explosion" and the "population bomb."
In a 1982 issue of *Columbia Journalism Review,* two anthropology
students said that the major media have mistakenly pointed to
overpopulation as the chief cause of hunger in the Third World.
They noted that many "respected social scientists" believe that the

[45]Dr. Malcolm Potts of the International Fertility Research Service, in a speech to
the National Abortion Federation (NAF), described how he had done this in the
Philippines. The writer's notes on NAF annual meeting, Washington, 28 May
1980. See also, Donald P. Warwick, "Foreign Aid for Abortion: Politics, Ethics
and Practice," in James T. Burtchaell, ed., *Abortion Parley* (Kansas City, Mo.:
Andrews and McMeel, 1980), pp. 301–322.

hunger problem has resulted from the development of cash-crop economies and the fact that "the vast majority of peasants were forced onto small plots in only marginally productive areas."[46] Rev. Richard Neuhaus had argued this point long before, saying that "the problem of world poverty is not created by the poor people but by the rich people" and that the population controllers serve "those interests that have a stake in maintaining the present maldistribution of the world's wealth."[47]

Economist Julian L. Simon suggested that the premises of the population controllers are factually wrong. Simon said that the world's food supply is increasing and that population growth has many long-term economic benefits, even for poor nations. He stressed the increase in knowledge and the technological innovation that result from having more people: "Writers about population growth mention a greater number of mouths coming into the world and more pairs of hands, but never more brains arriving."[48]

So much attention has been focused on the food problem in the Third World that problems of pollution are overlooked. We can be sure, however, that pollution will increase and that, like the hunger problem, it will be blamed on population growth. But it is instructive to look at what happened in our own country. Senator Alan Cranston, in dissenting from the 1972 report of the U.S. Commission on Population Growth and the American Future, said:

> Population pressures did not lead soap manufacturers to switch to detergents.
> Population pressures did not lead farmers to the use of pesticides and chemical fertilizers.
> Population pressures did not lead our cities to the abandonment of public transit systems nor to our public's dependence on the private automobile. . . .
> Population pressures did not bring about the switch to flip-top beer cans and nonreturnable bottles. . . .
> Most of our environmental disasters have been the technological successes of an economic system where the goal is to use technology to maximize profit. . . .[49]

---

[46]David Nugent and Michele Cros, "The Hunger Story: An Unbalanced Diet," *Columbia Journalism Review* (January–February 1982), p. 54.

[47]Richard Neuhaus, *In Defense of People: Ecology and the Seduction of Radicalism* (New York: Macmillan, 1971), pp. 309, 268.

[48]Julian L. Simon, *The Ultimate Resource* (Princeton, N.J.: Princeton University Press, 1981), p. 315.

[49]Alan Cranston, separate statements in U.S. Commission on Population Growth and the American Future, p. 150.

# THE HARDEST CASES

One can deal with hard cases individually, but it is more difficult to do so when circumstances are extreme or when several hard cases are combined. Suppose, for example, that a woman has six children, an alcoholic husband who beats her and abuses the children, and a contraceptive that fails. I would suggest that adoption is a better solution than abortion. Divorce might be another solution in this case; certainly, it makes more sense to remove the husband from the household than the child from the world. It is important to remember that a life is in the balance.

How about a case in which the child, if not aborted, seems destined for early death? Anencephalic children, who have only part of a brain or no brain at all, die hours or days after birth. Children with Tay–Sachs disease develop normally at first but then go into a long deterioration that leads to blindness, paralysis, and death at an early age. No cure seems possible for anencephaly, although there are indications that some cases of it may be prevented through better maternal nutrition.[50] No cure is in sight for Tay–Sachs disease; indeed, there appears to be little research for a cure, as selective abortion has been widely accepted as a remedy.[51]

The rationale for abortion in these cases is that the children are going to die anyway and that abortion saves the parents the emotional and financial cost of prolonged dying and (in the case of Tay–Sachs) saves the child from suffering. Yet, all of us are "going to die anyway," and many have diseases that are terminal in the short run. Cases of anencephaly and Tay–Sachs are devastating. But perhaps equally so are the cases of adults who die of amyotrophic lateral sclerosis (the disease that killed Lou Gehrig) or Huntington's chorea (the one that killed Woody Guthrie) or long and ultimately hopeless battles with cancer. Few now suggest that adults with terminal disease be killed in order to ease their families' suffering. Rather, the general response is to help patient and family through good medical care and, increasingly, through the compassion of the hospice movement.

This is not to suggest that we should be complacent about birth defects. One way to lower the incidence of genetically linked defects

[50]Jérôme LeJeune, "A General Theory of Retardation," in Dennis J. Horan and Melinda Delahoyde, eds., *Infanticide and the Handicapped Newborn* (Provo, Utah: Brigham Young University Press, 1982), pp. 79–80; Ronald J. Lemire et al., *Anencephaly* (New York: Raven Press, 1978), pp. 32–33.

[51]For example, see discussions in Michael M. Kaback, ed., *Tay-Sachs Disease: Screening and Prevention, Progress in Clinical and Biological Research,* vol. 18 (New York: Alan R. Liss, 1977).

is to encourage people at risk to marry outside their ethnic or racial groups. (Surely, one of the great ironies of human bigotry is that nationalist and racist theories of "pure blood" are so wrong from a genetic point of view. Marriage across ethnic and racial lines decreases the likelihood of genetic disease and birth defects.) And although genetic engineering may produce serious ethical problems, it may also solve some. That is, it may allow correction of genetic diseases by "switching on" or off certain genes.[52] It would be splendid, though perhaps too much to expect, if genetic engineering could be restricted to this area—and not used to produce superior heights, blue eyes, and so forth.

Finally, we should intensify research on the prevention and the cure of problems caused by defective genes, nutritional deficiencies, and drugs.

Children who have the most severe cases of Down's syndrome and spina bifida are profoundly retarded and cannot walk or care for themselves in any way. Although fairly rare, these are in some ways the hardest cases, because the children may live well into adulthood. They cannot enjoy life, as far as we know, and they are great burdens to their parents or to society, which often becomes their guardian. Amniocentesis cannot detect the severity of these problems, but parents who agree to amniocentesis tend to assume the worst and to opt for abortion if a defect is found.[53] Thus, many children with mild defects, or defects amenable to surgery and therapy, are aborted. This fact suggests that our operating principle should be not to assume the worst, but to assume that we do not know enough.

Even if we knew enough to say that one person would be mildly retarded, whereas another would be severely retarded and also badly crippled, we would not know enough to say that there is no meaning to the existence of the profoundly handicapped. People of religious faith are sure that there is a meaning; atheists are hard put to find any; but many must admit that they just do not know. But we can hope that medical research, which has solved many other problems that once seemed hopeless, will find a way to help these children.

A final note on the hard cases: Although it is essential to think about them and agonize over them, remember that they account for a very small proportion of the estimated 1.5 million abortions in the

[52]Victor Cohn, "Doctors Activate Dormant Gene to Treat Blood Disease Victims," *Washington Post* (10 December 1982), p. A-16.

[53]"Of the 113 fetuses who had chromosomal or biochemical abnormalities or who were male when the mother was at noteworthy risk of carrying an X-linked disorder, all but seven (93.8 per cent) were therapeutically aborted." Mitchell S. Golbus et al., "Prenatal Genetic Diagnosis in 3000 Amniocenteses," *New England Journal of Medicine* 300 (25 January 1979), p. 160.

United States each year. Often, in debates over ethics, people torture themselves with cases that are highly unlikely to occur. We ask, "Would I tell a lie to save the world" when we are far more likely to face the question, "Will I tell a lie to stay in someone's good graces?" We ask, "Would I have an abortion to avoid having a severely retarded child?" The question is more likely to be "Will I have an abortion to avoid social embarrassment or interference with my career?"

## WHERE PROLIFE AND PROCHOICE FORCES MIGHT AGREE AND WORK TOGETHER

Although there is strong conflict between the prochoice and the prolife camps on the philosophical and legal aspects of the abortion issue, there seems to be general agreement that no one really likes abortion. Many people on the prochoice side are troubled by the huge numbers of abortions performed in the United States today. While the two sides continue debating their differences, they should cooperate to keep hard cases to a minimum and to offer positive alternatives to abortion.

Here are several ways that the two sides could cooperate in preventing hard cases:

- Working together to prevent birth defects caused by hazardous chemicals in foods and drugs and working environments. A coalition of environmentalists, prolifers, and labor unions could have a major impact in this area.
- Supporting research on the prevention and cure of birth defects that are genetically linked. Many in the prolife movement cannot in conscience support the March of Dimes and other groups that fund amniocentesis, because of its link with abortion. But they are eager to support research that is directed solely toward the prevention and the cure of disease.[54]
- Cooperating on "Take Back the Night" marches, the teaching of self-defense techniques to women, and other efforts to prevent rape.
- Discouraging sexual activity among young teenagers. The goals here would be to avoid pregnancy in those too young to cope with it adequately, to prevent the psychological dam-

---

[54]The Michael Fund, based in Pittsburgh, was established by prolifers to fund research on the prevention or cure of Down's syndrome and related genetic problems. *Who's in Favor of Birth Defects?* (Pittsburgh: The Michael Fund, n.d.), 4 pp.

# Commentary to Chapter 6

## THEODORA OOMS

I find myself initially responding to Meehan's essay—as I have to other thoughtful prolife statements—with feelings of frustration and bafflement. Meehan and I appear to be looking at the same painting, but she sees only black and white colors and I see only varying shades of gray. The hard cases she discusses confront me with a conflict of values and create intellectual tension, doubt, and uncertainty. Yet, Meehan seems to find them easy to brush aside. Because she holds fast to the absolute value of the unborn life, these cases present her with no real moral dilemmas. She attempts conscientiously to balance the rights and interests of others against those of the unborn, but she discovers that, for her, one side of the balance scale is, after all, empty.

Meehan's argument rests on two basic premises: first, that life is the supreme human value, and second, that fetal life has the same value as born life and therefore needs equal protection in the law. As with other absolutist moral positions, Meehan's essay thus "seems to have the virtue of clarity and simplicity."[1] It is deeply felt and clearly argued. I like, and agree with, a number of her points: the fallacy of the "unwanted" child arguments; the denigration of a price-tag approach to valuing children (though I doubt that this approach is very prevalent); and her critique of the arguments for justifying the abortion of fetuses that amniocentesis reveals to be handicapped. Moreover Meehan's prolife position, unlike many, has the virtue of being consistent: She deplores violence in all its forms and does not

---

The views expressed in this commentary are solely those of the author and do not reflect those of her institutional affiliations.

[1]This phrase was applied to Immanual Kant's absolutist prohibition of all lies by Sissela Bok in her book *Lying: Moral Choice in Public and Private Life* (New York: Vintage, Random House, 1979), p. 41.

---

THEODORA OOMS ● Director, Family Impact Seminar, Catholic University of America, Washington, D.C. 20064.

believe in capital punishment or most war. And I admire her advocacy of a number of constructive actions that all of us should undertake to improve the quality of life for families and to help women avoid abortion.

My main difficulty with this essay, then, is that Meehan's absolutist moral vision simply does not correspond to the moral framework and the actual circumstances in which I, and most people I know, make moral decisions. I do not believe that any moral values are absolute standards that dictate the same answer to all relevant questions in all situations. Moral values—such as the need to preserve and protect life—are ideals to strive for. In concrete moral situations, they nearly always have to be weighed against other, conflicting moral values. They serve as principles to be applied differently to different situations, and the consequences of applying them also need to be taken into account.

## SHOULD ABORTION BE ILLEGAL?

Meehan believes that abortion should be "outlawed" politically. This outlawing would best be done, she says, with an amendment to the U.S. Constitution, but because this may be too difficult to accomplish, she will settle for legislation. Whereas some prolifers wish for a change in the law largely on symbolic grounds, Meehan clearly believes that the purpose of this legal ban would be to "protect" the lives of the helpless unborn. Would such a law achieve the purpose she desires? Meehan admits that the bill "would not by itself end abortion," but she does not ask what consequences this bill, if enacted, would have.

The extent to which laws shape attitudes and behavior rather than reflecting them is highly debatable, and it varies greatly depending on the issue. Undoubtedly, the 1973 *Roe* v. *Wade* decision reflected substantial changes that had already occurred in the public's attitude toward abortion. But also undoubtedly, such liberalization of the law did contribute to the rise in the number and the rate of abortion and has changed attitudes even further. (Some people may believe that, if abortion is legal, it cannot be morally wrong. Others can and do make this distinction.) But these changes in rates and attitudes cannot be reversed by legal fiat. If abortion were now made illegal, I believe that massive civil disobedience would follow. If abortions in hospitals and clinics were effectively stopped, I think it most likely that community-based, volunteer-operated, self-help abortion clinics would mushroom in communities all over the country. The great majority of those polled believe that abortion should be legal under some circumstances (see Lamanna, Chapter 1). The great majority of doctors insist that the abortion decision should remain in their hands. The experience of prohibition teaches that you cannot effectively legislate morality unless the dominant values of the community support you. (In Muslim countries, prohibitionist laws survive because the established Muslim religion forbids the consumption of alcohol.)

What penalties would accompany such a law? Who would enforce the law? Who would be prosecuted? The notion of prosecuting the more than a million women who seek abortion each year or even the thousands of doctors who assist them boggles the mind. Would you prosecute only the famous or the poor? And if they were not to be prosecuted, what would be the point of the law? What would be the effects on our respect for the political system of having yet one more law that so many would disobey?

Furthermore, if such a law were somehow passed, we would see an even greater polarization of the two sides. The energies of the prochoice movement would focus entirely on challenging, disrupting, or disobeying the law. Many whose sympathies lie with the prolifers' moral views would, on civil liberty grounds, become active supporters of the prochoicers. In such an atmosphere, there would be little progress on the collaborative and constructive actions for abortion alternatives that Meehan and others urge.

## IS ABORTION ALWAYS IMMORAL?

At this point, it may be the prolifers' turn to be baffled. If we believe that abortion is murder, they might say, then how can we *not* urge that it be made illegal? How can we possibly accept a situation where "murder" is legal, no matter what the consequences of making it illegal?

Here, I shall challenge the logic of Meehan's prolife argument, namely, that because fetal life is fully human, it should have the full protection of personhood under our laws. If this were correct—legally and morally—then there is no difference between a woman who aborts her 7-week-old fetus and another woman who kills her 7-year-old child. (The former may need the assistance of a doctor, but that doesn't make a moral difference.) And if both women have committed legal murder, then both should be submitted to the same degree of moral censure and legal punishment. Is this what prolifers believe? I do not think it is reasonable to believe that there is *no* moral difference between these two types of killing.[2] And if there is *some* difference, then it is appropriate for these two cases to be treated differently in the law. Just how differently is the important and very complex question that we are far from resolving.

There are a number of other points where Meehan over sim-plifies a complex world. I will mention two only briefly, as they are not central to her argument.

First, she firmly insists on the principle of equal protection for all handicapped born or unborn, no matter how severe their handicap or how serious the burden of caring for them. Meehan's real-life cases seem to imply that our society frequently violates the rights of the handicapped. She ignores the fact that probably at no time in the world's history have handicapped infants, children, and adults received as many resources and as much care or achieved as many rights as in the United States in recent decades. (In part, the reason is undoubtedly that many more survive with improved medical care). And although I would be among those who claim that we still have a long way to go in respecting and caring for the handicapped, I recognize that serious policy choices have to be made that restrict how far we *can* go. Policymakers, hospital administrators, and doctors have to make daily decisions about allocating scarce resources of time, skills, and money. Such decisions force them to weigh the value (or quality of life) of some individuals or groups against that of others. (Shall we establish a coronary-care unit for adults *or* an intensive-care unit for multiply handicapped preemies? Who should get the kidney of this new accident victim?) There must be some limits on how much protection society can afford for the seriously handi-capped—born or unborn.

Second, Meehan considerably oversimplifies and possibly mis-understands the feminist position. Her section on the value of chil-dren is written from the position of an observer. It detaches children from their families and ignores the impact of being a parent. The prochoice argument for permitting abortion is not based on disliking children, undervaluing them, or putting a cost tag on them. In fact, it is sometimes precisely because women do value children so highly, both the unborn and the children already born, that they are so

[2]In an article, Bok discussed a number of ways in which killing a fetus is morally different from killing persons who are already born. Among those she cited is the loss and suffering to those who know and care for the born victim. Although I think she underestimates the degree to which abortion, too, can be experienced as a loss by the woman or others in the family, there does seem to me a clear qualitative difference here. See Bok, "Ethical Problems of Abortion," *Hastings Center Studies* 2, no. 1 (January 1974), pp. 42–43.

reluctant to enter into parenthood lightly, by mistake, or without sufficient resources.

Feminists cling to their right to choose when and whether to be parents, in part, because they are preoccupied with the fact that historically motherhood has been their only identity, their sole contribution to society. Congressman Hyde has made impassioned reference, which Meehan quotes, to the great problems of our time (and the great artistic achievements) that might have been solved by a "somebody" who was aborted. Feminists could turn this argument on its head. What about the women over the ages who might have become Einsteins, Picassos, Beethovens, or Salks if they had not been tied down to enforced years of motherhood? Our present struggle as a society to find ways to balance the demands and the rewards of work and family, and to gain greater opportunity and equality for women, may not be solved by free access to abortion and may not be worth the moral costs of easy abortion, but Meehan will not dispose of these problems by blaming abortion on men's desire (not women's?!) to have trouble-free sex, exhorting us to value housewives more and to love children or to institute the marginal change of flexitime.

In spite of my many differences with her presumptions and arguments, Meehan and I share a broad common ground. We both believe that the present abortion rate is unacceptable, and that too many abortions are being performed for insufficient reason and without adequate consideration of the alternatives. (I would also add that too many people take the risk of unprotected sex.) Meehan and others in the prolife movement have done an enormous service in challenging prochoice people to think more deeply about the moral issues of abortion, to question some unexamined assumptions, and to realize the interlocking ways in which society expresses or denies respect for dependent and vulnerable lives. But their main policy solution is too simple. Those of us who think that making abortion illegal would be a grave mistake need to accept the challenge: to find other policy and program initiatives that will help women *and* men to grapple with the moral gravity of the abortion decision, to consider alternatives to abortion, and to be more responsible about preventing unwanted pregnancies.

CHAPTER 7

# Abortion and Equality

## MARY B. MAHOWALD

### AUTOBIOGRAPHICAL STATEMENT

*In an article written about nine years ago, I characterized myself as ideologically feminist, socialist, and Christian. Although I still identify with that description, I regard these as acquired rather than genetic traits, and I acknowledge continuing discrepancies between my ideological principles and the way I live my life.*

*Born a Catholic and raised in an individualistic, middle-class environment, I was converted to a more communal orientation by living in a community, teaching in a Puerto Rican ghetto, and studying Marx. I came to see the social criticisms and ideals of the young Marx as a valid and convincing interpretation of Christianity, as expressed in Bonhoeffer's definition of Christ as one who lived fully and freely for others.*

*My conversion to feminism followed my attraction to Marxism; I suppose it began shortly after by marriage, when I noticed legal and social differences in the way I was treated. This discovery spurred me to do some remedial work in the history of philosophy, that is, to reexamine what philosophers have had to say about woman in light of what they have said about "man," and to become more knowledgeable about contemporary feminist criticism. Over the years, while continuing to study and teach this material, and having three children, I have attempted to bridge the gap between my own and others' understanding of "man" and woman, in order to develop a less inadequate and better justified concept of human nature.*

*During the same period, I have taught and studied ethics, both theoretical and applied, in an attempt to extend my interest in human nature to a critical examination of practical questions relevant to women. My*

MARY B. MAHOWALD • School of Medicine, Case Western Reserve University, Cleveland, Ohio 44106.

*interest in the abortion issue parallels this development. Some years ago, I remember objecting to treatments of abortion as a "women's issue" rather than a social problem. For example, Mary Anne Warren's article "On Moral and Legal Aspects of Abortion" was first published in a special issue of* The Monist *devoted to "Women's Liberation." However, as I experienced, read, and reflected on the fact that women are much more drastically affected by pregnancies than are men, and as I noticed that male authors, no matter what their viewpoint on the morality or the legality of abortion, tended to ignore the pregnant woman and to focus exclusively on the fetus, I became more willing to accept that emphasis.*

*Recently, I have found myself resisting articles by men who write about abortion unself-consciously. I just wish there were some acknowledgment of the limitation of their perspective. Of course, my perspective is limited, too; which is why the way in which this book was put together was so appealing. I was delighted that most of the contributors are women, and that their views are so diverse; these factors added breadth, critical awareness, and confirmation to my own thinking. I hope it provides a similarly remedial service to a wider audience.*

Although views on abortion are typically treated as if there were only two opposing positions, "prochoice" and "prolife," these terms are often used uncritically and simplistically. The diversity of the contributions to this book attests to the inadequacy of such labels. Our subtle as well as obvious differences argue that there is actually a complicated continuum of positions stretching from total rejection to total support of abortion.

The complications derive from different conditions introduced as justificatory, for example, early stage of fetal development, fetal defect, danger to the health or life of the pregnant woman, economic or emotional hardship, and the unwanted nature of the pregnancy. They also derive from differing views about legality and morality: Some distinguish clearly between these, whereas others see them as integrally related. In the former group are those who approve of the legality but not the morality of abortion, as well as those who construe the moral dimensions of abortion as being irrelevant or nonexistent in a pluralistic society. The latter group includes those who seek to establish legal definitions of the morality or the immorality of abortion.

If the human fetus is to be respected, regardless of whether it counts as a fully human being or person, the claim that abortion decisions are morally neutral or irrelevant is clearly insupportable. Still, the history of the question, as well as current studies, provides convincing evidence that social disagreement on the morality of abortion will continue, and that laws will change because they reflect that disagreement.[1] Accordingly, I think it more useful to focus on the morality than on the legality of abortion. Insofar as the law coerces an individual to choose or to refuse abortion, the decision is amoral, even though the abortion itself has a moral or an immoral character. Both the freedom to make moral decisions, and the likelihood that such decisions will be correct, can only be enhanced by a careful, rational analysis of the moral alternatives.

In this essay, I develop a position on the morality of abortion that falls somewhere between the extreme positions of total condemnation and total permissiveness. I regard this view as consistent with feminist and egalitarian principles, which are integrally related. In order to describe my position adequately, however, I need first to do "battle against the bewitchment of our intelligence by means of language," with which debate about abortion has been beset.[2]

## FIVE BASIC AFFIRMATIONS

One way to reduce the bewitchment is to consider five basic affirmations embedded in the available arguments. Some are prochoice, others are prolife, and others still are proabortion, prowoman, or profetus. On analysis, each of these positions reveals implications that might startle their advocates. For example, a genuinely proabortion position emphasizes abortion itself as either morally neutral or positively recommended because the fetus is in reality an invasive growth, like a wart or a tumor, that may better (in some cases, at least) be expelled than preserved. Indeed, even without assuming that status for the fetus, one might argue that abortion is morally obligatory in some situations, for example, where world hunger and overpopulation threaten to deny the necessities of life to those already born. But a proabortion position could not logically argue the converse, namely, that in situations of depleted populations, abortions ought not to be permitted.

A genuinely prochoice position would impute to the pregnant woman the right to decide whether to terminate a pregnancy regardless of her reasons. If this position were consistent, however, it

[1]Cf. Kristin Luker Chapter 2, this volume; Daniel Callahn, *Abortion: Law, Choice and Morality* (New York: Macmillan, 1970); and John T. Noonan, *A Private Choice* (New York: Free Press, 1979).
[2]Ludwig Wittgenstein, *Philosophical Investigations,* trans. G. E. M. Anscombe (New York: Macmillan, 1968), p. 109.

would also take account of the choices of others affected by abortion decisions, for example, the prospective father and health professionals who might assist in the procedure. It might further be argued that individuals whose taxes or insurance premiums contribute to the support of seriously defective newborns deserve to have their choices weighed in decisions regarding abortion. Needless to say, those popularly labeled as prochoice advocates are not usually concerned about the autonomy of others in addition to the pregnant woman.

A prowoman position would clearly stipulate that the interests of the pregnant woman are the exclusive determinant of whether her pregnancy should be terminated or continued. Obviously, one need not be proabortion to be prowoman, as one may actually view abortion as morally wrong while endorsing the right of the pregnant woman to choose it. This position is more clearly related to a prochoice view because it affirms the right of the pregnant woman to choose her own interest over that of the fetus. However, in cases where those who are pregnant are children, or mentally retarded, or insane or comatose—that is, where the autonomy of the pregnant person is questionable or lacking—affirmation of her interests is obviously not equivalent to an affirmation of her choice.

A profetus position would stand at the opposite end of the spectrum from a proabortion view. It basically affirms that the interests of the fetus are the primary determinant of the morality of abortion decisions. Typically, this view entails a belief that the right of the fetus to continue developing *in utero* supersedes the rights and interests of all others affected by the decision—regardless of developmental immaturity, possible or actual defect, or threat to the life or health of the pregnant woman. If fetal life is to be preserved even at the cost of the pregnant woman's life, one might characterize this position as antiwoman. In some cases, however, a profetus position might entail the acceptability of abortion for severe fetal defect, justifying it in the name of fetal euthanasia.

In contrast to the popular view that is typically labeled prolife, a genuinely prolife position would reject all of the preceding views as unjustifiably limited in their affirmation of human life. The proabortion position negates the value of fetal life outright; the prochoice position makes life, at least fetal life, subordinate to liberty; and both the prowoman and the profetus positions ignore the relevance of other lives affected by abortion decisions. Because life is not lived by individuals in isolation from one another, but as an ongoing, complex system of interpersonal relationships, a really prolife position does not affirm the life of the fetus alone or the pregnant woman alone; it affirms the life of the community in which they both participate.

What has startled me in my own reexamination of the abortion issue is a recognition that arguments for all of the preceding affirmations have some validity. Because all five factors obviously cannot be affirmed simultaneously, some principle needs to be introduced as a criterion by which to order them. To that end, I propose a concept of equality, which I will subsequently describe and defend. In order to represent that concept adequately, however, I first must explain the concepts of human nature and woman on which it rests.

## UNDERLYING CONCEPTS OF WOMAN AND HUMAN NATURE

A further reason is pertinent to the discussion of these concepts, and it concerns the two individuals most affected by abortion decisions. Although the moral status of the fetus has remained a pivotal point of disagreement despite numerous attempts to clarify and justify its status, the status of the pregnant woman as a person is generally uncontested. If we assume that a valid argument concerning abortion entails a concept of woman consistent with a corresponding concept of human nature, then both of these concepts are crucial to understanding and assessing the argument. Yet, most of the leading arguments have either focused exclusively on the fetus, ignoring the concept of woman, or assumed a concept of woman that in my view is ultimately unacceptable.[3] Although I cannot here develop my criticisms of these two types of argument, I can at least avoid the points criticized by specifying and defending the concepts that underlie my alternative approach.

I shall begin, then, by defining woman as a biologically mature human being, typically capable during some portion of her life of conceiving, bearing, and nursing children. In contrast, man is a biologically mature human being, typically capable during part of his life of fertilizing human ova. Based on these definitions, the only significant difference between women and men is their distinctive biological capabilities.

Obviously, other male and female mammals have similar bio-

[3]E.g., Baruch Brody, Michael Tooley, and Judith Thomson, in Joel Feinberg, ed., *The Problem of Abortion* (Belmont, Calif.: Wadsworth, 1973); Mary Anne Warren, "On the Moral and Legal Status of Abortion," *The Monist* 57 (1973), pp. 42–62; John T. Noonan, "An Almost Absolute Value in History," in John T. Noonan, ed. *The Morality of Abortion* (Cambridge: Harvard University Press, 1970).

logical capabilities. What distinguishes human beings from other mammals, as Aristotle and Aquinas suggested, is a known capability for rationality and autonomy.[4] Thus, human beings are unique in that they are typically, during part of their lives, capable of exercising reason and choice. However, just as biological capabilities may not be exercised by specific members of a species, so the capability of reason and choice may never be exercised and may even be absent in some individuals. The specific meaning of human nature nonetheless depends on the presence of these developmental capacities in most members of the species.

Whether and when such capacities are present may be impossible to determine in some instances. Clearly, biological maturity is not compelling evidence of rational maturation. Nor is biological impairment or immaturity compelling evidence of its lack. The very meaning of *capacity* is controversial because it may or may not be identified with the potentiality of a healthy fetus or a newborn. But the certainty that such capacities are present in specific individuals is not crucial in determining whether they are human beings. A sufficient and necessary condition is that the individual belong to a class whose members typically possess those capabilities. Surely, one's womanhood (Freud to the contrary) is not negated by the fact that one has never become a mother, whether that "never" is determined by choice, by inability, or by circumstance. A similar point may be made about manhood and humanhood.

As they occur in individuals, capacities for reproduction, reason, and choice are developmental rather than sudden, all-or-nothing achievements. In other words, they develop (i.e., progress and/or regress) gradually from fertilization until death, whether these occur uterinely or extrauterinely. Such capacities vary within the same individual as well as among different individuals, and each is relative to some ideal of its complete fulfillment or realization.

Thus far, I have avoided the term *person* in characterizing human beings because it seems hopelessly controversial—and unnecessary. Its controversial quality is amply illustrated by popular as well as philosophical debate over the issue of criteria for personhood.[5] It is unnecessary because we can deal with the issue of whether it is moral to end a pregnancy or to terminate fetal life without settling the personhood question. Our household pets are not persons, but it is

[4]See Aristotle's *De Anima* and Thomas Aquinas on intellect and will, *Summa Theological* I, Questions 75–83.
[5]Cf. Tooley, Warren, and Noonan, *The Morality of Abortion;* Joseph Fletcher, "Humanness," in *Humanhood: Essays in Biomedical Ethics* (Buffalo, N.Y.: Prometheus Books, 1979).

surely wrong to cut off their food supply or to poison them need-lessly. Similarly, even if a human fetus is not a person during any point in its development, deliberately expelling it from the uterus is not a morally indifferent matter. Neither is the deliberate contin-uation of a pregnancy a morally indifferent matter.

Because human life is a developmental continuum it is also morally relevant to advert to the level of development that an in-dividual has reached or can reach, both physically and mentally, in determining the morality of that person's decisions.[6] Thus, just as the fact that a patient is near death is relevant to the morality of decisions regarding treatment, so the fact that a fetus is nearly viable, or seriously defective, is morally relevant to a decision regarding abortion.

Another morally relevant factor about human individuals is that they are interacting entities. Although their interactions may be min-imal or inadvertent, they occur at every level of development. For example, a fetus interacts with a pregnant woman through biological and nutritional dependence on her, and many pregnant women (and others, sometimes) interact emotionally with fetuses, even before the final stages of pregnancy. Because human lives are inextricably related, these relationships are pertinent to moral decisions regarding individuals. Moreover, an analysis of such relationships provides the basis for determining how advantages and disadvantages are distrib-uted among such individuals. That determination, in turn, constitutes an account of the meaning and the degree of equality that exists in the society. If equality is a good to be promoted, or even if it is simply an essential means to some good end, it represents a criterion by which to order the competing values relevant to abortion decisions.

## THE CONCEPT OF EQUALITY

But the term *equality* is notorious for its diverse interpretations. Among its political and economic meanings, we might subscribe to a literal interpretation that entails a distribution of the identical share of resources available to every individual, regardless of her or his different needs and capabilities. Alternatively, we might maintain a *laissez-faire* view by which equality is defined as leaving all individuals

---

[6]Noting the impact of such knowledge on actual abortion decisions, two physicians who have operated an abortion clinic in New York wrote the following: "About 25% of our patients decide not to have the procedure done when they learn that a formed fetus will be aborted." Selig Neubardt, M.D., and Harold Schulman, M.D., *Techniques of Abortion* (Boston: Little, Brown, 1977), p. 69.

equally alone or "free" to pursue their own interests according to their different talents. Or, we might assume a Marxist notion, by which resources are to be equally distributed according to the distinctive traits of individuals, "from each according to ability, and to each according to need."[7] We will return to this point later.

Because none of these meanings defines the "individual" to whom equal shares (of material goods or liberty) are due, we might also distinguish concepts of equality on the basis of those defined as candidates for distribution. From a purely biological perspective, the term *equality* might apply to every living, distinct human organism, no matter what its level of development, functional capacity, or health status. From a psychological perspective, it might apply only to those who have achieved—or have the potential to achieve—consciousness, rationality, and/or autonomy. The key questions, then, for determining the meaning of equality that underlies various accounts of human relationships or interactions are: On what basis are individuals declared comparable, and how is that reflected in a policy of distribution?

Here, we are obviously dealing with the broader concept of justice. In effect, whenever we grapple with problems of fairness or equity, we argue on the basis of specific concepts of justice *and* equality, so that it seems impossible ever to speak of one without the other. This is particularly evident where distributive justice is the theme invoked, as in John Rawls's treatment of justice, which calls for equal liberty and a minimization of the inequities that arise because of that liberty (cf. "the difference principle").[8] It is also evident in the recent treatment of "distributive equality" by Ronald Dworkin.[9] In such discussions, the terms *equality* and *justice* are often interchangeable, although the former may also be construed as a means to the latter.

Without attempting to explore further the conceptual and practical relations between equality and justice, I would like to suggest that either or both are means rather than ends in themselves. They

[7]Cf. Karl Marx, "Critique of the Gotha Program," *The Marx-Engels Reader*, ed. Robert C. Tucker (New York: Norton, 1972), p. 388. Although all of these concepts of equality have to do with treating people in the same way, their diversity shows that the "same way" may be interpreted quite differently in different political or economic contexts. Cf. R. Flathman, "Equality and Generalization: A Formal Analysis," *Nomos IX: Equality*, ed. J. R. Pennock and J. W. Chapman (New York: Atherton Press, 1967), p. 38.

[8]John Rawls, *A Theory of Justice* (Cambridge: Belknap Press of Harvard University Press, 1971), p. 60 ff.

[9]Ronald Dworkin, "What Is Equality?" *Philosophy and Public Affairs* 10, nos. 3, 4 (Summer and Fall 1981), pp. 185–246, 283–345.

are necessary means to the promotion of an ideal society, that is, a community in which the potentials of all individuals and their inter-relations are maximally supported and supportive. Although such an ideal of community is unattainable, it remains approachable. As approachable, it represents a moral paradigm in light of which alternative decisions may be assessed by individuals. The ethical framework in which the ideal is embodied is one of virtue or invitation rather than an ethics of obligation.[10]

In contrast with an ethics of obligation, this framework does not provide—or attempt to establish—a clear line of demarcation between right and wrong. Rather, it allows that there are various paths to, and degrees of, achievement of a common moral ideal. Most of the moral decisions that human beings make, I believe, are of this type. In other words, we more often struggle to discern which is the better course of action among given alternatives, than we attempt to determine what is morally necessary or obligatory. This is particularly true with regard to abortion, where circumstances sometimes force an option among tragic alternatives, several of which may be moral. Accordingly, the notion of equality that I regard as most helpful in addressing the abortion issue is one that provides the possibility of applying a moral ideal to practical situations.

Consistent with the preceding account of human nature, I propose a concept of equality that respects both biological and psychological differences as these apply to human beings throughout their lives. Such a conception focuses primarily on individuals as such, insisting that advertence to the differences between them is the only possible way of establishing genuinely egalitarian relations among them. It is thus a conception that eschews generalizations based on sex or gender, or even on developmental stage, as adequately defining the moral status of individuals.

In this view of equality, each pregnant woman ought to be regarded not only as *a* pregnant woman, but as *this* pregnant woman, with such-and-such a set of abilities and desires regarding her pregnancy, her life, and so on; and every human fetus ought to be regarded not only as human and as *a* fetus, but as *this* fetus, with such-and-such a health status, potentiality, capability for pain, and so on. Moreover, where equality is invoked as a principle to be observed in an abortion decision, it entails regard for all the differences, present and anticipated, in those affected by the decision.

In his two-part article entitled "What Is Equality?" Dworkin

---

[10]I am thinking here of an Aristotelian ethic of virtue such as that developed by Bernard Mayo in *Ethics and the Moral Life* (New York: St. Martin's Press, 1958).

distinguished between equality of welfare and equality of resources, and he elaborated the difficulties involved in the former view. Although he did not advert to a biological view of equality, that notion generally represents a form of (his concept of) equality of welfare, one in which welfare is defined as biological fulfillment. The notion of psychological equality is clearly another form of equality of welfare, one that Dworkin usually identifies with the fulfillment of one's preferences. A useful and relevant vantage point from which to criticize both conceptions, as well as any other concept of equality of welfare, is Dworkin's proposed conception of *equality of resources*.

From that perspective, the unrestricted fulfillment of each one's preferences is an impossible and unjust goal. Not only are the resources inadequate, but individual and group interests are bound to clash, introducing new restrictions for some. As for the biological model, which proposes that all living human individuals ought to be supported without regard to limitations in social resources, it is unrealistic and possibly unjust. Surely, the quality as well as the quantity of human lives deserves to be considered in making decisions regarding human reproduction. However, despite these and other problems raised by an equality of welfare, the ideal need not and ought not to be dismissed entirely. A possible and desirable alternative is a notion of equality that determines the extent to which we can adhere to equality of welfare in the face of the limited resources available. In the next section, I describe such an alternative.

## TOWARD AN EGALITARIAN ETHIC

The following principles are basic to the egalitarian ethic that I propose to apply to abortion[11]:

1. Individual lives should not be destroyed.
2. Those that can suffer should not be caused to suffer.
3. Those that can think and choose should not have their thoughts or choices ignored or impeded.
4. Individuals should not be misused or abused, that is, treated as other than who or what they are.

[11]To provide a complete survey of plausible principles, I might have proposed the following, as preliminary even to the first: What already exists should not be destroyed. This principle would have extended my argument to nonliving entities, while suggesting that responsibilities to nonliving beings are less binding (in the application of conflicting principles) than those to living entities. For instance, I do believe that we have a *prima facie* responsibility not to deface a work of art or destroy natural resources.

All but one (Number 3) of these principles are clearly applicable to others besides human beings, even (in Number 4) to nonliving individuals. I believe that all four principles are self-evident, as long as we acknowledge their status as *prima facie* rather than absolute responsibilities on the part of the moral agent. Any one principle may thus be subordinated to the others if adequate reasons are offered.

In order to resolve the conflicts that inevitably arise for moral agents who wish to pay due regard to all of these principles, a fifth principle is needed:

> 5. Equality demands that all individuals be given an equal share of the resources available, insofar as these are pertinent to their needs, desires, capabilities, and interests.

The obvious advantage of applying this principle is the avoidance of merely literal equality, that is, the distribution of the same resources to everyone, regardless of their relevance to the individual. Instead, the equal shares entail the equal distribution of the resources relevant to those among whom (which) they are distributed. Admittedly, the criteria of relevance are complicated and overlapping; for example, one might claim that a particular virgin forest should not be destroyed, but one may also claim that a group of poor human beings who need its lumber for their homes may destroy it. It is therefore necessary to introduce a sixth principle that acknowledges a priority among different kinds of individuals. The sequence of Principles 1–3 already suggests that Principle 1 is subordinate to Principle 2, and Principle 2 to 3, so that Principle 6 may be described as follows:

> 6. Human beings have a primary responsibility to distribute equal shares of pertinent resources to human beings, a secondary responsibility to distribute equal shares of pertinent resources to other sentient beings, a tertiary responsibility to distribute equal shares of pertinent resources to other living beings, and a quartiary responsibility to distribute equal shares to nonliving beings.

Lest this principle evoke the charge of speciesism, I would respond to that anticipated objection by insisting that speciesism, like other chauvinisms, occurs only where irrelevant reasons are used as a basis for discriminatory behavior toward individuals of a particular group.[12]

---

[12]Radical proabortionists such as Tooley and Warren are likely to level the charge of speciesism, as they view membership in the human species as irrelevant to the morality of abortion decisions. A more recent attack on speciesism is in Peter Singer's *Practical Ethics* (New York: Cambridge University Press, 1979), pp. 48–69.

I believe that there are relevant reasons sufficient to justify the claim that human beings have a primary responsibility for distributing equal shares of pertinent resources to other human beings rather than to other members of other species. Among these are the following possibilities:

a. A natural, perhaps biologically rooted, inclination.
b. An *a priori* moral obligation toward one's kin.
c. Laws and customs.
d. Religious views.
e. Objective superiority of the species.

Regarding (a) we need not go as far as Edward O. Wilson's thesis that the members of every species are determined to preserve one another.[13] If a strong form of that thesis is true, then there is no question of moral obligation with regard to such behavior. Short of sociobiological determinism, however, we can acknowledge what seems manifest: That human beings, like members of some other species, are naturally inclined to value members of their own species more highly than members of other species. Actually, there seems to be a natural inclination based on proximity of blood, cultural, and affective ties, so that one is most inclined to preserve one's own life, then the lives of one's closest kin, friends, less close kin or friends, neighbors, other citizens of one's own country, and so on. Concerning (b), the natural inclination of (a) suggests a basis for ordering one's responsibilities toward others: One does have a graver responsibility to one's children, spouse, friends, and so on, than one does toward those to whom one is totally unrelated by blood, affection, or acquaintance. Duties of fidelity are thus directly linked to kinship with one's family, race, species, and so on.

As for (c), clearly laws and customs support Principle 6. In our own country, as in others, legislation is not directed toward nonhumans, except insofar as its influence on them might affect human beings. Further, although those who live in modern cities may scarcely realize it, use of the environment to fill the needs of human beings has been generally sanctioned throughout history and prehistory. Regarding (d), religions and religious teachings have reinforced the notion that the world and everything in it (except other human beings) were created for the benefit of humankind.[14] But justification for the *use* of nonhuman by human creatures does not constitute justi-

---

[13]Cf. Edward O. Wilson, *Sociobiology* (Cambridge: Harvard University Press, 1975); Edward O. Wilson, *On Human Nature* (Cambridge: Harvard University Press, 1978).
[14]E.g., cf. Genesis 1.

fication for their abuse or misuse; accordingly, although raising or hunting and killing animals for necessary food is surely moral, it is probably wrong to kill or to inflict pain on them needlessly (cf. Principles 2 and 4). I shall return to this point later.

Perhaps the most convincing support for the claim that human beings have graver responsibilities to other human beings than to members of other species is the objective superiority of human over other species (e). Since we cannot preserve everything, surely we ought to focus our efforts on what is most worth preserving. In that context, it seems clear that no other species, on the whole, possesses worthier characteristics than our own. Some chimpanzees have been educated to a remarkable degree, and dolphins seem to have a rather impressive mode of communication, but human beings are generally not only educable but educated and educating to a high degree of sophistication, and human beings have devised and practiced ex-tremely advanced, complicated, and diverse modes of communica-tion. This is not to say that an individual chimp or dolphin may not be more intelligent than a particular (say, profoundly retarded) hu-man adult. The important point is that the average chimp or dolphin (and probably the most precocious or educated chimp or dolphin) is surely greatly inferior to the average human being in its ability to reason and communicate.

If we value such competencies as intelligence and speech, then we ought also to value—to a lesser degree of course—the probability of such competence that the average human fetus represents. I use the word *probability* here instead of *potentiality* to connote a stronger meaning than the latter. A potentiality may remain permanently un-fulfilled unless certain steps are initiated in order to actualize it— for example, my potentiality for learning Russian, which I do not intend to actualize even though ability and opportunity for doing so are already present. A probability is likely to be actualized unless impeded from doing so. The application of this probability-poten-tiality distinction to the abortion issue is clear enough. Under normal circumstances, without the active intervention of abortion, a human zygote, embryo, or fetus will develop to term, will be born, and will eventually reach undisputable personhood. In contrast, human ova and spermatazoa may have the potentiality but not the probability of similar development. Although alive and human, germ cells do not develop into persons without the initiative of fertilization.

Another distinction between the human germ cell (egg or sperm) and a human zygote, embryo, or fetus is also relevant to the abortion issue: The former does not constitute *a* human life, whereas the latter does. (A fertilized ovum constitutes at least *a* human life; it may, of course, constitute more than one, as twinning remains possible until about two weeks after fertilization.) Of itself, a human germ cell is no more *a* human being than is any other human cell, such as skin or blood cells; in fact, we might say it is less human because it represents only half the chromosomal endowment of normal human somatic cells. If human cloning from nongerm cells ever becomes feasible, then we might argue that every human cell represents a possible human life, but it would not constitute a probable human person until initiation of development in that direction through the technology of cloning, which is thus comparable to the initiative of fertilization.

Although it seems clear that a human life is of greater value than mere parts of a human life (e.g., blood or germ cells), this does not imply that every human life, at every stage of its development, is of greater value than the life of any or even every member of other species, at any point in their development. We might consider, for example, the way human beings treat other sentient animals as well as human fetuses in light of Principles 6 and 2. In Principle 6, we acknowledged a primary responsibility to distribute equal shares of pertinent resources to other human beings, and a secondary responsibility for doing so with regard to other sentient beings. Principle 2 implies a responsibility not to cause suffering to sentient beings. Our capability (resources) of reducing or eliminating pain is not pertinent to a zygote or an embryo as it is to later-stage fetuses and other sentient animals. Accordingly, an early abortion whose aim is to reduce or eliminate the pain or suffering (physical, mental, or both) of a pregnant woman may be justifiable, whereas a later abortion—that is, one that occurs after the fetal nervous system has developed to a degree sufficient for the experience of pain (surely during the third trimester, and possibly during the second trimester)—may be unjustifiable if the fetus's pain would be greater than that of the pregnant woman.

Just as a permissive view of capital punishment does not imply the moral acceptability of any means of inflicting that punishment (e.g., torture), so the fact that abortion is probably justified in certain cases does not imply that a specific abortive procedure is morally justified. Accordingly, the available techniques need to be assessed in light of Principle 2, as this principle applies to those affected by the procedure. Hysterotomy (removing the fetus intact from the uterus through surgery) is probably the least painful for the fetus, but the least safe for the woman. In contrast, dilatation and evacuation (D & E) involves mutilation and removal of the parts of the fetus by means of instruments inserted into the uterus through the vagina of the anaesthetized woman. In addition to the obvious violence and probable pain inflicted on the fetus, assisting clinicians report that this is an anguishing experience for them; nonetheless, it is probably the safest among the available techniques for the pregnant woman. Saline infusion and prostaglandin injection are less extreme in their effects; both induce premature labor and the delivery of a nonviable fetus. Of the two, prostaglandin is probably both safer for the woman and less painful for the fetus (saline causes toxicity *in utero*).[15]

The moral relevance of these different techniques will probably be more fully appreciated as the understanding of fetal development increases, and as reproductive technology advances to the point at which artificial wombs are a reality. Even now, however, consideration of the moral justifications for alternative procedures is not only consistent with Principle 2 but also with the landmark U.S. Supreme Court decision of 1973 (*Roe* v. *Wade*)—which legalizes premature termination of pregnancy, but not necessarily the termination of fetal life.[16] If it were prevalently possible to end a pregnancy safely without seriously injuring the fetus, procedures such as D & E might well be outlawed.

## FURTHER APPLICATIONS

Although I believe that the preceding account supports the claim that we have responsibilities toward human fetuses as (at least) probable persons and as sentient beings at some stage of their development, it does not constitute adequate justification for a profetus or an antiabortion position. It merely sets up the framework in which the principle of equality (whose meaning I have specified in Principles 5 and 6) may be applied to the controversy so as to provide a genuinely egalitarian solution.

In order to interpret that framework correctly, we need also to recall our concept of human beings as developing, psychosomatic entities. Typically, uterine development, as well as development during infancy and childhood, is almost exclusively progressive, con-

[15]Cf. *CDC* (Center for Disease Control) *Abortion Surveillance Annual Summary 1978* (Washington: U.S. Department of Health and Human Services, 1980), p. 49, Table 23.

[16]This distinction is critically elaborated in my "Concepts of Abortion and Their Relevance to the Abortion Debate," *Southern Journal of Philosophy* 20, no. 2 (Summer 1982), pp. 195–207.

sisting mainly of increments in one's physical and mental powers. After a certain point (the "prime of life"?), however, human development involves a larger component of regression or the deterioration of one's powers. The life lost through an abortion is therefore likely to be a more progressive stretch of life than that lost in practicing euthanasia toward an elderly comatose patient. Nonetheless, there is more than individual development to be concerned about, because important interactions occur constantly among all developing individuals. In other words, human beings, like other species, are essentially social animals. One could further argue that the early, painless abortion of the healthy fetus of a woman whose pregnancy places her life or health in jeopardy is justified because the pregnancy also threatens the developing lives of those who depend on her.

Although both pregnant woman and fetus are developing, psychosomatic individuals, the responsibility of giving due regard to others' thoughts and choices (cf. Principle 3) is clearly applicable to the pregnant woman but not to the fetus. This, of course, is the point at which the debate over abortion often seems most heated, since woman's choice is pitted against fetus's life as irreconcilable values. One possible way of resolving the dilemma is through the egalitarian route of Principle 5, which maintains that equal shares of *pertinent* resources ought to be distributed to both fetus and pregnant woman. Health and life are pertinent resources to both fetus and pregnant woman, but autonomy is pertinent only to the pregnant woman. Hence, the woman's autonomy ought to be respected to the extent that this respect is compatible with her and the fetus's equal share of health and life. The autonomy of the woman in circumstances where both she and the fetus are at risk thus tips the scale in favor of the woman. If those circumstances are not present, however, the woman's autonomy alone does not seem to justify the termination of fetal life. In other words, abortion justified solely on the basis of the woman's choice at any stage of pregnancy cannot be defended on egalitarian grounds as long as we allow the reach of equality to include nonautonomous human individuals.

Other lives besides those of the pregnant woman and the fetus are obviously influenced by abortion decisions, as we all are affected by the lives and deaths of others. The prospective father, other family members, and close friends are often significantly affected by such decisions. Although it may be difficult to assess the impact, in some instances we can predict with a high degree of certitude that no one, including the fetus, will benefit by declining an abortion. Consider, for example, fetuses diagnosed through chromosomal or biochemical assays as having Tay-Sachs disease, trisomy-13, or trisomy-18.[17] In all of these cases, where the prognosis includes not only failure to survive infancy, but also a painful and painfully slow dying process, Principle 2 seems clearly applicable.

Beyond families and friends, clinicians are not only affected by, but at least partially responsible for, abortions or births in which they assist. And others who are totally uninvolved in specific cases are influenced by such decisions, for example, by contributing voluntarily or involuntarily to the support of some children who are not aborted, or through the enjoyment of the subsequent social contributions of those children. Nonetheless, the impact of abortion decisions on clinicians or other autonomous individuals is so much less than the impact on the pregnant woman herself that their contrary input could hardly justifiably override her choice. If we lived in an ideal world, where the responsibilities of pregnancy, abortion, childbirth, and child rearing were shared by all, the situation would be otherwise, because then the autonomy of everyone would be an equally pertinent resource.[18]

The fact that we live not in an ideal world—but in one in which the pregnant woman is overwhelmingly more affected by these events than anyone else (except the fetus)—is itself a gross affront to egalitariansim. And the affront is scarcely reduced by legalizing abortion. In fact, the law's insistence on the (practically) exclusive right of the pregnant woman to decide the fate of her fetus places a great and ultimately solitary burden on many women, some of whom are still children. For that right is not one that can be exercised or not; rather, as an unavoidable option, it also represents an unavoidable and absolute responsibility. To impute to the pregnant woman such exclusive responsibility is not sufficiently justified on the basis of her biological role—because there are surely social factors that greatly affect the decision and may severely limit the autonomy of the individual making it. If society were welcoming toward unwed mothers and defective infants as well as supportive of the option of abortion in certain cases; if fathers and others really shared in child raising; if extrauterine means of reproduction were available; if overpopu-

---

[17]Cf. Richard M. Goodman and Arno G. Motulsky, eds., *Genetic Diseases among Ashkinazi Jews* (New York: River Press, 1969), pp. 217–231, 285–301; Jean de Grouchy, *Clinical Atlas of Human Chromosomes* (New York: Wiley Medical Publications, 1977), pp. 127–132, 160–164.

[18]An excellent elaboration of this argument is in Alison Jaggar, "Abortion and a Woman's Right to Decide," in Carol Gould and Marx Wartofsky, eds., *Women and Philosophy* (New York: Putnam 1976), pp. 347–360.

lation were not a matter of world concern—then we would have at least some of the conditions necessary for a genuinely egalitarian approach to the abortion issue.

We do not live in an egalitarian society, however, and therefore, we have to deal with the inequities that exist, while working toward an egalitarian, communal goal. Because that goal represents a moral ideal by which individuals may assess their own choices, a woman might decide whether to terminate her pregnancy (and how) by considering to what extent equal shares of pertinent resources will thereby be distributed to those affected. Or a couple might decide together whether, when, and how to have a child and to share in the responsibility for its rearing—in light of the same principle. Obviously, the more individuals and couples base their decisions on this egalitarian ideal, the more society in general will approximate the ideal, reflecting a recognition by others besides pregnant women and parents of the responsiblity for uterine as well as extrauterine life.

## FEMINISM AND EGALITARIANISM

At the outset, I indicated that I regard the position developed here as consistent with feminist as well as egalitarian principles. As there are different concepts of equality, however, there are different versions of feminism. Accordingly, I would like to conclude my thoughts on abortion by briefly considering alternative versions of feminism, their corresponding views about sexual equality, and their implied or explicit positions on abortion.[19]

A liberal version of feminism is one that supports social structures that maximize individual liberty, and that criticizes the present system insofar as it fails to treat women on an equal basis with men. The notion of equality reflected here is essentially individualistic, where the main or the only benefit to be distributed equally in the name of justice is that of liberty. Unfortunately, this view generally applied would serve to increase disparities other than liberty among individuals. Applied to abortion, it implies the absolute right of individual women to terminate pregnancy at any stage for any reason.

Some radical feminists view the relationship between the sexes

---

[19]These ideas are more fully developed in my "Feminism and Abortion Arguments," *Kinesis* 11, no. 2 (Spring 1982), pp. 57–68. Alison Jaggar discussed alternative theories of feminism, distinguishing between Marxist and socialist views, and between radical and lesbian separatist views, in her "Political Philosophies of Women's Liberation," in Sharon Bishop and Marjorie Weinzweig, eds., *Philosophy and Women* (Belmont, Calif.: Wadsworth, 1979), pp. 258–265.

as essentially unequal because women are superior to men. Lesbian separatism tends to endorse this approach, which represents a reversal of the traditional antifeminist view that women are naturally inferior and subservient to men. Applied to abortion, such a position would also support the absolute right of women to choose abortion at any stage of pregnancy for whatever reason. However, one would think that female fetuses have a counterclaim consistent with radical feminism, namely, that *they* have a right to survive, whereas male fetuses do not.

As readers may have surmised, the version of feminism to which I am ideologically committed is essentially socialistic, in the sense described by the young Marx in his "Critique of the Gotha Program." In that construal, equality between the sexes means that women and men have equal shares of pertinent rewards and social services. Those functions undertaken by women because they are able and choose to do so (e.g., pregnancy, childbirth, and lactation) are thus valued equally with other socially necessary or enriching functions—and are appropriately rewarded. Equality is thus an indispensable means to a communal ideal by which different needs and capabilities are equally respected, and social progress is maximized. The achievement of this ideal depends on the autonomy of individuals to build a society in which the benefits and deficits of its members are constantly adjusted so as to ensure as egalitarian a situation as possible. Autonomy is thus a crucial, yet not the only, factor to be considered in promoting equality among all individuals. Others' fundamental needs, such as life or health, may justify overriding individual autonomy. The liberation of women, then, like human liberation and equality generally, is not an end in itself, but a necessary means to the communal ideal in which the potentials of all individuals may be maximally, simultaneously fulfilled.

Applied to abortion, this version of feminism insists that the fetus is morally relevant to abortion decisions, but not exclusively determinative of their morality. At the same time, it insists that the mere assertion by law or social attitude that individual women are "free" to choose abortion does not mean that they are actually free to do so. In fact, until and unless men as well as women share equally in the responsibilities for children, there shall be no equality between the sexes, and no genuine liberation for women. Moreover, until and unless the fulfillment of those responsibilities is generally esteemed by others, and rewarded accordingly, the decisions of couples regarding the option of parenthood will be less than fully free. In general, under present circumstances, decisions to have children often place a greater burden on individuals than decisions not to have them—at least as far as the material situation is concerned. As feminist and egalitarian, I wish we might transform that situation into one where reproductive decisions were truly free, and so possibly moral, both subjectively and objectively.

Admittedly, such a transformation would constitute a radical shift in our way of viewing and valuing the "private" and the "public" spheres of life.[20] Minimally, it would require the dissolution of the prestige and power gap between the two. Those who are better at nurturing than others might continue to be women, but they would then not need to leave the workplace of their home to achieve equality with men. Some might combine roles of nurturing and material productivity; others would engage primarily or exclusively in the latter. And men might choose to be primary nurturers without suffering the disesteem of others. In such a turned-around world, feminism would no longer be necessary because sexual equality would be a reality. Abortions might still be moral in certain cases, but they would be an expression of, rather than a means of promoting, an egalitarian society. Moreover, because both men and women would take advantage of contraception or sterilization more consistently, and because the care of children would be more widely shared, there would actually be fewer abortions.

I would like to end by citing the suggestion of a daughter who recently learned that her favorite baby-sitter, an unmarried college coed, had just had a baby. When told that the new mother had quit school, needed financial assistance, and would now be less available to play with her, the little girl spurted out with enthusiasm, "I know what we should do. We should take the baby, because we have room, and could pay for what he needs, and could take care of him. And his mom could go back to school and come here anytime." In terms of the egalitarian criterion that we have here elaborated, the child was surely on target. Unfortunately, none of those concerned were "free" or virtuous enough to implement her suggestion. So much for the gap between our own ideals and practices.

---

[20]Cf. Jean Bethke Elshtain's ideas in *Public Man, Private Woman* (Princeton, N.J.: Princeton University Press, 1981).

# Commentary to Chapter 7

MARY C. SEGERS

Mary B. Mahowald has rightly chosen to tackle one of the most difficult aspects of the abortion controversy, namely, the relation between abortion and equality. In this controversy, both sides invoke the egalitarian imprimatur: prolifers, who stress the equal value of human life at every stage of development from womb to tomb,[1] and abortion rights advocates, who see abortion as one of many planks in a platform designed to realize sexual equality and human equality. How is it that the same concept of equality can be used to justify diametrically opposite views?

It can be so used because *equality* is such an ambiguous term. As J. L. Lucas pointed out, there are many, often competing, equalities[2]; note, for example, the notions of equal representation in the U.S. Congress, in which Senate seats are assigned on the basis of arithmetical equality (two to each state), and House seats are allocated on the basis of proportional equality (according to population). When different concepts of equality conflict, trade-offs must be made. The principles of Mahowald's egalitarian framework provide a method for reconciling competing equalities and for making such trade-offs.

---

[1]The following is an example of the prolife argument based on equality: "If we are to oppose discrimination for age, sex, race or religion consistently, on the grounds that all humans have equal rights just because they are human, then we must also grant that to admit that from the moment of conception the new organism inside a pregnant woman is another human being is to admit without qualification that it has rights equal to those of the woman who mothers it. Both are human and have equal rights, which implies that the rights of the human being who is the fetus cannot be sacrificed to those of the other human being, who is its mother, even in cases where their rights seem to be in conflict." Benedict Ashley, *Ethics and Medics* 7, no. 4 (April 1982), pp. 1–2.

[2]J. L. Lucas, "Equality," in Richard E. Flathman, ed., *Concepts in Social and Political Philosophy* (New York: Macmillan, 1973), pp. 347–351.

---

MARY C. SEGERS • Department of Political Science and Director of Women's Studies, Rutgers University, Newark, New Jersey 08903.

Mahowald recognizes that there is a complicated continuum of positions on the legality and the morality of abortion. Characterizing her own position as egalitarian, feminist, and prolife, she attempts to support the claim that we have obligations to human fetuses as (at least) probable persons and as sentient beings at some stage of their development. Her argument is very subtle, nuanced, balanced, and appreciative of the complexities of the abortion dilemma. I suspect that I am basically more in agreement than in disagreement with her views. I shall comment on the positive aspects of her arguments and then raise some questions concerning the substance and the political implications of her views.

## CONCEPTS OF HUMAN NATURE

In the early section of the essay, there is a splendid linking together of basic issues: human nature, the nature of woman, and the status of the fetus. Without getting bogged down in sterile, futile arguments about the humanity of the fetus, Mahowald develops two basic arguments as the framework for her egalitarianism. She contends that (1) human life is a developmental continuum; and (2) human beings are social, rational, and volitional creatures who are interrelated and interdependent. She then draws out the implications of these arguments. First, the fact that human life is a developmental continuum means that the stage of development is relevant to determining the morality of decisions regarding a person:

> Just as the fact that a patient is near death is relevant to the morality of decisions regarding treatment, so the fact that a fetus is nearly viable, or seriously defective, is morally relevant to a decision regarding abortion.

Second, if human beings are by definition social, interdependent creatures, then already-existing human relationships are pertinent to moral decisions regarding individuals:

> One could further argue that the early, painless abortion of the healthy fetus of a woman whose pregnancy places her life or health in jeopardy is justified because the pregnancy also threatens the developing lives of those who depend on her.

Third, the conception of human life as a developmental continuum enables Mahowald to avoid fixation on the status of the fetus; at the same time, it enables her to distinguish—with her potentiality–probability distinction—between human germ cells (spermatozoa and ova), which constitute "human life," and a human embryo, which is "*a* human life, *a* human being." Still a fourth advantage of Mahowald's developmental emphasis is that she is able to argue implicitly for the equal dignity and the common humanity of imbeciles, the handicapped, and the retarded (a feat that has eluded most philosophers of egalitarianism, who, for the most part, simply ignore this problem). Fifth, she is able to avoid controversies over personhood. In sum, Mahowald's developmental approach enables her to move beyond some bioethical questions and difficulties that have consumed much time and energy in discussions of abortion.

## THE CONCEPT OF EQUALITY

Mahowald's conception of equality is rich and multidimensional. She avoids reducing the concept of equality to identity or similarity; in fact, she goes the opposite way, stressing differences and individual characteristics. Clearly, she is not a "leveler." Her conception of equality "focuses primarily on individuals as such, insisting that advertence to the differences between them is the only possible way of establishing genuinely egalitarian relations among them." She seeks to avoid generalizations based on sex or gender, or even on developmental stage, as adequately defining the moral status of individuals. And her notion of equality applies to living and nonliving individuals (human beings, animals, forests, stones, things).

This broad notion of equality implies that decisions regarding the morality of abortion cannot be of the character of general rules but will take into account the individual circumstances and characteristics of the woman and the fetus and others who will be affected by the decision. Thus, Mahowald's notion of equality permits *ad hoc* determinations and the exercise of discretionary judgment—and this seems appropriate and fair in abortion decision-making.

## TOWARD AN EGALITARIAN PROLIFE ETHIC

Although this nuanced, subtle analysis of abortion and equality is said to be written from a "genuinely prolife" perspective, it seems far more reasoned and reasonable than anything yet heard from right-to-life advocates in public debate. For Mahowald's view allows for early abortion in some circumstances, abortion for severe fetal indications, and abortion in life- or health-threatening pregnancies. And because women are more seriously affected by involuntary pregnancies than almost anyone else, Mahowald supports the right of a woman to decide—with the additional proviso that "abortion justified solely on the basis of the woman's choice at any stage of pregnancy cannot be defended on egalitarian grounds as long as we allow the reach of equality to include nonautonomous human individuals." This "genuinely prolife position" is not, in other words, "profetus" or "antiabortion" (to use Mahowald's terms).

Finally, Mahowald's argument contains the crucial qualification that most feminists insist on: the distinction between the ideal and the real—between the egalitarian ideal (in which the life of the fetus would be accorded equal concern with the life of the mother) and the antiegalitarian reality of everyday life for most women. She insists, however, that women begin to make abortion decisions in accordance with her broadly egalitarian criteria as a step on the way to an ideally communal society.

## CRITIQUE

The ideal society that Mahowald has in mind is a community "in which the potentials of all individuals may be maximally, simultaneously fulfilled." This ideal community is just, egalitarian, and respectful of the autonomy and the dignity of all:

> Autonomy is thus a crucial, yet not the only, factor to be considered in promoting equality among all individuals. Others' fundamental needs such as life or health may justify overriding individual autonomy. The liberation of women, then, like human liberation and equality generally, is not an end in itself, but a necessary means to the communal ideal.

I have a few quibbles with this egalitarian, communitarian ideal. It seems that Mahowald is placing too much weight on the concept of equality, that is, making equality do the work of other basic concepts such as justice, fraternity, mutual aid, and community. This becomes clear if we ask ourselves the question: Why *should* we struggle to achieve this ideal society? One answer might be that we should work toward a society of equals because gross inequalities in wealth, status, and power erode the mutual respect that should obtain in human relations. Or because, as Aristotle wrote long ago, friendship is possible only between equals (and the ideal community is one of friends). In other words, equality may be valued because it leads to other ends (liberty, fraternity, community). Now, if equality is simply a means to these other goals, then perhaps it is incorrect to describe the ideal society as egalitarian; to the extent that social inequalities are more efficient means to these other ends, perhaps such inequalities should be embraced.

In short, I think Mahowald is interested more in fraternity and community and less in equality. Her principles create or acknowledge a presumption in favor of equal treatment of both fetuses and women—because of basic equal dignity and common humanity. In creating an initial presumption in favor of equality, Mahowald places the burden of justifying departures from this rule on those arguing for abortion. This stance is acceptable. But I wonder if one can call it an egalitarian ethic.

My second objection concerns Mahowald's sixth principle, which acknowledges a priority among different kinds of individuals (within a broad egalitarian framework that encompasses all individual creatures):

> Perhaps the most convincing support for the claim that human beings have graver responsibilities to other human beings than to members of other species is the objective superiority of human over other species. . . . Because we cannot preserve everything, surely we ought to focus our efforts on what is most worth preserving. In that context, it seems clear that no other species, on the whole, possesses worthier characteristics than our own.

Here, Mahowald's egalitarian position sanctions a quality-of-life ethic that seems rather utilitarian. That is, the very argument for ranking humans above all other creatures seems to undermine the attempt to protect fetal life because fetal life is more or less human, depending on its stage of development.

Elsewhere Mahowald writes, "If we value such competencies as intelligence and speech, then we ought also to value—*to a lesser degree, of course*—the probability of such competence that the average human fetus represents." (italics added). But in an abortion situation, wouldn't this scheme of values almost always weight the case in favor of the pregnant woman? And if this is true, then perhaps Mahowald's egalitarian account does not (as she claims) support "the claim that we have responsibilities toward human fetuses as (at least) probable persons." For although she suggests that the fetus is a value to be respected, her argument for the superiority of the human to other species seems to undermine her attempt to respect fetal life.

Mahowald's developmental approach would probably not sit well with abortion opponents in the larger society. Perhaps, one cannot really respect fetal life without ascribing to the fetus complete personhood. Yet, I suspect that Mahowald's balanced, nuanced developmental account is a more plausible, a truer, and a more accurate reflection of life's gradual beginnings and endings. I applaud her "genuinely prolife position"; it is more subtle and qualified and more sensitive to the realities of women's lives than either the profetus or the antiabortion positions that prompt the restrictive legislation currently before Congress.

## CHAPTER 8

# Beneath the Surface of the Abortion Dispute

## Are Women Fully Human?

SANDRA HARDING

### Autobiographical Statement

*After receiving an undergraduate degree in literature from a women's college in the mid-1950s, I worked for 10 years in the entertainment industry in New York City. After my second daughter was born, I returned to graduate school, first in sociology and then in philosophy; at this time, I commuted back to New York University in Manhattan from Albany, New York. Thus, during the period when many of my earlier and later friends were active in the civil rights movement and the radicalism of the 1960s, I was busy changing diapers, maintaining a style of living suitable for a faculty household, and going to graduate school. When the women's movement arrived in Albany in the early 1970s, I was more than ready for it. In 1973, I began teaching at The Allen Center, an interdisciplinary college (which no longer exists) within the State University of New York at Albany. Since 1976, I have been in the philosophy department at the University of Delaware and have taught many women's studies courses. Since 1981, I have been, by joint appointment, also in sociology. I have been a single parent since 1974, and my two daughters are now heading off on their own.*

*In philosophy, I began examining the problems created by positivist inheritances in current American epistemology, philosophy of science, and philosophy of social science. During the last five years, my research and publications have focused on how the most abstract and formal aspects of*

SANDRA HARDING • Department of Philosophy, University of Delaware, Newark, Delaware 19711.

*Western thought reveal the distinctive "fingerprints" of the social groups that created this thought.* Discovering Reality: Feminist Perspectives on Epistemology, Metaphysics, Methodology, and the Philosophy of Science, *which I coedited with Merrill Hintikka, was published in March 1983 by Reidel; I am currently completing a monograph, (supported by the National Science Foundation and a Mina Shaughnessy Fellowship from the U.S. Department of Education's Fund for the Improvement of Post-Secondary Education) that examines the problems for mainstream liberal and Marxist theories of knowledge created by the new research on women and gender in the social sciences and biology.*

*The opening paragraphs of the second section of my paper indicate some of the ways in which I suspect that my experiences have influenced my beliefs about the politics and the social values that lie beneath the surface of the abortion dispute.*

Feminist theory and politics have emerged from within two great traditions in Western moral, political, and social thought.[1] They have emerged from liberalism, which assumes that conflicts between the timeless and universal natural rights of rational individuals should be adjudicated within the free market of social contracts. And they have emerged from Marxism, which assumes that conflicts between the socially determined needs of "animals who labor" are created by divisions of labor in the social relations of production.

Until recently, feminists have tried to fit into these traditions their fundamental insights that women are fully human and that the sexual order is a fundamental component of the social order. By "fully human," feminists mean that women's activities, too, are *as* social—as consciously, intentionally, historically organized—as men's. Thus, reproduction—which includes sexuality, family forms, and domestic life, as well as the consciously mediated process of birthing that continues the species—is a fully human activity; it is not "merely natural."[2] By "the sexual order" is meant sexual politics, the way in which social meanings of sex differences are fundamental variables

---

[1]Both the issues and the arguments of the first draft of this paper were developed with Shakuntla Bhaya, now at Northeastern Law School. I have tried to keep hearing her insistence on focusing clearly on the issues central to achieving recognition of full personhood for women of all classes and races. I have greatly benefited from comments by Sarah Begus, and from the responses to the first draft by Lisa Cahill and the other participants in the Hastings Center Conference on Abortion.

[2]Mary O'Brien, *The Politics of Reproduction* (Boston: Routledge and Kegan Paul, 1981); cf. review by Sandra Harding and Shakuntla Bhaya, *Signs: Journal of Women in Culture and Society,* 8 no. 2 (1982), pp. 361–363.

in the organization of both social life and social thought. Thus, the sexual order has both an "ideational" or belief component and a "material" or concrete social-practice component: Culturally variable meanings of sex differences are used to organize social practices, and these social practices make the sexual meanings of practices appear "natural." Noticing the sexual order makes possible the recognition that sex/gender is perhaps *the* most significant social variable in determining life opportunities and belief characteristics for individuals within any particular culture, and often even across cultures: There are identifiable commonalities in women's activities and beliefs and in men's activities and beliefs that are not attributable to "the natural."

These considerations are leading to the emergence of an "autonomous feminist standpoint." Such a theoretical, empirical, and political perspective begins with the assumptions that women are fully human and that the sexual order fundamentally structures the social order. It uses these assumptions to evaluate critically our inherited liberal and Marxist theoretical discourses, the adequacy of existing empirical understandings of the social order, and the moral and practical consequences of public policy.

The abortion dispute provides a good example of how and why the feminist standpoint is basically in conflict with the moral and the political assumptions of the liberal and Marxist discourses. Feminists are coming to understand that neither prolife nor prochoice women should expect to have their needs met or their rights granted by the various solutions to the abortion issue proposed in the current political arena. Although I would not underestimate the important differences in the immediate needs and values of prolife and prochoice women, I propose that many of these differences are entirely the consequence of different strategies that the patriarchal state and economy use in different classes and races to prevent women from exercising full human personhood. Prolife and prochoice women implicitly share the understanding that the solutions to the abortion dispute proposed in the public arena do not begin to address our fundamental needs as humans who exist in female bodies and in a society organized by racism, classism, and sexism. We are forced to fight against each other on a terrain foreign to our needs, perceptions, and values as women, lest we join together to reorganize social life in ways that would accommodate our full membership in the species.

Thus, from the feminist standpoint, there are important commonalities in prolife and prochoice women's actual needs, perceptions of their needs, and values. These commonalities are distorted or ignored in the current abortion dispute and often by women on both sides of the dispute. Beneath the surface of the abortion dispute can be detected women's shared recognition that we are fully human, and that the sexual order—the sexual politics of the social order—refuses to recognize our fundamental humanity. Can women come to articulate and act on the recognition that there may be more that binds us together than that separates us?

## THE SOCIAL ORIGINS OF BELIEF

I will forgo the usual intellectual pretension to political neutrality in the service of a dispassionate, disinterested, "objective" analysis of this conflict. Clearly, my own social experiences have contributed to making the prochoice position reasonable to me as public policy in the United States at this moment in history. However, reflecting on my experiences has also helped me to appreciate the social circumstances that I do and do not share with women for whom the prolife position appears reasonable. No woman, I think, would select abortion as the most desirable way to exercise choices about how her own sexuality and ability to reproduce are to be expressed. Thanks to access to contraceptives and to luck, I have never had the occasion to consider having an abortion, though I know very few women my age who have not had one. When I wanted to bear children, my pregnancies were easily begun, and my children were born healthy. I have been full time in study or in the wage-labor market for virtually all of my adult life. I am a female head-of-household with children under the age of 18—one of the 20% minority in that U.S. Census Bureau category able to live above the poverty level. Furthermore, I am a highly educated professional for whom wage-labor and the rest of my social relations are difficult to separate; at any rate, merely staying in place in an occupation structured to suit men's administrative-class work patterns requires devotion considerably above and beyond the call of a 40-hour work week. (There are, however, benefits in not having an adult male in my household: Evidently, I perform eight hours less per week of domestic labor than do women with a resident adult male—whether or not those women also perform wage-labor, and regardless of the age and the number of children in the household and the amount of time those males contribute to "domestic labor"![3]) Finally, my parents' family histories are full of tales of women and children socially and economically abandoned by husbands and fathers, of women dying young from childbearing

[3]Heidi Hartmann, "The Family as the Locus of Gender, Class, and Political Struggle: The Example of Housework," *Signs: Journal of Women in Culture and Society* 6, no. 3 (1981), pp. 383–385.

and farm labor, of men marrying for the third and fourth times. I also come from a long line of strong and self-willed women who were forced by economic and social circumstances to give far less to their children and to themselves than they thought right—a claim that could be made about far fewer of my male ancestors.

What significance does this confession of personal history have? Does it make the claims of this paper merely subjective? My reading of history suggests that my families' experiences are by no means uncommon. Whatever else political theorists and historians may say about the popular tendency to reminisce about the happy families and contented wives and mothers of the past, clearly these families—and women's contented role in them—are more often figments of socially regressive sentiment than facts of history. Furthermore, it is one of the assumptions of this paper that *all* ideas, beliefs, and knowledge claims are grounded in particular, historical, social experiences. Our grasp of the issues in the abortion dispute is distorted if we understand these issues only through the distinctively sexist and also anachronistic social experience grounding liberal and Marxist discourses. One epistemological project of feminism is to reason as best we can while keeping clearly in focus the social origins of all human belief—our own as well as our opponents. This approach is preferable to relegating our historically specific lived experiences to the underground of our unconscious, or to the "merely personal" and "merely subjective." The directives of the dominant discourse, which supposedly produce objectivity, merely make it more difficult to locate the precise social origins of false universalizations about man, humankind, the social welfare, human rationality, scientific belief, and the like.[4] So from the perspective of this paper, everyone's personal confessions are not only in order, but epistemologically important. In lieu of hearing personal confessions from the liberal and Marxist theoreticians about the social experience that made their assumptions reasonable to them, we shall have to "read the text" of their assumptions anthropologically in order to reveal what these social experiences must have been.

---

[4]For key discussions of the feminist epistemological issues, see Jane Flax, "Political Philosophy and the Patriarchal Unconscious: A Psychoanalytic Perspective on Epistemology and Metaphysics"; Nancy Hartsock, "The Feminist Standpoint: Developing the Ground for a Specifically Feminist Historical Materialism"; Sandra Harding, "Why Has the Sex/Gender System Become Visible Only Now?"; all in S. Harding and M. Hintikka, eds., *Discovering Reality: Feminist Perspectives on Epistemology, Metaphysics, Methodology and the Philosophy of Science* (Dordrecht: Reidel, 1983); Dorothy Smith, "Women's Perspective as a Radical Critique of Sociology," *Sociological Inquiry* 44 (1974), pp. 7–13.

Although liberalism, Marxism, and feminism have had different meanings for their proponents at different times in their histories, the central assumptions mentioned have remained relatively constant. We need to keep in mind the social origins of these belief systems. Liberalism originated in seventeenth- and eighteenth-century justifications for legal, political, and economic reform in Europe during the transition from feudal to early capitalist formations. Liberalism has been intimately involved in the transformation of the role of the economy and the state, and in modern, scientific modes of producing and justifying belief-claims. Liberal assumptions originated centuries ago in the needs of a new class of public policy administrators. The understanding of what exactly are the political, social, and moral policies that liberalism requires has obviously varied in liberalism's long history. Nevertheless, one can trace through this history the administratively useful assumptions that human beings are essentially rational individuals possessing timeless and universal natural rights, and that, when such rights conflict, they should be adjudicated through the free market of social contracts. Liberal theory was created within a society structured by the sexual order. But the fact that men constructed liberal theory and that men administer public policy is presumed by liberals to be neither peculiar nor interesting.

Marxism emerged in the mid-nineteenth century in Europe as an attempt to reconceptualize the vast social disorder created by the industrial stage of capitalist expansion, so as to provide the rapidly increasing number of wage-laborers—the primary producers and victims of that expansion—with strategies for bettering their condition. Marxist assumptions are based on the needs of those whose labor is primarily wage-labor. A century and a half of struggle to guide social life within Marxist understanding in Asia, Africa, and South America, as well as in Europe, has created vast differences in the way Marxism and socialism are understood today. Nevertheless, common to all these understandings are the beliefs that humans are essentially socially laboring animals, that human needs are thus socially determined, and that conflicts in these needs are primarily created by divisions of labor in the public realm of production. Marxism, too, was created within a society structured by the sexual order. But the fact that men constructed Marxist theory, and that men control both proletarian and bourgeois labor, is presumed by Marxists to be neither peculiar nor interesting.

Finally, although isolated feminist insights can be detected even in antiquity, feminism as a significant social force emerged only in the nineteenth century in Europe and the United States, and within liberal and Marxist political struggles. We have begun to understand only in the last few decades that feminism must be an autonomous moral, political, and social perspective. The beginnings of this new understanding can be detected in Simone de Beauvoir's observation that women are neither a natural biological category (a sex) nor understandable entirely in economic terms (as a part of classes); women are a socially created "other."[5] Feminist assumptions are based on the social experiences of women as women—of a group increasingly relegated to the sole responsibility for privatized domestic labor controlled from the public sphere, and to the least powerful and lowest-paid jobs in wage-labor. Today, what feminism means to its proponents varies widely across classes, races, and cultural settings. Nevertheless, common to all varieties of feminism are the assumptions that women are fully human, and that the sexual order prevents the acknowledgment of women's humanity. The fact that feminist theory and politics are constructed by women and men critical of at least some aspects of the sexual order is presumed by both men and women to be significant.

One challenge that feminists have faced is to convince men and women that beliefs legitimated in male-dominated cultures are just as much the product of men's subjective social experience *as men* as the beliefs produced by women are the product of their social experiences as women. As de Beauvoir noted:

> A man never begins by presenting himself as an individual of a certain sex; it goes without saying that he is a man. The terms *masculine* and *feminine* are used symmetrically only as a matter of form, as on legal papers. In actuality the relation of the two sexes is not quite like that of two electrical poles, for man represents both the positive and the neutral, as is indicated by the common use of *man* to designate human beings in general. . . . It is understood that the fact of being a man is no peculiarity. A man is in the right in being a man; it is the woman who is in the wrong.[6]

If women, too, are fully human, then being a man is a peculiarity. Men's ideas are as subjective as women's. Liberal and Marxist moral, political, social, and epistemological claims that do not recognize the peculiarity of masculinity are unable to recognize women as fully human.

The epistemologically alert reader will see two possibilities at this point: cognitive relativism, or the need for a more adequate formulation of cognitive absolutism than the liberal epistemology of

[5]Simone de Beauvoir, *The Second Sex* (New York: Knopf, 1953).
[6]Ibid., p. xv.

modern science has provided.[7] Taking the relativist alternative, feminists would hold that sexist and feminist experiences are equally reliable groundings for adequate belief, and hence, that sexist beliefs are as true as feminist beliefs. Obviously, this is not the feminist epistemological stance, nor should cognitive relativism be the stance of anyone who thinks that humans can sort beliefs into those more and less likely to be true. How to develop a formulation of cognitive absolutism more adequate than the liberal epistemology of modern science is an issue of concern today to feminists as well as to epistemologists generally. Common to many of these projects is the understanding that not all social experiences provide equally desirable grounds for belief, as well as the understanding that beliefs produced by the dominating groups in socially stratified societies are grounded in epistemologically undesirable social experience. From the perspective of these understandings, the peculiarity of masculinity would have to be judged epistemologically disadvantageous in sexist societies such as ours.

In discussions of the abortion issue, there is a markedly ahistorical flavor in claims made about the state's obligations in regulating abortion, "the family," and the value of children. It is worth reminding ourselves that abortion became illegal in this country only during the late nineteenth century:

> In 1880 no jurisdiction in the United States had enacted any statutes on the subject of abortion; most forms of abortion were not illegal and those American women who wished to practice abortion did so. Yet by 1900 virtually every jurisdiction in the United States had laws upon its books that proscribed the practices sharply and declared most abortions to be criminal offenses.[8]

Furthermore, we need to avoid references to such a nonexistent entity as *the* family, unless we mean by this term strictly the abstract sociological category of the unit in every culture, whatever its members and structure, within which the young are raised. In the abortion dispute, *the family* usually refers to the nuclear family. But families consisting of a wage-earning male, a female engaged in full-time domestic labor, and young children have functioned as a political, social, and/or economically significant unit only in a very limited number of class, racial, and cultural formations. As we shall see later, such families now constitute a rapidly shrinking minority of households in the United States for reasons that have little to do with

[7]For key arguments favoring these alternatives, see Jack W. Meiland and Michael Krausz, eds., *Relativism: Cognitive and Moral* (Notre Dame, Ind.: Notre Dame University Press, 1982).
[8]James C. Mohr, *Abortion in America: The Origins and Evolution of National Policy, 1800–1900* (Oxford: Oxford University Press, 1978).

feminism and much to do with the changing needs of the economy.[9] Furthermore, such families have functioned as "a haven in a heartless world" within which individuals (men?) can find their "true selves" only in late industrial societies, where production and reproduction take place in separate spheres.[10] Finally, the social values attached to having children have varied widely cross-culturally and have clearly been influenced by socail needs originating in the economy, the state, and other institutions of public life.[11]

With these preliminaries out of the way, let us turn to the abortion issue as a good example of how the feminist standpoint conflicts fundamentally with the moral and political assumptions of the liberal and Marxist discourses.

## LIBERAL PHILOSOPHERS AND ABORTION

### IS THE FETUS A PERSON?

Most philosophers today work within the liberal theory of human nature, human knowledge, and the social order. The assumptions of this theory are those of modern science. As one reviewer of the philosophical literature on abortion has pointed out, moral philosophers have attempted to solve the abortion problem by locating a "crucial question," the answer to which would solve once and for all the moral issues that abortion raises.[12] They have been "almost unanimous"[13] in deciding that this crucial question is "Is the fetus a person?"[14] Furthermore, they claim to be able to provide arguments to convince us that their answers to this question are plausible. Some have claimed to be able to determine that a fetus is

---

[9]Data supporting and explanations of this claim can be found in the papers in Martha Blaxall and Barbara Reagan, eds., *Women and the Work-place* (Chicago: Chicago University Press, 1976); Rosalind Pollack Petchesky, "Antiabortion, Antifeminism, and the Rise of the New Right," *Feminist Studies* 7, no. 2 (1981), pp. 206–246; Hartmann.

[10]Eli Zaretsky, *Capitalism, The Family, and Personal Life* (New York: Harper and Row, 1976).

[11]Phillippe Ariès, *Centuries of Childhood: A Social History of Family Life* (New York: Knopf, 1970); Carol Brown, "Mother, Fathers, and Children: From Private to Public Patriarchy," in L. Sargent, ed., *Women and Revolution* (Boston: South End Press, 1981).

[12]David Solomon, "Philosophers on Abortion," in E. Manier, W. Liu, and D. Solomon, eds., *Abortion: New Directions for Policy Studies* (Notre Dame, Ind.: Notre Dame University Press, 1977), p. 162.

[13]Ibid.

[14]A notable exception is Judith Jarvis Thomson, "A Defense of Abortion," *Philosophy and Public Affairs* 1, no. 1 (1971), pp. 47–66.

a person from the moment of conception[15]; at the other end of the scale, one philosopher claims that not even infants are persons.[16]

There are a number of problems with this approach to the abortion issue. First of all, there is clearly no way to establish when and if a fetus is a person on the basis of appeals either to biological evidence or to a consensus on the social recognition of "personhood."[17] This should surprise no one, if only because it is widely understood that there is a similar lack of consistency in the biological or the social criteria for the end of "personhood," as, for instance, the euthanasia dispute has long made clear. Life and death are fundamentally philosophical concepts, not biological givens. Thus, the meanings of and the referents to life and death will vary from culture to culture and often from group to group within a heterogeneous culture as do the meanings of and the referents to all concepts: All concepts are the product of culturally varying human social experience.

This "crucial-question" approach to resolving moral issues borrows whatever plausibility it can muster from its presumed usefulness in the physical sciences. However, as the French physicist Pierre Duhem pointed out long ago, there are no crucial experiments even in the physical sciences.[18] During the last few decades, the development of Duhem's insights by Quine, Kuhn, and others has lead to the widespread recognition that the beliefs about the entities constituting "nature" that the most rigorous of the "hard sciences" propose are as much a product of our explicit hypotheses and our implicit world views as they are of Nature herself.[19] Thus, even the distinction between philosophical and biological concepts drawn above is suspect because biological concepts, too, are created by culture as well as by nature.[20]

Furthermore, this crucial-question approach clashes with another tenet of liberal epistemology, namely, that one can't conclude

[15]John Finnis, "The Rights and Wrongs of Abortion," *Philosophy and Public Affairs* 2, no. 2 (1973), pp. 117–145.

[16]Michael Tooley, "Abortion and Infanticide," *Philosophy and Public Affairs* 2, no. 1 (1972), pp. 37–65.

[17]Cf. Solomon.

[18]Sandra Harding, ed., *Can Theories Be Refuted?: Essays on the Duhem-Quine Thesis* (Dordrecht: Reidel, 1976).

[19]W. V. O. Quine, *Ontological Relativity and Other Essays* (New York: Columbia University Press, 1969); T. S. Kuhn, *The Structure of Scientific Revolutions* (Chicago: Chicago University Press 1970).

[20]Donna Haraway, "Animal Sociology and a Natural Economy of the Body Politic," *Signs: Journal of Women in Culture and Society* 4, no. 1 (1978), pp. 21–60, shows how cultural influences have shaped both the best and worst of biology; Alison Jaggar, "Human Biology and Feminist Theory: Sex Equality Reconsidered," in Carol C. Gould, ed., *Beyond Domination: New Perspectives on Women and Philosophy* (Totowa, N.J.: Littlefield Adams, 1983), criticizes the nature–culture dichotomy itself.

an "ought" on the grounds of an "is." Thus, even if one could determine once and for all the facts about when a fetus becomes a person, for liberal epistemologists nothing at all should follow about morals or social policy. I would be among the last to underestimate the importance of the well-known problems with the claim that values cannot be the consequence of facts: I have argued elsewhere that they always and necessarily mutually influence each other in ways that can be scientifically and morally progressive or regressive.[21] But it is inconsistent for liberals to argue both that the facts about when a fetus becomes a person can be distinguished from the social values fetuses and motherhood do or do not have for individuals and cultures, *and* that, if we know these facts, then everything will become clear about moral and policy issues.

Finally, regardless of what liberal philosophers claim is the answer to the question "Is the fetus a person?", their writings support New Right political forces in the United States today not just on the issues of how to best repress and control female sexuality and women's "personhood," but also on the whole array of New Right economic, political, and social directives, which are inseparable from issues concerning the control of women's sexuality.[22] We can understand this surprising consequence of liberal writings on the fetus as a person by noting the following reasonable response to liberal arguments: if *this* is the key to solving the moral issues about abortion, and if it cannot be proved once and for all that the fetus is *not* a person, then moral prudence would suggest that the state should not permit these possible persons to be "killed." From this line of reasoning does follow, "naturally," an array of state policies proposed by the New Right that must—alas—forgo recognizing women as fully human.

## ABSTRACT INDIVIDUAL RIGHTS VERSUS CONCRETE SOCIAL RESPONSIBILITIES

Seen from another perspective, the selection of *this* as the crucial moral issue arises from liberal concerns with establishing when individuals have formal, abstract rights that articulate and organized

[21]Sandra Harding, "Does Objectivity in Social Science Require Value-Neutrality?", *Soundings* 60, no. 4 (1977), pp. 351–366; "Four Contributions Values Can Make to the Objectivity of Social Science," in P. D. Asquith and I. Hacking, eds., *PSA 1978*, vol. 1 (East Lansing, Mich.: Philosophy of Science Association, 1978); "The Norms of Social Inquiry and Masculine Experience," in P. D. Asquith and R. N. Giere, eds., *PSA 1980*, vol. 2 (East Lansing, Mich. Philosophy of Science Association, 1980).

[22]Petchesky makes clear the inseparability of these issues. See also Zillah Eisenstein, "Antifeminism in the Politics and Election of 1980," *Feminist Studies* 7, no. 2 (1981), pp. 187–205.

special-interest groups can then ask state administrators to defend. Moral preoccupation with when the fetus should be regarded as a person diverts liberal and New Right eyes from concrete moral and political issues about who should be responsible for satisfying the needs prerequisite for an infant of any race, sex, or class to become a *real* moral agent, that is, a competitor in the liberal "free market" of adult social relations. Even a staunch defender of free-market economic relations pointed out, "Liberalism always justifies society's abandonment of a group unable to articulate or defend its own claim,"[23] and women, existing children, citizens of color, and the poor already constitute groups abandoned by our liberal state. For liberalism, where "tastes" differ, matters are left to "free decision in the market place . . . and the class whose humanity is in dispute is treated with legal indifference."[24]

Necessarily invisible within this moral discourse about the possible personhood of the fetus are the moral, social, and political issues that feminists take to be central. From the feminist perspective, the central question should not be about the abstract individual rights of fetuses, but about broader reproductive responsibilities and how to create the social conditions that would make possible the fulfillment of these responsibilities. These women's questions about reproductive responsibility concern the politics of sexuality and the politics of economic life. Why are adult women not treated by law or custom as full social persons with equal rights and needs to articulate and defend claims to social personhood for themselves and for the children whom they bear or wish to bear? How can a woman or a child exercise her or his "right to life" or "freedom of choice" in the face of poverty, unemployment, racism, legal and individual sexism, and the whole gamut of material conditions attributable to these material restrictions on social personhood? Why are women's and children's rights and needs systematically regarded as less important than "the stability of the family" (read "The stability of men's control of family life"), to which both the pro- and antiabortion liberal thinkers appeal as a crucial limit on their recommendations about abortion? The family of concern here, we are discovering, is the locus of training in racism, classism, and especially sexism. It is also the social setting among all classes for the heretofore hidden but widespread incidence of incest, wife battering, marital rape, child abuse, and gender-stratified "lifestyles," as well as the battleground for war between the sexes on many issues of public policy. "The family" to which liberals appeal appears to be a crucial foundation of women's

[23]Milton Friedman, quoted by Solomon, p. 171.
[24]Ibid.

oppression and of white, bourgeois, male domination in both public and private life.[25]

These two kinds of conflicts between liberal assumptions and the beliefs that women are fully human reveal the underlying contradiction within liberalism between its commitment to ruling-class men's control of reproduction, female sexuality, and women's labor, and hence of both public and private life, and to the liberal ideology implying that a legitimate social order must be committed to supporting democratic decision-making and equality of opportunity *for all*.[26] Contrary to the liberal assumption that humans are essentially disembodied and inherently rational individuals (that is, that our bodies are accidental features of our personhood), humans come embodied, and in (roughly) two sexes. In our culture, embodied sexuality is a mainstay of our identity as persons.[27] The refusal to permit women to participate in the design of social life within which female sexuality and reproduction are expressed systematically restricts the personhood of women while encouraging distinctively masculine meanings of sexuality to permeate social life. Furthermore, only those who are in the material and political position to compete in the free market of social contracts can articulate their rights. Even were it decided that fetuses should be granted human rights, they would remain unable to articulate and defend those rights. They would join women, existing children, people of color, and the working class in this country, all of whom satisfy any criteria for personhood proposed in the abortion dispute, and all of whom must depend on others to articulate and defend their rights as human beings. We should not have to pit these groups against each other with regard to their inability to articulate their rights, as the liberal insistence on understanding reproductive responsibility in terms of abstract rights in the abortion issue forces us to do.

Thus, we can begin to glimpse how liberalism restricts its understanding of human personhood and social life to those categories that are plausible and useful from the perspective of a distinctive minority of human experiences: the experiences of existing or would-be administrators who constitute the ruling class in the kind of society idealized in the West since Hobbes's and Locke's day. Administrators

---

[25]Zillah Eisenstein, *The Radical Implications of Liberal Feminism* (New York: Longmans, 1979); Susan Moller Okin, *Women in Western Political Thought* (Princeton, N.J.: Princeton University Press, 1979).

[26]Cf. Sandra Harding, "Is Equality of Opportunity Democratic?", *The Philosophical Forum* nos. 10, 2–4 (1979), pp. 206–223.

[27]Esther Spector Person, "Sexuality as the Mainstay of Identity: Psychoanalytic Perspectives," *Signs: Journal of Women in Culture and Society* 5, no. 4 (1980), pp. 605–630.

have no obligation to nurture or help others, or to design social arrangements that satisfy anyone's fundamental needs as human beings. Their obligations are restricted to adjudicating the conflicting rights that are, in fact, "rationally" articulated to them, and to legitimating their own existence. The liberal insistence on articulating the competing rights between fetuses and women reinforces the legitimacy of administrative ruling while it successfully avoids giving priority to satisfying the needs that differently embodied humans beings have. The assumption that the administrative mode of resolving conflicts is a desirable human mode prevents our understanding how deeply administering itself is grounded in masculine meanings of the sexual order.

## MARXISM AND WOMEN'S CONDITION: CONFLICTING CONCEPTIONS OF WOMEN

If the feminist assumption that women are fully human but that social life is structured by the sexual order cannot be accommodated within a liberal discourse, it fares not much better within the assumptions of the classical Marxist discourse. It is the Marixst discourse within which social life is conducted for close to two thirds of the world's inhabitants today. (Significantly, whereas many nonfeminist liberals discuss the abortion issue, few nonfeminist Marxists do. On the other hand, Marxists have often addressed questions of population control, pointing out how issues of political economy, not of morality, underlie population control policies.) Feminist problems with the Marxist discourse have been widely discussed, and I cannot take time to review these criticisms here.[28] Instead, I want to draw attention to the two conflicting conceptions of "women" within the Marxist discourse from which the feminist criticisms of Marxism can be understood to originate. Both make it difficult to understand how the human needs of women can be recognized, let alone satisfied, within the Marxist discourse. On the one hand, for Marxists, human beings are the one species with no timeless, universally observable nature. Our interactions with our natural/social surround, through the production of food, shelter, clothing, and the other materials that we need to survive, transform us as we are busy transforming our surround: "The hand is not only

[28]See the essays in Lydia Sargent, ed., *Women and Revolution* (Boston: South End Press, 1981).

the organ of labour, it is also the product of that labour."[29] Thus, observable differences between men and women, like so many other observable differences between individuals, are as much a product of the past and present social practices of production as they are of nature.

On the other hand, key aspects of reproduction and sexuality are treated in Marxist thought and politics as exceptions to this understanding of human nature as socially created. First of all, it is the division of labor in the "sex act" itself that is claimed as the fundamental natural resource used to transform preclass into class societies. The differences between human beings required for the "sex act" alone are inferred to lie outside the prior intervention of culture. However, what Marxists take to be the necessary and biologically given aspects of the "sex act" extend far beyond the sexual (vs. asexual) reproduction required to continue the species. Marxists have often understood that particular historical elaborations of the "sex act," which are socially created and oppressive to women, have become the means of structuring kinship, marriage, and social relations between the sexes. But they have failed to notice that what distinguishes our species from others here, too, is the plasticity of our natures in the hands of culture, and thus the extent to which the sexual order and other components of the social order organize each other. Thus, the "sex act" is a totally socially mediated and fully human interaction. The social influences on sexuality and the sexual influences on differing forms of sociality remain in fundamental respects outside the Marxist critique of the liberal nature-culture dualism. Even when revisionist Marxists notice that social arrangements do have origins in the sexual order (as did the Freudian Left), they fail to notice these origins in distinctively masculine experience of the sexual order. The fact of being a man is no peculiarity for Marxists.

Second, although the division of labor by sex is for Marxists the natural prime mover of uniquely human history, it never appears subsequently as an actor in distinctively human drama. Sexual reproduction is the precondition for human history, but its elaboration as human sexuality exists only as an object for human (economic) history to act on.

In the third place, and consequently, Marxist theory envisions no end to the general social division of labor by sex, nor to the sexual meanings of sociality; the practices of socialist countries are just one

---

[29]Frederick Engels, "The Part Played by Labour in the Transition from Ape to Man," in Karl Marx and Frederick Engels, *Selected Works* (New York: International Publishers, no date), p. 359.

kind of evidence of this failure. The Marxist solution to the "woman problem" is to industrialize women's domestic labor. In both theory and practice, this labor remains labor by women, whether industrialized or not. As one critic noted, Marx

> takes for granted women's responsibility for household labor. He repeats, as if it were his own, the question of a Belgian factory inspector: If a mother works for wages, "how will (the household's) internal economy be cared for; who will look after the young children; who will get ready the meals, do the washing and mending?"[30]

And Marx's vision of social life "after the revolution," in which each person fishes in the morning, hunts in the afternoon and philosophizes after dinner, leaves curiously unaddressed how the fish and the products of the hunt get on the dinner table in the form of a meal, let alone who's tending the babies during the philosophy sessions. Reproducing Marixst man is assumed to be a natural labor for women.[31] Sociality remains intimately structured by masculine sexual meanings for Marxists to the extent that the social relations of public life are envisioned as essentially productive relations among men, and as the only relations that must be fundamentally restructured if everyone is to achieve unalienated personhood.

Thus, within the Marxist discourse, women cannot be recognized as fully human without undercutting the validity of the Marxist conceptions of distinctively human nature and of distinctively human social activity. These conceptions are appealing only from the perspective of men who expect to hold one job in wage-labor, to do no domestic work, and to have no responsibilities for child care. Regardless of divisions of labor by class, women all perform sex-divided labor in both public and private life. Thus, although Marxists are correct in understanding state policies on abortion, sterilization, and population control as issues of class maintenance, these are fundamentally issues involving the maintenance of male dominance. The "proletariat" has felt no need to share in reproductive responsibility and thus to create the social conditions in which "the female man," too, can hunt in the morning, fish in the afternoon, and philosophize in the evening. The Marxist insistence on theoretically and politically fixating on the social needs of men in the workplace successfully avoids giving priority to, or even noticing, the needs of women that arise from their assigned roles in the social division of labor by sex.

[30]Hartsock, p. 291.
[31]Mary O'Brien, "Reproducing Marxist Man," in Lorenne M. G. Clark and Lynda Lange, eds., *The Sexism of Social and Political Theory: Women and Reproduction from Plato to Nietzsche* (Toronto: Toronto University Press, 1979). See also Note 2.

It also prevents our understanding how both "men's work" and "women's work" are structured by masculine assumptions of the naturalness of the sexual order.

From the perspective of Marxism, the abortion dispute appears merely as a typical bourgeois attempt to obscure the fundamental class organization of social life. There are no *social, human* needs, perceptions, or values that women across the class spectrum can share, because class divisions drive women into antagonistic relations with each other as firmly as they separate the proletariat and the bourgeoisie to which women fundamentally "belong." The assumption that the class struggle mode of resolving conflicts is the desirable human mode prevents our understanding how deeply class relations—with their insistent focus on production—are themselves grounded in masculine meanings of the sexual order.

## THE FUTURE: EMERGING TRENDS, IMPLICIT RECOGNITIONS

I have been suggesting that the needs that will be met and the rights that will be defended by politics originating within Marxist and liberal discourses are not human needs and rights, but only the felt needs and claimed rights of the men who control the racial and class hierarchies. Unfortunately, the oppressed can never afford the luxury of refusing to fight on any terrain defined by their oppressors. Women will have to continue to assert their needs and rights as human beings within existing politics simply in order not to lose ground. No doubt the racist, classist, and sexist interests that make reasonable prolife versus prochoice policies in churches, the medical professions, the state, and the economy will continue to keep abortion on the public agenda as long as possible, forcing women to struggle against each other and to beg for the different kinds of crumbs of human dignity that this social order offers. No doubt, in socialist countries, policies on reproduction and domestic labor will continue to be influenced only by percieved and changing production needs. However, I want to point to some emerging socioeconomic trends in the United States that might increase profeminist recognitions by women, and to some recognitions shared by pro- and antifeminist women that, if politically activated, could transform the goals of the feminist political agenda. Both of these possibilities have implications for our future understanding of the abortion dispute.

Kristin Luker has formulated the notions of androgynous and

sex-specific life resources for women.[32] Androgynous life resources are created through the kinds of education, income, and occupations outside the home that have heretofore been reserved for men. Sex-specific life resources for women are created within the "traditional" family model that has been the middle-class ideal: a lifetime of economic support by a single husband in exchange for a lifetime of domestic labor bearing and caring for children, husband, and often extended kin in other generations.

Sociologist Rosalind Petchesky has summarized in the following way the data indicating the rapid disappearance of the kind of family model that traditionally offered sex-specific (vs. androgynous) social resources for women. First, "by 1975, husband-wife families with two or more children in which only the husband worked outside the home constituted only 13.5 percent of all husband-wife families." Second, within the steady rise of labor force participation by women since World War II, the rate of participation of married women "and particularly those with young children" has risen fastest: "by 1977, three-fourths of all married women were working outside the home, and well over one-half of all those with school-age children." Third, "divorce rates have doubled since the 1960's, and one out of three marriages ends in divorce." Fourth, "by 1977, one out of seven of all households in the United States was headed by a single women," and the number of such households had "more than doubled since 1960." Fifth, "the total fertility rate has reached its lowest point in this country's history, reflecting more than anything else a reduction in average family size." Sixth, "while the overall birthrate has declined, the rate of births to unmarried women under twenty-five has risen, particularly among teenagers, who account for one-half of all 'illegitimate' births."[33] Thus, shifting patterns of labor-force participation, of marriage, of household constitution, and of childbearing all reveal the near extinction of the domestic support system within which women could have a reasonable chance of gaining access to sex-specific social resources. As this family model disappears, increasing proportions of women attain greater access to androgynous life resources: education, independent wages, and occupations outside the home. And those women whose life resources remain contained within the older family model can no longer afford to bet that they will be able to continue to exchange lifelong domestic labor for economic and social support.

[32]Kristin Luker, *Abortion and the Politics of Motherhood* (Berkeley University of California Press, 1984).
[33]Petchesky, pp. 235, 236.

However, the availability of androgynous life resources is not distributed evenly over the female political spectrum. For instance, Luker pointed out that prolife and prochoice activists do not share the same life resources. Prochoice activists tend to have relatively high access to androgynous resources: Their education, occupations, and income are more similar to men's. The prolife activists whom she interviewed faced significantly greater social barriers to the education, the occupations, and the income that would create real alternatives to economic and social dependency on family resources.[34]

Luker's correlations are supported by Petchesky's analysis correlating life resources with pro- and antifeminist attitudes more generally.[35] Petchesky pointed out that antifeminists are found primarily in two groups, located at opposite ends of socioeconomic status scales. But what these women share besides antifeminist attitudes is access only to sex-specific life resources. Both groups of women tend to begin child bearing relatively early, to have more children than women in the middle of the socioeconomic status scales, and to enter the wage-labor market only temporarily and as part-time workers. Petchesky pointed out that struggles for equal pay for equal work do not address the economic needs of these women; that liberalized divorce laws make it easier for husbands to end the arrangements that have supported them economically and socially; that even if the wife gains court-awarded alimony and child support, a divorce will still mean a severe lowering of lifestyle for both groups of women; and that struggles for specifically sexual equality simply enable the husbands of these women to justify escaping the restrictions that monogamy supposedly imposes on them. For these women, the existing liberal feminist agenda aimed at providing equal rights exerts subtle and not so subtle pressures to substitute limited access to androgynous resources for the considerably more attractive, if more fragile, access that they have to sex-specific resources. (However, for antifeminists, there is an inherent contradiction between the relatively androgynous lifestyles of the Anita Bryants, the Phillis Schaflys, and the other professional antifeminist activists, and the sex-specific social resources that these activists idealize. If the medium is the message, antifeminist activists are giving a profeminist message.)

If antifeminist politics seem reasonable mainly to women restricted to sex-specific life resources, and if increasing proportions of women are gaining more androgynous life resources, one would

[34]Luker.
[35]Rosalind Pollack Petchesky, presentation at *The Feminist and the Scholar*, Barnard Conference, New York City, March 1980.

expect increasing proportions of women to share profeminist politics. This prediction might appear to imply that more women will come to adopt the faulty liberal understandings. Or it might appear to support the Marxist understanding that the "woman question" will be resolved through the industrialization of domestic labor: That economic changes are the fundamental cause of all social changes. However, if we think as archaeologists do and look beneath the surface of the pro- and antifeminist "texts," we can discover an implicit recognition of the inadequacy of both the liberal and the Marxist understandings of women's situation that both groups of women share. If this recognition can be politically activitated, the public feminist political agendas can be transformed in ways that undermine their perceived compatibility with liberal and Marxist agendas.

First, both pro- and antifeminist women recognize that mothering is a far more socially valuable and distinctively human activity than is recognized in liberal and Marxist discourses. Both understand that important aspects of personhood and of social life are developed and maintained only through the kinds of activities and relationships that are absent in men's conduct of public life, that is, through expressions of female sexuality in mothering. "Maternal thinking" and expressing responsibility for particular relationships through nurturing and caring for others hold human social life together wherever it *is* together.[36] Where individuals and social life fall apart—in violent war mentalities, impersonal administrative bureaucracy, the war against nature, and the "fair" creation of human misery—one can detect the absence of concern for human relationships, the absence of responsibility for dependent others, for nurturing, and for contextual thinking. These are the concerns traditionally relegated to women's work.

Second, both groups of women understand that children—and human beings generally—have social value in themselves, that human value is not measurable only in the rationalistic and economic terms assumed by both liberal and Marxist discourses. For both groups, human beings are valuable not merely as rational competitors whose rights may or may not be recognized in the freemarket, or merely as workers whose labor can be controlled by themselves or by their employers. The human potentiality of both adults and children has value because it is human, not merely insofar as it is used in one legitimated social mode or another.

[36]Sara Ruddick, "Maternal Thinking," *Feminist Studies* 6, no. 2 (1980), pp. 342–367; Nancy Chodorow, *The Reproduction of Mothering* (Berkeley: University of California Press, 1975); Carol Gilligan, *In a Different Voice: Psychological Theory and Women's Development* (Cambridge: Harvard University Press, 1982).

Third, both groups assume that women's life needs, whether assessed sex-specifically or androgynously, are fully human. Both understand that women should not be victimized by public policy that directly or indirectly bars them from adequate material resources, from an equal say in the social/sexual relations of reproduction, and from an equal say in social decision-making generally. Pro- and antifeminist women assess these human needs differently—as do any people with differing life resources. But they share the belief that women's needs are legitimate human needs, and that access to satisfaction should not be closed off either by public policy or by the social legitimation of men's socially created irresponsible impulses and needs.

Finally, both groups of women implicitly take the existing socially legitimated expressions of male sexuality to be inherently in conflict with the "normal," desirable expression of female sexuality. Antifeminist women express their advocacy of constraints on male sexuality through appeals to the state to lodge sexual responsibility in the family. It is in the family that antifeminist women's life resources are located and that they have the greatest power to negotiate with men. The family is seen as a place where women can negotiate protection against men's otherwise intrusive sexuality. Profeminist women want the state to constrain men collectively and to support women as a group against such phenomena as economic inequity, rape, incest, wife battering, and default on alimony and child support, as well as enforced sterilization and restrictions on contraceptives and abortion, all of which maintain the dominance of male over female sexuality. Thus, the conflict here is not so much whether or not male sexuality is now legitimated in ways that are oppressive to women, but what strategies will effectively control male sexuality.

I am arguing that not far beneath the surface of the politics of prolife and prochoice women lies a shared recognition of the inadequacy of liberal and Marxist understandings of human nature and of women as fully human. What I perceive as the distinctively women's issues in the abortion dispute could transform the feminist political agenda, thereby revealing the illegitimacy of the entire social order. I do not mean to suggest that the abortion issue itself is destined for a quick demise, or that transforming the classist, racist, and sexist social order into the human social order will be an easy task. I do mean to show that the presence of the abortion issue on the public agenda can reveal to women what has often been hidden from our understanding: Issues of who should control sexuality and reproduction and of how it should be controlled are inextricably linked with the broadest economic, political, and social issues about what kinds of persons we want to be and what we want human social life to look like.

Human sexuality is incredibly plastic: It is easily shaped in different ways in different societies. But the social order is plastic too, and is shaped in differing ways by the meanings of human sexuality. The importance of the feminist agenda is that it focuses on how both sexes are fully human, it explores how the sexual order is a fundamental component of the social order, and it dismantles the edifices built on the assumption that *human* goals, desires, and ways of structuring social relations are identical with the masculine forms of these goals, desires, and relations. In both liberal and Marxist circles, the politics of abortion and of reproduction have generally been constructed out of distinctively masculine social experience. Whether this situation will change depends on whether women come to believe that we share more than separates us from each other.

# Commentary to Chapter 8

LISA SOWLE CAHILL

Sandra Harding's essay presents an illuminating critique of liberalism and Marxism, and a persuasive call for social reorganization. Perhaps its major contribution is its stress on the social context in which the assumptions of any belief system necessarily originate. Many of us tend to construe in an abstract, ahistorical way the vantage points from which abortion is analyzed and to impute to them as "philosophical positions" a logical integrity and autonomy that prescind from the social interests of their progenitors. In fact, we often use the tags *liberal* and *Marxist* without very full-blown or even adequate definitions of what or whom we mean. Harding has clarified the background of the abortion discussion, to the advantage of all its participants.

In brief, it still remains unclear to me why the feminist concerns expressed in Sandra Harding's analysis of abortion entail the pro-choice position. Although she addresses many issues worth further attention, two are salient to what I have to say: The status of the fetus in the human community, and that of women as "fully human," yet distinctively "female."

It seems to me that a coherent position on abortion (or on the status, value, or rights of any class of members of the species *Homo sapiens*) needs to involve two moves. The first is some normative definition of the moral order of human community (for example, feminism, utilitarianism, liberalism, or Marxism); the second is a definition of the class of humans in question, as it is included in or excluded from participation in that order. I take it that the feminist position Harding convincingly espouses is premised precisely on the definition of a moral order that includes, for all its members, at least access to the minimal material conditions requisite for equal participation in domestic and social life, as well as a definition of women

LISA SOWLE CAHILL • Department of Theology, Boston College, Chestnut Hill, Massachusetts 02167.

as "fully human," that is, as being included as members in that egal-itarian community. Granting that the question of whether fetuses also are included should not be pursued in the abstract "personhood" and "rights" language in which it often has been framed in liberal philosophy, I am unconvinced that that question can be circumvented altogether. If the title and the text of Harding's essay urge us rightly, as I believe they do, to recognize women as fully human, and to enhance the social conditions of their full humanity, then it follows either that a parallel exhortation about other members of the species (for example, fetuses) is implied, or that some criteria of "full" hu-manity include women and exclude fetuses (if not absolutely, then in some developmental phases or in some circumstances). But what are these criteria for determining who receives recognition as "fully human"?

Harding states that, contrary to the liberal assumption, "there is clearly no way to establish when and if a fetus is a 'person' on the basis of appeals either to biological evidence or to a consensus on the social recognition of 'personhood.'" I do not disagree, if "estab-lishment of personhood" means incontrovertible *proof* that unborn humans have from conception the full value, status, and rights of born humans. However, I am convinced that there is in our society (and in others) a "softer" social consensus based on "softer" evidence, partly biological (the human genotype, the increasing resemblance of fetus to a baby, the mother's experience of the fetus as a growing and moving "other"), that the interests of fetuses, especially in their lives, deserve more consideration than is guaranteed to them by the legal protection of their mothers' nearly unimpeded right to choose autonomously the fetuses' deaths.

A further important problem is whether there are, among human individuals, differences contingent on the particular characteristics of their own embodiment and whether these are relevant to moral decision-making. A very difficult and controversial question in fem-inist theory (anthropology, sociology, psychology, and ethics) is whether the physical differences associated with the reproductive roles of men and women are paralleled by differences in cognitive and af-fective traits or tendencies, and whether these have or do not have any implications for social roles. Harding certainly presupposes that sex differences should not be a basis for exclusion from full partic-ipation in social life; this is what she means by referring repeatedly to women as "fully human." On the other hand, she suggests that "social experience" can be "distinctively" masculine or feminine. Al-though some differences in male and female experience obviously are attributable to the social mediation of reproductive roles and to the institutionalization of a sexual hierarchy, it is unclear from Harding's paper whether she takes gender-related differences to have some more permanent foothold in male and female "natures."

For instance, she appeals for recognition of the needs of women "as women," "as humans who exist in female bodies," and asserts, again against liberalism, that "humans come embodied, and in (roughly) two sexes." In addition, in stating her thesis that in the feminist view "women's activities" are as "social" as men's and thus "fully human," she surprisingly offers "reproduction" as an example of a socially mediated *women's* activity. Although I am certain that Sandra Harding would never endorse crass biological determinism, she seems not to exclude the possibility that being embodied as male or female provides a certain perspective on the world that permits distinctive experiences and contributions. Both feminist and antifeminist women, for example, are said to recognize that "important aspects of human personhood and of social life are developed . . . through expressions of female sexuality in mothering." Among these are "nurturing and caring for others," "concern for human relationships," "responsibility for dependent others," and "contextual thinking." Although these concerns are "traditionally relegated to women's work," Harding does not say that men are innately incapable of them. What needs clarification here is the relation between full humanity, particular embodiment as a male or a female, male and female reproductive roles, cognitive and emotional capacities or special skills, social roles, and any peculiar interests or rights that may derive from the concrete expression of humanity as male or female.

This question of the moral implications of peculiar forms of embodiment within full humanity connects with the morality of abortion in two ways. First, one of the characteristics that clearly sets fetuses as a class apart from other humans is their special sort of embodiment. It is as an *unborn* human that the fetus is defined; *fetus* refers to certain physical characteristics, just as *male* and *female* do. Fetuses as a human class are distinguished not only by developmental immaturity, but also by a necessary, definitive dependence for survival on the bodies of their mothers. When they are no longer so dependent, they are by definition no longer fetuses. This dependence on the womb can be either contingent or necessary, realized or unrealized. (For example, even a viable fetus is known as a *fetus* while still *in utero,* and thus as *de facto* but contingently dependent on its mother. Human beings aborted before viablity usually are called *fetuses* also, a label indicating that although they have ceased to be sustained by their mothers, they were nonetheless necessarily dependent on them for continued life. The conditions of actual, realized dependence were revoked.[1]) If it is true that the embodiment of peculiar classes of humans creates both special needs on their parts and special obligations of other humans toward them, then it is difficult to see why this principle does not apply to fetuses as well as to women (and men).

Second, if embodiment is to be taken seriously, it must be understood as a source not only of assets and benefits due, but also of obligations. Children, I would assert, do, in fact, have an obligation to honor the parents who bore them, which they are expected to act on when they are of an age to do so. Parents have similar obligations to promote the welfare of their children. For better (in some ways) and worse (in others), the *maternal* obligation to the unborn child takes the special form, derived from the embodiment of *both,* of corporeal support. This is not to say that on the whole women are more responsible for children than men are; nor that the burdens of pregnancy are to be supported by women alone (especially by pregnant women); nor yet that the duty of adults to sustain unborn humans *never* can be overridden by other duties, in situations of conflict. But it *is* to say that all members of the human community have obligations to support those special needs of fellow humans that are contingent on the very form that their embodied humanity takes.

I will conclude with two questions, one posed from the perspective of fetal embodiment, the other from that of female embodiment. If, as Sandra Harding claims, the morality of abortion is related to the social justice issue of recognizing marginal classes, ought that recognition to include fetuses? Does the social practice of abortion itself represent a restriction of women's sexuality and humanity insofar as it represents and institutionalizes the unwillingness of society to give pregnant women real options, and to require that other human beings meet their obligation to support, with material resources, the exercise of those options?

---

[1]There is a further semantic and conceptual question of whether, if unborn human beings were sustainable outside the womb by some "womb substitute" early in the developmental process (for example, in the first trimester after conception), they would still be called *fetuses* by virtue of their dependence on the substitute, or *babies* by virtue of their physical independence from their parent. More important than the issue of vocabulary would be how the mother's moral relation to the fetus would change as a result of severing the bond of physical dependence.

## CHAPTER 9

# Abortion and the Culture
## Toward a Feminist Perspective

MARY C. SEGERS

## Autobiographical Statement

*Labels are poor ways to characterize a person, but if pressed, I suppose I would have to describe myself as a left-of-center liberal who is Roman Catholic and a feminist. In less pretentious moments, I say that a good many of my waking hours are spent in teaching political philosophy and political science, and in doing the traditional tasks of being a wife and the mother of two young children.*

*I first began to think and write about the abortion issue when pregnant with our first child nine years ago. Although the experiential basis of such a concern seems obvious, other factors led me to write about abortion. I was interested in jurisprudence, and abortion seemed a timely, problematic case illustrating the general relation between law and morals. I was also somewhat taken aback by the persistent characterization, in the press and in public debate, of Catholic right-to-lifers as dogmatic extremists and fanatical rightwingers. My sense of fairness aroused, I sought to articulate the more plausible elements of a right-to-life position—while at the same time disagreeing with the political and legal implications of Catholic prolife views. My sense of fairness was also aroused by the tendency of Catholic and other right-to-lifers to ignore the complexities of women's lives and to focus almost entirely on the status of the fetus in their discussions of abortion. This position, too, seemed to require correction and adjustment.*

*I attribute my own views on abortion to family, religious, and broadly educational influences and experiences. I think specifically of a period of*

MARY C. SEGERS ● Department of Political Science and Director of Women's Studies, Rutgers University, Newark, New Jersey 07102.

*psychotherapy (individual and group) in which I came to appreciate the value of individual freedom in a pluralistic society. The women's movement has reinforced a concern about equality and justice and has demonstrated the continuing need for articulating a woman's perspective on these issues. I am undoubtedly influenced by a Catholic religious upbringing. Although the church's specific moral teaching on abortion has not figured prominently in my thinking, Catholicism as a general tradition has influenced me greatly, often in a subliminal way. It has provided a kind of world view, a value orientation, an elemental atmosphere of basic assumptions and presumptions, a cultural sensibility.*

*However, the most influential factor in my thinking about abortion was, I believe, my father's illness and death. When I was 12, my father suffered a stroke that left him speechless, semiparalyzed, and bedridden. His recovery being impossible, he lingered on for 14 months, and we, his family, had to make several difficult choices regarding his care. His illness left me with several convictions of relevance to the abortion issue. I came to realize in an immediate way that persons are not to be valued according to their use or abandoned when they are "useless" (or cannot function normally). I need not spell out how this conviction has made me sympathetic to the "sanctity-of-life" ethic of those who oppose abortion. Like them, I am distinctly uncomfortable with "quality-of-life" notions that separate the healthy from the unhealthy, the useful from the useless.*

*At the same time, my father's illness taught me that there are limits to what we can do for others and that there are times in life when hard choices have to be made. Eventually, we (his family) could not care for him and had to entrust his care to others who might not be as sympathetic to his plight. With respect to the abortion dilemma, I believe that this experience has given me some feeling for and sympathy with those who say that they do not have the resources and the energy to bring new life into the world and to care for it.*

*For a variety of reasons, I favor the legal availability of abortion. As to the morality of abortion, I believe that abortion may at times be morally permissible. Nevertheless, abortion seems a poor solution to the problems that women face: poverty, lack of support and assistance in parenting, and constant career interruptions because of childcare responsibilities. Because it is such a poor solution, the increasing cultural acceptability of abortion is troubling. As a society, we should be able to do better than this.*

The continuing abortion debate in American society mirrors deeper cultural attitudes on such basic matters as the role of women in society, the use of law to solve social problems, and the priority given to individual freedom and responsibility in a liberal society. In one way or another, our attitudes and beliefs on these matters are expressions of a liberal cultural ethos. Indeed, the liberal character of the American cultural experiment is what has most influenced how we as a society have dealt with the abortion issue. For better or worse, our society is a liberal democratic polity in a heterogeneous, pluralistic culture. Our political-philosophical commitments are liberal, and they include an emphasis on individual freedom, where liberty is understood not as license but as, among other things, freedom from governmental restraint; an insistence on the separation of law and morals, associated with nineteenth century utilitarian liberal reformers such as Jeremy Bentham and John Austin; and a distinction between state and society, a distinction that led thinkers such as John Locke and J. S. Mill to favor limited government while relying on a resourceful citizenry to police itself, thereby preventing the excesses of an untrammeled exercise of individual freedom.[1] In the ideal of a liberal society suggested by writers such as Mill, L. T. Hobhouse, and even a liberal egalitarian such as R. H. Tawney, human conduct would be the result of spontaneous voluntary action rather than governmental coercion, and the limits of liberty in the area of private, self-regarding conduct would be set less by bureaucratic regulation than by a vast array of intermediate institutions—religious, social, educational, and familial—that would monitor and shape the moral standards of the culture.[2]

How do the values of this liberal ethos relate to the abortion controversy? I am concerned that, in the absence of inhibitory laws, abortion will become casual, commonplace, routine, and culturally acceptable. My basic premises should be made explicit. I assume that, in itself, abortion is a negative event, not something we joyfully celebrate with cigars and champagne, as we celebrate the birth of a baby. Nevertheless, abortion seems necessary, given the kind of world we live in and the devastating impact of pregnancy and moth-

---

[1] Left liberals, such as L. T. Hobhouse, T. H. Green, A. D. Lindsay, and perhaps Mill himself and R. H. Tawney, would, of course, insist that there is a major difference between nongovernmental intervention in the economy and nongovernmental intervention in the sphere of morals. The difference is that a laissez-faire free-market economy works to undermine freedom for most individuals, so government must intervene to curb monopolies and "hinder the hindrances to freedom" (to quote Lindsay, *The Modern Democratic State* [New York: Oxford University Press, 1947]). However, governmental intervention in the sphere of private morality does not promote or maximize freedom; it only reduces it.

[2] See J. S. Mill, *On Liberty,* ed. David Spitz. (New York: Norton, 1975); L. T. Hobhouse, *Liberalism* (New York: Oxford University Press, 1964); R. H. Tawney, *Equality* (London: George Allen and Unwin, 1964), especially Chapter 1; D. J. Manning, *Liberalism* (New York: St. Martin's Press, 1976).

erhood on involuntarily pregnant women. So I believe that abortion should be legally permissible. At the same time, we as a society should try to reduce the frequency of this negative event. Thus, my question: How can we reduce the incidence of abortion without coercing women? And if we cannot use the force of law to reduce abortions, what other means are open to us? Before addressing that question, however, I will discuss why a liberal democracy such as ours should not make abortion illegal once again.

## JURISPRUDENTIAL ARGUMENTS FOR LEGALIZED ABORTION

Some arguments for legalized abortion originate in jurisprudential considerations of the relation between law and morality. These arguments are compatible with a view of abortion itself as a negative event, whose prevention is best entrusted to institutions of social cooperation rather than to mechanisms of governmental coercion. These arguments are also in part contingent, based on empirical evidence. As the empirical evidence changes, so they could change. Yet, under present circumstances in American society, they comprise some of the stronger arguments for the legality of abortion. These arguments stress the pluralistic character of American society and the importance of tolerance and respect for others in a liberal democracy; they also emphasize the uniqueness of abortion and adopt a consequentialist approach to the evaluation of antiabortion laws.

Prochoice and prolife views on the relation between law and morals differ to such an extent that they seem to inhabit separate jurisprudential worlds. Prolife advocates share affinities with an older tradition of classical and medieval philosophy that views law and morality as closely interrelated (though not coterminous). They see the moral and the legal as "tightly tied together, for the moral decision determining who is human is decisive for constitutional adjudication."[3] Moreover, the necessity of laws restricting abortion is predicated on the belief that moral valuations depend on the law to a substantial degree and that society cannot continue to regard abortion as wrong in the absence of a law against it.

By contrast, prochoice advocates seem to share affinities with a more modern jurisprudential tradition, especially that associated with

---

[3]John T. Noonan, "Introduction," in John T. Noonan, Jr., ed. *The Morality of Abortion: Legal and Historical Perspectives,* (Cambridge: Harvard University Press, 1970), p. x.

Anglo-American legal positivism. The separation of law and morals is emphasized; the fact that abortion is legal is not held to be conclusive of its morality. The law is viewed simply as a system of coercive sanctions keeping the citizen from external actions harmful to the community. Relatively little stress is placed on law as a shaper of behavior and an inculcator of internal beliefs, norms, and dispositions. Greater recognition is given to the limits of the criminal sanction in shaping behavior; legislators are cautioned not to "confuse crime with sin."[4]

As applied to public policy on abortion, this refined form of legal positivism lead abortion rights advocates to make the following kinds of arguments. First, prochoicers claim that they are not against "legislating morality" as such. In the absence of any public consensus on the morality of a practice such as abortion, however, they are understandably reluctant to use the commanding powers of the law to control social behavior. Rather than employing coercive sanctions to impose a particular view, abortion rights advocates maintain that the law should leave decision making in this area to the individual citizens most concerned.

This view stresses the absence of societal consensus and the presence of deeply divided public opinion on the abortion issue. Since 1972, surveys have consistently shown small clusters of prolife and prochoice adherents at either end of the spectrum of public opinion (20% favor strict legal prohibition of abortion while another 20% support a policy of abortion on request). Almost 60% of the public (in the middle of the spectrum) favor first trimester abortions but then differ on the legality of abortion depending on the time of gestation and the reasons proffered for terminating the pregnancy.[5]

"Dissensus" seems to characterize public opinion on the morality as well as the legality of abortion. Between prolife and prochoice activists, major philosophical differences indicate a polarization of values. Abortion proponents and opponents seem to differ on such basic issues as the determination and ascription of value, the relation between law and morals, the uses and limits of politics in solving

[4]A prominent exponent of this view is H. L. A. Hart, who, in various debates—with Patrick Devlin and Lon Fuller—over the enforcement of morals and the implementation of moral precepts in the law, has defended the liberal-utilitarian insistence on the separation of law and morals. See H. L. A. Hart, "Positivism and the Separation of Law and Morals," *Harvard Law Review* 71 (1958) p. 593, reprinted in Joel Feinberg and Hyman Gross, eds., *Philosophy of Law* (Belmont, Calif.: Wadsworth, 1980). See also H. L. A. Hart, *The Concept of Law* (London: Oxford University Press, 1961), especially Chapter 9.

[5]For a detailed analysis of public opinion on the legality and the morality of abortion, see the account given by Mary Ann Lamanna, Chapter 1, this volume.

social problems, the use and control of science, and the value of scientific progress.[6] Sociological analyses of activists confirm how isolated each side is from the other side and how profound are the differences separating them.[7]

Given the differences in worldviews between abortion proponents and opponents, it seems unlikely that any consensus other than "we agree to disagree" can inform law and public policy on abortion. Such a libertarian consensus implies the necessity of tolerance and respect for the opinions, beliefs, and moral judgments of others who differ with us on the issue. Moreover, in a pluralistic society deeply divided over the morality of abortion, coercing an involuntarily pregnant women to bear a child when, in conscience, she thinks she should not is held to be objectionable when no substantive harm would be done to the common good by removing legal compulsions. According to Daniel Callahan:

> A conviction that abortion for less than good and serious reasons is morally wrong cannot serve as a rationale to *coerce* someone else *with different convictions* unless it can be shown that the actions following upon a recognition of their convictions threaten the whole of society.[8]

Now prolifers argue that abortion does threaten the common good because it is the first step down the "slippery slope" to a moral abyss in which euthanasia and infanticide become commonplace. However, whether a legal policy of abortion on request threatens the peace, security, and safety of the whole society is in part an empirical question requiring evidence to support an affirmative answer. If we ask what evidence there is that legalized abortion threatens the common good, we find very few supporting data. Though abortion has been practiced for centuries, it has not been shown to have led to calloused attitudes toward the aged and the infirm in other societies. More important, in Eastern Europe and Japan, where abortion has been legalized for over 30 years, these results have not been observed. Although induced abortion is a form of killing, it is *sui generis* in being the killing of prenatal life. Abortion, in short, seems to be unique; as Callahan stated, "It is all but impossible to extrapolate from attitudes towards fetal life attitudes towards existing human life."[9]

[6]For a more detailed explanation of these differences, see my "Can Congress settle the Abortion Issue?," *Hastings Center Report* 12, no. 3 (June 1982), pp. 20–28.

[7]See Kristin Luker's analysis in Chapter 2, this volume. See also James R. Kelly, "Beyond the Stereotypes: Interviews with Right-to-Life Pioneers," *Commonweal* (20 November 1981), pp. 654–59.

[8]Daniel Callahan, *Abortion: Law, Choice and Morality* (New York: Macmillan, 1970), p. 474.

[9]Ibid., p. 475.

In the absence of evidence that permissive abortion laws jeopardize the common good of a society, prochoicers ask: Why compel women to bear children simply in order to satisfy those whose consciences are offended by abortion? Prochoicers support the repeal of restrictive antiabortion laws, which compel involuntarily pregnant women to continue their pregnancies, often in violation of their consciences. Abortion should be legalized, so the argument runs, because

1. Permissive laws are not injurious to the common good.
2. Permissive laws enhance the freedom of those who believe that they should be able to elect abortion in accordance with conscience.
3. Restrictive laws do offend the consciences of many in American society.
4. Restrictive laws do in fact injure, threaten, and jeopardize the common good.

On this last point, abortion rights advocates stress the undesirable political and social consequences of reinstating laws restricting abortion. Given the permissive atmosphere that has developed in the decade since *Roe* v. *Wade,* such laws would probably not be enforced and might well be unenforceable; they would therefore invite disrespect and contempt for law. Moreover, such laws would be *de facto* discriminatory against poor women, who often lack the financial resources to pay discreet, respectable physicians for their services. Finally, they would probably not significantly reduce the incidence of abortion; instead, they would increase the number of illegal, unsafe, unhygienic abortions, with high risks to the women involved. These costs seem too high a price to pay for using the criminal law to register our moral convictions.

Prochoice advocates thus have a realistic sense of the limits of the criminal sanction; citing Prohibition in the United States, they emphasize that laws recriminalizing abortion will not achieve their intended effect of reducing the incidence of abortion and will result in more harm than good. These jurisprudential arguments about the relation between law and morals suggest that a society should not have laws prohibiting abortion in the absence of any consensus about the morality or the immorality of this practice. These arguments for a policy of legalized abortion are made by a wide variety of prochoice advocates and are not specifically feminist arguments. There is, however, considerable overlap between the prochoice movement and the movement for women's rights; and it is worth exploring feminist arguments for legalized abortion to see if they add anything distinctive to the prochoice case.

# A FEMINIST PERSPECTIVE ON THE LEGALITY OF ABORTION

A feminist perspective on abortion gives high priority, if not paramount importance, to the interests, claims, and rights of women. Such a perspective emphasizes what motherhood and pregnancy mean for women who have life-plans to realize. A feminist approach is not oblivious to the claims of the fetus or of other interested parties (fathers, doctors, healthcare professionals, society). But these claims are considered in the context of a society that still does not accept women as full, equal citizens and that seems remarkably unsympathetic to the plight of involuntarily pregnant women.

A feminist perspective on abortion compensates for the lack of attention to women's interests in previous philosophical and political discussions of abortion.[10] As Jane English noted, prior to 1971 male philosophers tended to discuss abortion from the perspective of a physician who is asked to choose between two equally "innocent" lives, rather than from the pregnant woman's point of view. Only when female philosophers began to write about abortion did the interests of women receive anything approaching full consideration.[11]

The phrase "a woman's right to control her own body" has perhaps had unfortunate connotations of an excessively individualized independent role in reproduction, implying no right to the assistance of others in childbearing and child rearing. Later feminist writings have rejected this privatization of maternity. As Rosalind Petchesky has written, "Reproductive freedom—indeed the very nature of reproduction itself—is irreducibly social and individual at

[10]Though there is a large prochoice literature available, not all arguments for legalized abortion originate in a perspective that holds the interests of women to be paramount or even of high priority. The variety of groups that have been active in the movement to reform abortion laws in the United States include demographic planners concerned about population control; doctors seeking to practice medicine free from governmental intervention; social workers and public health administrators worried about problems of housing, poverty, and child abuse; and civil libertarians concerned with tolerance, the uses of law, and the limits of the criminal sanction.

[11]As English put it, "Before Judith Jarvis Thomson's landmark article, "A Defense of Abortion," in 1971, the philosophical debate was dominated by such male-oriented questions as 'How can you decide between two innocent lives? and Isn't it better to let a woman die than by your actions to kill a fetus?' As late as 1972, Richard Brandt defined abortion as an operation on a woman; let us rather follow Mary Anne Warren and take it as the action a woman takes to terminate an existing pregnancy." Jane English, *Abortion,* unpublished paper, 1973 p. 1.

the same time."[12] Although feminists did not want to isolate women in some quasi-Lockean, private world, they did want to stress the importance of being free to decide whether to undertake the joys and cares of maternity. Thus, the crucial feminist goal with respect to law and public policy on abortion has been to retain the legal right to decide in the hands of women themselves. At the same time, feminists have always stressed the creation of genuine conditions of choice, "For a real choice about abortion requires that a woman should be able to opt to have her child as well as to abort it."[13]

In her classic essay "Abortion and a Woman's Right to Decide,"[14] Allison Jaggar attempted to provide a moral justification for the claim that each woman should have the sole legal right to decide whether or not, in her own case, an abortion should be performed. Jaggar did not base her argument on alleged privacy rights, on utilitarian claims, or on "the unclear and dubious 'right to one's own body.'" Rather she appealed to two relatively uncontroversial principles: first, that the right to life for a human being "means the right to a full human life and to whatever means are necessary to achieve this"; and, second, "that decisions should be made by those, and only by those, who are importantly affected by them." According to Jaggar, the first principle suggests that if an individual or an organization does not make a genuine attempt to guarantee all of a child's needs, both before and after birth, it cannot be viewed as the protector of that child's right to life. Right-to-life groups or the state itself, acting as defenders of the unborn's right to life, must be prepared to fulfill all the conditions necessary to the child's achieving a full human life if they are to legitimately prohibit abortion. Since, as society is now constituted, the responsibility for fulfilling a child's needs falls primarily on the mother, the state has no grounds for compelling an involuntarily pregnant woman to bear this responsibility. Rather, the decision must rest with her.

Applying the second principle—that the abortion decision should be made by all those whose lives are to be importantly affected by that decision—Jaggar argued that, in the present social situation, the woman is most significantly and permanently affected by abortion decisions and should therefore be the ultimate locus of the right to

[12]Rosalind Petchesky, "Reproductive Freedom: Beyond 'A Woman's Right to Choose,'" *Signs* 5, no. 4 (Summer 1980), p. 661.
[13]Alison Jaggar, "Abortion and a Woman's Right to Decide," in Carol C. Gould and Marx W. Wartofsky, eds., *Women and Philosophy: Toward A Theory of Liberation* (New York: Putnam's, 1976), p. 357.
[14]Ibid.

decide whether or not, in her own case, abortion is justified. Though Jaggar concluded that, in our society, no individual or group has a justified claim to restrict a woman's right to decide, she strongly emphasized the contingent character of this right, which depends on certain conditional features of women's social situation:

> These features include the inadequate pre- and post-natal health care provided by the state, the fact that the main responsibility for raising a child is laid on its biological mother, and the small proportion of the national resources devoted to welfare.[15]

Were these conditions to change, in Jaggar's view, a woman's right to decide might be overridden by the social needs of the larger community, though she would never lose her right to participate in collective societal decision-making. Revolutionary social changes (for example, cheap or free medical care for all children and a deemphasis on the nuclear family as the ideal living arrangement) would be a necessary condition of such a diminution of women's rights, however. If women were to be compelled to carry pregnancies to term, society would have to assume virtually full responsibility for the health and welfare of mothers and children.

What does a feminist perspective add to the prochoice case for legalized abortion? First, it considers the abortion dilemma from the vantage point of involuntarily pregnant women living in societies that do not always value highly or support adequately the tasks of child-bearing and child rearing. Prochoice writers other than women have tended to neglect this perspective.

Second, a feminist perspective stresses the asymmetrical impact of pregnancy. Daniel Maguire noted the obvious and profound differences between women's and men's experience of reproduction:

> In the sexual encounter man can inseminate and ride off dreamfully into the sunset, but for woman a biological drama of symbiosis may begin which, through pregnancy and nursing, will tie her to the moment for many months. Indeed, by historical role assignment it may link her there for a good chunk of a century immersed in child care and "homemaking."[16]

The impact of conception and pregnancy is asymmetrical not only because of the traditional (in the West) sexual division of labor between women as child rearers and men as providers. As Petchesky has pointed out, female health and sexuality are also involved:

---

[15]Ibid., pp. 348, 352.
[16]Daniel Maguire, "The Feminization of God and Ethics," in *Christianity and Crisis* 42, no. 4 (15, March 1982), pp. 59–67.

> Because pregnancies occur in women's bodies . . ., the continued pos-
> sibility of an "unwanted" pregnancy affects women in a very specific
> sense, not only as potential bearers of fetuses, but also in their capacity
> to enjoy sexuality and to maintain their health.[17]

Moreover, the social consequences of childbearing in women's lives may vary widely, depending on the culture involved. Adrienne Rich described some of these consequences:

> A man may beget a child in passion or by rape, and then disappear;
> he need never see or consider child or mother again. Under such cir-
> cumstances, the mother faces a range of painful, socially weighted choices;
> abortion, suicide, abandonment of the child, infanticide, the rearing of
> a child branded "illegitimate," usually in poverty, always outside the
> law. In some cultures she faces murder by her kinsmen. Whatever her
> choice, her body has undergone irreversible changes, her mind will
> never be the same, her future as a woman has been shaped by the
> event.[18]

Given these sex differences in the meaning and the impact of conception, we may better understand why a feminist perspective on abortion always emphasizes the consequences of conception for women's lives.[19]

Third, a feminist perspective emphasizes the conditions of so-ciety and the "social relations of reproduction." "We live immersed in patriarchy," Virginia Held suggested,[20] and this elusive term is meant to encompass the many forms of domination by men over women in late-stage industrial America. The variety of feminism that focuses on the power wielded by men over women in a patriarchal society tends to see reproductive control as the central issue in the abortion controversy. In this view, opposition to abortion is seen as only one aspect of a broader opposition to female autonomy generally.

One need not be a radical feminist to see elements of truth in this analysis. Despite the gains made by the women's movement in the last decade, the general political and economic situation of women in American society is not encouraging. Women constitute a majority (51.3%) of the population, yet few hold public office. Of the 535 members of Congress, only 23 are women. Of 50 governors, none are women. Women represent less than 7% of the federal judiciary

---

[17]Petchesky, p. 666.

[18]Adrienne Rich, *Of Woman Born: Motherhood as Experience and Institution* (New York: Norton, 1976), p. xiv.

[19]As Petchesky has written, "Reproduction affects women as women, in a way that transcends class divisions and that penetrates everything—work, political and com-munity involvements, sexuality, creativity, dreams." (p. 666).

[20]Virginia Held, book review, *Signs* 7, no. 3 (Spring 1982), p. 696.

and only 11% of federal appointees. Only 13% of state legislators and 11% of mayors and councillors are women.[21] These statistics mean that men dominate political decision-making on the issue of abortion. Women are simply not confident that male-dominated legislatures, courts, and agencies will always be knowledgeable about women's lives or sympathetic to women's interests.

With respect to economic power, the position of American women is not optimistic either. Full-time year-round working women earn, on the average, 59 cents for every dollar earned by men. Job segregation by sex remains a major characteristic of the workplace; 80% of the women in this country work in 25 job categories that are overwhelmingly "women's jobs" (secretaries, clerks, librarians, nurses, retail salespeople, household workers).[22] Sexual harassment of women in the workplace continues to be a significant problem. Two thirds of poor people in this country are female. As the National Organization of Women has pointed out, since 1980 the burden of federal budget cuts in social services has fallen disproportionately on women. This direct and indirect sex-based discrimination helps to explain why involuntarily pregnant women support ready access to legal abortion. Many find themselves too financially constrained to carry their pregnancies to term. It also supports the feminist argument that genuine choice in reproductive matters requires public support and assistance for women.

Gross discrepancies in wealth, status, and power between the sexes are not, strictly speaking, arguments for the legality, much less the morality, of abortion. However, they do situate the plight of involuntarily pregnant women in context and make their abortion decisions more understandable.

There is a fourth dimension that a feminist perspective adds to prochoice arguments for legalized abortion, namely, the insistence that abortion is unique and that, moreover, pregnancy terminations are rarely undertaken lightly, frivolously, or casually. The uniqueness of abortion—its dissimilarity from rather than its similarity to other ethical dilemmas involving killing—has been discussed above. With respct to casual abortion, those who work closely with involuntarily pregnant women insist that abortions are never chosen "for convenience' sake" but are undertaken "in necessity and sorrow" and in

[21]These statistics were supplied by the National Women's Political Caucus and by the Center for the Study of the American Woman and Politics at Rutgers University. They obtained as of January 1983.

[22]Wendy Kahn and Joy Ann Grime, "Pay Equity: Beyond Equal Pay for Equal Work," in Ellen Boneparth, ed., *Woman, Power and Policy* (New York: Pergamon Press, 1982), p. 76.

many cases with considerable ambivalence. Some thought has been given to deciphering what exactly it is that women mean to do when they have abortions. This approach is, in part, a reaction to arguments that blame women for having become involuntarily pregnant and that suggest that they are selfish, amoral, and socially irresponsible. Mary B. Mahowald has elaborated a distinction that helps to clarify women's intentions in abortion decision-making:

> Although it may be the case now that a decision for abortion is practically inseparable from a decision to end the life of a fetus, this will not be so in the future due to continuing developments in reproductive technology. Even at this point in time, the two decisions are not only conceptually separate but also intentionally separable. If what one intends to do makes a morally relevant difference, the decision to end a pregnancy must be distinguishable from the decision to end fetal life.[23]

A feminist perspective emphasizes these aspects of abortion decision-making in an effort to counter apparently profound fears that women will abuse their reproductive freedom. Feminists recognize that this fear of women as rapacious creatures is part of the problem, namely, a misogynistic culture characterized by fear and hatred of women, resentment of their reproductive capacities (powers), and refusal to take women seriously as autonomous moral agents. Barbara Hayler has suggested that fears of casual abortion for selfish reasons may derive from "the most deadly anti-woman bias of them all, namely: that unless women are carefully controlled they will kill their own progeny without reason because they are not fully rational creatures."[24]

There is a fifth dimension that a feminist perspective adds, namely, the insistence that arguments for legalized abortion can be understood properly only in light of the larger aims and purposes (justice, liberty, and equality) of the women's movement. According to Gloria Steinem, "Feminism is the belief that women are full human beings. It is simple justice."[25] In all its varieties feminism insists that women be taken seriously as moral agents. An instrumentalist conception of women is rejected by all feminists, no matter what their ideology. As the late Dame Rebecca West wrote in 1913, "I myself have never

---

[23]Mary B. Mahowald, "Concepts of Abortion and Their Relevance to the Abortion Debate," *Southern Journal of Philosophy* 20, no. 2 (1982), p. 199.

[24]Barbara Hayler quoting Marvin Kohl, *The Morality of Killing: Sanctity of Life, Abortion and Euthanasia* (New York: Humanities Press, 1974), in *Signs* 4, no. 2 (Winter 1979), pp. 322–323.

[25]Gloria Steinem, "Reflections," in Lynn Gilbert and Gaylen Moore, eds., *Particular Passions* (New York: Clarkson Potter, 1981), p. 167.

been able to find out precisely what feminism is: I simply know that people call me a feminist whenever I express sentiments that differentiate me from a doormat or a prostitute."[26]

In addition to justice and equality, feminism is, of course, concerned with freedom: Women's moral autonomy remains a fiction as long as their lives are determined by factors (for example, biology, politics, the workplace, and cultural attitudes and expectations) over which they have no control. Minimal freedom and autonomy are ultimately dependent on each woman's full and free control of her procreative life. Moreover, through social and economic assistance, this freedom must be made meaningful for all, so that both poor and well-to-do women may have genuine options in making decisions about childbearing. Of course, reproductive freedom (like political and legal freedoms) must be exercised responsibly. But first it must be achieved and must be seen in relation to the larger goals of the women's movement.

Finally, a feminist view contributes to the prochoice case a conviction that the rights of the woman and of the fetus in the abortion dilemma are contingent rather than absolute. The moral right to abortion for which Jaggar argued

> is not a universal or absolute one enjoyed by all women regardless of their social situation. Rather it is a right whose existence depends on certain contingent features of the social situation in which women find themselves.[27]

Similarly, although Jaggar did not dwell at length on the rights of the fetus, it is clear that these are contingent, not absolute. She assumed that fetuses "do not have a right to life so absolute that the question of abortion may never be raised."[28] At the same time, Jaggar takes seriously the fetus's right to life and bases the first of her two principles on it. More important, the whole tenor of Jaggar's essay is that, as social conditions improve, the balance between the contingent rights of mother and unborn child may change so that the right to life of the fetus may outweigh the involuntarily pregnant woman's right to decide.

Petchesky also insisted that the right to reproductive freedom is not absolute and unconditional:

> Recognizing a situation of real conflict between the survival of the fetus and the needs of the woman and those dependent on her, the

---

[26]Dame Rebecca West, quoted in *New York Times Book Review* by John Leonard, 28 May, 1982, p. 25.
[27]Jaggar, p. 348.
[28]Ibid.

feminist position says merely that women must decide, because it is their bodies that are involved, and because they still have primary responsibility for the care and development of the children born.

But determining who should decide—the political question—does not tell us anything about the moral and social values women ought to bring to this decision, *how* they should decide. Should women get an abortion on the grounds that they prefer a different gender (which amniocentesis can now determine)? Such a decision, in my view, would be blatantly sexist, and nobody's claim to "control over her body" could make it right or compatible with feminist principles. That is, "a woman's right to control her body" is not abstract or absolute, but we have not yet developed a morality . . . that would tell us what the exceptions should be.[29]

Both Jaggar and Petchesky see a genuine conflict between the contingent rights of fetus and mother, and both hold out the possibility that the balance may be struck in favor of fetal rights. Both insist on the legal right of women to decide, and both invite women to ethical reflection on how conflicting rights and needs may be balanced. The legality of abortion is not conclusive of its morality, these feminists insist; moreover, "to say that each woman in our society has the moral and legal right to decide whether or not she should terminate her pregnancy is not to say that abortion is always justified."[30]

But ethical reflection by feminists on *how* women should decide abortion dilemmas has been stymied by the continuing political controversy over *who* should decide. Forced by the fierce opposition and tactics of antiabortion groups, feminists have focused on the political and legal aspects of abortion rather than on moral questions about when, under what conditions, and for what purposes abortion decisions should be made. Fortunately, materials are now available on women's ethical thinking and judging that may help feminists to give moral content to the phrase "reproductive freedom."

## A FEMINIST PERSPECTIVE ON THE MORALITY OF ABORTION

Developing a feminist perspective on the morality of abortion involves reconsidering notions of liberty and individual rights in light of some recent scholarship on the ethical thinking and the moral development of women. Articles and books published within the last five years, including Sara Ruddick's essay "Maternal Thinking" and

[29]Petchesky, pp. 668–669.
[30]Jaggar, pp. 355–356.

Carol Gilligan's "In a Different Voice: Women's Conceptions of Self and of Morality,"[31] illuminate different ways in which men and women view moral decisions in general and abortion decisions in particular; they are also suggestive of women's moral sensibilities. They exemplify provocative, fascinating scholarship on questions such as: How do women construe moral problems and ethical dilemmas? Is there such a phenomenon as a feminine moral sensibility? And (my question) if so, what would such a sensibility imply in abortion decision-making? If, for example, women's moral judgment differs from men's in emphasizing compassion, care, and responsibility for others, how might these values be preserved and encouraged in abortion decision-making?

One argument supporting a permissive legal abortion policy is that women should be able to decide such significant matters (as whether to bear a child) free of the heavy hand of governmental coercion. Employing Isaiah Berlin's distinction concerning two types of liberty,[32] we may say that the conception of liberty underlying this argument is "negative"; that is, liberty is construed as freedom from external restraints, especially political, economic, and social restraints applied to women through law and public policy. But feminists have always been quick to emphasize the inadequacies of such a limited conception of reproductive freedom, which isolates women in their private decision-making and deprives them of all social supports. The tendency is to move toward a more "positive" conception of liberty, which views reproductive freedom as freedom from necessity in order to be available for moral action (as defined by a particular individual). But what are the moral ends (service to others? self-realization? both?) for which women are to be free? A more intelligible defense of reproductive freedom seems to require women to attempt to specify imperatives that might guide abortion decision-making.

If reconsidering the concept of liberty is necessary, rethinking the notion of individual rights is even more so. Conceiving of the abortion dilemma as a question of competing rights has more often than not functioned in the way that H. L. A. Hart's "definitional

[31] Sara Ruddick, "Maternal Thinking," *Feminist Studies* 6, no. 2 (Summer 1980), pp. 342–367. Also, Carol Gilligan, "In a Different Voice: Women's Conceptions of Self and of Morality," *Harvard Educational Review* 47, no. 4 (November 1977), pp. 481–517. There is also Gilligan's subsequent book, *In A Different Voice: Psychological Theory and Women's Development* (Cambridge: Harvard University Press, 1982).

[32] Isaiah Berlin, "Two Concepts of Liberty," in *Four Essays on Liberty* (New York: Oxford University Press, 1969), pp. 118–172.

stop" has functioned in discussions of punishment: to cut off all further conversation between the two sides. Moreover, rights language has often proved misleading because the rights that are stressed are conceived of as being formal, abstract, absolute, and indivdual—with little attention given to notions of duty and responsibility. As Larry R. Churchill and Jose Jorge Siman pointed out, appeals to the "right to life" or the "right to control one's own body" neglect the fact that "rights are social in origin and make sense only in the context of a larger communal order of living."[33]

A feminist perspective on the morality of abortion recognizes that the assertion of rights does not settle an issue such as abortion. Rights are, rather, the beginning of ethical reflection, a "first step in moral discernment."[34] A feminist perspective also reiterates the basic ethical notion that a moral right—for example, the right to control reproduction—involves moral duties. Women who have the legal right to decide also have moral rights and duties to choose responsibility and with consideration for the others affected by reproductive decisions.

Churchill and Siman maintained that neglect of the more complex moral notion of rights has crippled the abortion debate in the United States. They recommended the substitution of a more expanded notion of rights for the narrow, individualized, abstract version now in use; they also urged that discussions of the morality of abortion focus partly on the motives and intentions of actors:

> It is important whether an abortion is sought reactively and thoughtlessly, or deliberately and with due regard for alternatives and their relative costs. It matters whether persons initiate actions out of selfishness or out of duty, with malice or with beneficence. The moral meaning of abortion is contingent upon whether abortion is a last resort or a matter of convenience.

These authors insisted that

> moral theory strives to understand the unity between the self and its acts. The goodness of acts is related to (though not determined by) the goodness of the actor and the circumstances in which he or she is given to act.[35]

Here, Gilligan's interviews with women contemplating abortion are relevant, for they illuminate the ways in which women actually struggle with the moral dilemmas. Gilligan concluded on the basis

---

[33]Larry R. Churchill and Jose Jorge Siman, "Abortion and the Rhetoric of Individual Rights," *Hastings Center Report* 12, no. 1 (February 1982), pp. 9–12.
[34]Ibid, p. 9.
[35]Ibid., p. 12 (emphasis in the original).

of these lengthy interviews, that the feminine construction of the moral domain relies on a language different from that of men, a language of care and responsibility as opposed to a language of individual rights.

Gilligan's research flowed from her work with Lawrence Kohlberg on stages of moral development and was an effort to adjust and remedy the inherent limitations of Kohlberg's work (she noted, for example, that Kohlberg derived his conception of moral development from all-male longitudinal research data).[36] She maintained that the morality or the responsibility that women described to her stands apart from the morality of rights that underlies Kohlberg's conception of the highest stages of moral judgment. In contrasting the moral judgment of men and women, Gilligan noted that Kohlberg's conception of moral development,

> which has consistently found the development of woman to be either aberrant or incomplete, has been limited insofar as it has been predominantly a male conception, giving lip-service, a place on the chart, to the interdependence of intimacy and care but constantly stressing at their expense, the importance and value of autonomous judgment and action.[37]

Kohlberg's emphasis is on separation, the resolution of moral dilemmas in some hypothetical manner by individual agents who stress abstract rights. The moral man

> thinks formally, proceeding from theory to fact, and defines both the self and the moral autonomously, that is, apart from the identification and conventions that had comprised the particulars of his childhood world.[38]

By contrast, Gilligan maintained, women bring to the feminine experience and construction of social reality a distinctive voice and a different moral conception. Their perspective on the construction and the resolution of moral dilemmas emphasizes care and responsibility. They tend to construe, understand, and judge moral problems in terms of conflicts between self and other. The feminine voice speaks in contextual terms; there is a relational bias in women's thinking that leads them to reconstruct moral dilemmas in terms of their effect on others. And they tend to reconstruct hypothetical moral dilemmas in terms of the real, and to insist on additional

[36]Gilligan, "In a Different Voice," p. 483.
[37]Ibid., p. 509.
[38]Ibid., p. 481. The vision of Martin Luther, "journeying from the rejection of a self defined by others to the assertive boldness of 'Here I stand,'" is held up by Gilligan as the model of the complete moral man: separate, individualized, autonomous.

concrete information about the nature of the people involved. According to Gilligan, the insistence by women on the concrete, the particular, and the contextual seems to reflect the view that

> only when substance is given to the skeletal lives of hypothetical people is it possible to consider the social injustices which their moral problems may reflect and to imagine the individual suffering their occurrence may signify or their resolution engender.[39]

Of course, Gilligan was charting the development of women's moral judgment and the process of abortion decision-making rather than assessing the objective action of abortion itself. Yet, how we resolve moral conflicts has to do with how we perceive them; and Gilligan's interviews show how women construe—and then resolve—such problems differently from men. She noted that, "When women begin to make direct moral statements, the issues they repeatedly address are those of exploitation and hurt."[40] Using Kohlberg's progression from preconventional through conventional to postconventional levels of moral conceptions, Gilligan maintained that, at the higher levels of moral judgment, women tend to subsume both societal conventions and individual needs under the moral principle of nonviolence (nonviolence to self and to others). In situations such as the abortion dilemma, where the choice is between a variety of possibilities for hurt, the resolution may entail choosing the lesser of two evils. As she pointed out, many women decide for abortion because they feel a sense of responsibility toward new life (caring for the baby) and also feel that they cannot undertake that responsibility now without seriously hurting others and/or themselves.

Sara Ruddick is also convinced that there are female traditions and practices out of which a distinctive kind of thinking has developed. Maternal thought, in her view, is rooted in maternal practice and has distinct interests, namely, the preservation, growth, and development of children. In attempting to express and respect maternal thought, Ruddick identified among its characteristic features (1) a maternal humility and acceptance of the reality of conflicting interests; (2) the recognition of the priority of holding over acquiring; (3) a resilient good humor; and (4) respect for persons, respect for the growth process, and flexibility in adapting to change:

> Women are said to value open over closed structures, to eschew the clear-cut and the unambiguous. . . . these may well be interwoven responses to the changeability of a growing child.[41]

---

[39]Ibid. p. 512.
[40]Ibid., p. 514.
[41]Ruddick, p. 352.

Ruddick was not saying that mothers are especially wonderful people; like all human beings, they are a mixture of noble and ignoble. But in doing the work of attentive love that is child rearing, a different mode of thinking develops:

> My point is that out of maternal practices distinctive ways of conceptualizing, ordering, and valuing arise. We think differently about what it means and what it takes to be "wonderful," to be a person, to be real.[42]

The maternal conception of human achievement is different. This means that ends, goals, priorities, and purposes are weighted differently.

For Ruddick, maternal thinking is a discipline and a logic of inquiry that transcends gender: "maternal" is a social, not a biological category.[43] This type of thinking—attentive love and loving attention—is a value for all to emulate. Ruddick herself has recently sought to broaden maternal thought to encompass women's political expression and to consider ways in which maternal thought might transform feminist and peace politics.

Finally, another source of reflection on women's nature is Daniel Maguire's provocative essay "The Feminization of God and Ethics," in which he argued that "the experience of women has given them certain advantages in their moral perceptivity," advantages we would do well to incorporate into our general ethical inquiry.[44] Citing Gilligan and also the work of women scholars in scriptural studies, Maguire claimed that

> something profound is going on in our culture, and feminization is its name. It is shaking foundational categories of awareness, striking at long regnant myths and metaphors, affecting not just the splashing waves of issues debates, but actually shifting the deep-running affective and symbolic tides that carry our thought in ways that argument often does not even know.[45]

According to Maguire, the moral sensitivity of women is *generally* enhanced in at least four basic ways:

> (1) Women are less alienated from bodily existence and are thus less seducible by abstractions; (2) the affective component of moral judg-

---

[42]Ibid., p. 359.
[43]To illustrate, we might note Ruddick's definition of "fathers": "I look forward to the day when men are willing and able to share equally and actively in transformed maternal practices. . . . On that day, there will be no more 'Fathers,' no more people of either sex who have power over their children's lives and moral authority in their children's world, though they do not do the work of attentive love " (pp. 361–362).
[44]Maguire, pp. 59–67.
[45]Ibid., p. 59.

ment is less suppressed in women; (3) women have historically had more opportunity to "go to school" as children and thus to be more identified with the moral rhythms of minimally corrupted human life; (4) women enjoy the wisdom that accrues to the alienated.[46]

Like Ruddick, Maguire does not believe that women have a monopoly on this "advantageous femininity," nor did he suggest that sin is a masculine prerogative. He claimed that women's experience in childbearing and child rearing gives rise to a mode of thinking and to refined moral evaluative capacities: "Women are less likely to do what Sartre called the greatest evil in the human repertoire, to treat as abstract that which is concrete.[47] A feminine sensibility, informed by this rootedness in the concrete, emphasizes the inseparability of theory and experience/practice. Moreover, Maguire claimed that the moral judgments of women are more closely tied to feelings of empathy and compassion than those of men, and that this heightened affectivity makes women more reliable, more integral to, and more fit for public life (than men).

Like Ruddick and Gilligan, Maguire emphasized that confining this feminine ethics and maternal thinking to merely one sex is damaging for both sexes. In this view, the old saying that "Women's liberation means men's liberation" takes a new twist, applying not only to external activity (the liberation of women and men from traditional sex roles and work) but also to internal styles of thinking, judging, and feeling. According to Maguire, we should all welcome the feminization of culture.

Assuming that these authors are correct in their description of this feminine moral sensibility what would such a sensibility imply concerning responsible choice in cases of involuntary pregnancy? That is, how is it possible to integrate the relational thinking and caring aspects of women's traditional experience into feminism in general and into feminist thinking about reproductive freedom in particular?

To move from the developmental process to the substantive content of women's moral thinking would be to take as normative the values of caring, nurturing, and preserving life and to use them as the foundation of an ethics of reproductive freedom. A responsible feminist morality of abortion might begin by acknowledging the humanity of the fetus and accepting the burden of having to justify the decision to abort. The next task would be for feminists to think jointly about what count as good reasons for having or not having

[46]Ibid., p. 61.
[47]Ibid.

an abortion. We might try to elaborate a spectrum of reasons, ranging from the trivial through the serious to the compelling—a trivial or insufficient reason being the sex of the child (as Petchesky suggested) or fear of loss of attractiveness on the part of the pregnant woman.[48] As we move toward more compelling reasons, we might consider the so-called soft reasons for terminating pregnancy (poverty; mother unmarried; mother married but wants no more children because of age, existing family, or career). Finally, we would have to think about the "hard" reasons (threat to the mother's life or health, fetal defects, or pregnancy being the result of rape or incest). The idea would be to develop a set of moral considerations that individual women might use in thinking and deciding about abortion—subject to the proviso, of course, that each women has to decide according to her perception of her situation and the alternatives open to her. Thinking about the reasons for having or not having an abortion is meant to promote (not hinder) reproductive freedom and respect for the moral agency of women as subjects.

Feminists need to recognize the negative cultural trends that abortion signifies to many in our contemporary society. They need to say more about the morality of abortion and about the ethical dimensions of reproductive freedom in its broadest sense—encompassing contraception, sex education, abortion and sterilization, and family life. As one feminist wrote, "To allow antiabortionists to be the only ones to question ethical and psychological aspects of abortion is to anoint them as the sole protectors of morality."[49] Why can't this be a joint effort?

## ABORTION, LIBERALISM, AND FEMINISM

I began this essay with a question: How can we reduce the incidence of abortion without coercing women? To put this question another way: How can we arrive at a situation in which abortion, though legally permissible, is morally and socially discouraged?

The first part of this essay sought to show why the law should not be used to reduce the number of abortions. To summarize briefly, the prolife solution of reinstating restrictive laws would not work,

[48]Leslie Savan, "Abortion Chic: The Attraction of 'Wanted-Unwanted Pregnancies,'" *The Village Voice* (4 February 1981), p. 32, suggested some other trivial or insufficient reasons for having an abortion (abortion as rite of passage, as a desirable tinge of tragedy, and so on.)
[49]Ibid.

would do great injustice to women, and, moreover, would bring about a state of affairs worse than that preceding the enactment of such laws. Furthermore, using the law to enunciate society's moral standards regarding abortion seems inadequate because law is too blunt an instrument of social control. Legal rules do not adequately take into account the complex dilemmas confronting the involuntarily pregnant woman.[50]

But if the law should not be used to reduce the incidence of abortion, must a liberal society acquiesce in a kind of moral anemia regarding abortion? As Hart and others have insisted, the legality of a practice is not conclusive of its morality. The positivist separation of law and morals was intended to heighten our awareness of this important truth. An ideal liberal society relies on mediating institutions, rather than the law-enforcement agencies of government, to educate, transmit, and preserve moral values.

Now, there is no reason why various feminist groups cannot undertake the task of shaping the moral views of our society with respect to abortion. Indeed, I would argue that they should do this because they will presumably be most sympathetic to the plight of involuntarily pregnant women. Moreover, as Ruddick, Gilligan, and Maguire have suggested, women's moral sensibilities and perspectives—the emphasis on compassion, care, and responsibility for others—can provide valuable moral guidance on the abortion issue. Further, it is not a departure from the values of liberalism to hold that individuals can be taught, encouraged, educated, exhorted, urged, entreated, and persuaded—but not legally compelled—to use their freedom (including reproductive freedom) wisely and with due care for others.

There is, of course, an obligation to respect the moral autonomy of individual women regardless of their final decisions. Gilligan's interviews show how the morality of good reasons is operative even when women ultimately decide for abortion. Feminism and liberalism demand of us that we respect the rights of others to make basic, life-determining decisions. But they also impose on both prochoice feminists and prolife feminists the obligation to think about responsible reproductive freedom.

I have sought to show how women's moral sensibilities and perspectives can provide moral guidance on the abortion issue. A

[50]See Stephen Toulmin, "The Tyranny of Principles," *Hastings Center Report* 11, no. 6 (December 1981), pp. 31–39, where Toulmin reflected on the inadequacies of abstract general rules and principles in solving problems regarding ethics, administration, and law. Urging that law must be balanced by equity, he argued for a discretionary approach to practical moral dilemmas such as abortion.

commitment to the availability of legalized abortion need not bind
one to a kind of casual ethical relativism. As one author has written:

> Civil tolerance is hardly tolerance at all if one moral choice is in principle
> as good as another. It can only make sense, and show its full strength,
> when there are standards against which to measure behavior.[51]

I believe that feminists can and should define the moral standards
and principles against which to measure our behavior with respect
to abortion. Otherwise, those who want to use the law to coerce
women may succeed in realizing their goal.

## ACKNOWLEDGMENTS

I wish to thank Nancy Holmstrom, Marie Collins, Jerome Travers, and Mary Meehan especially for helpful comments, questions, and suggestions in the writing of this essay.

---

[51]Daniel Callahan, "Minimalist Ethics," *Hastings Center Report* 11, no. 5 (October 1981), p. 25.

# Commentary to Chapter 9

MARY MEEHAN

## INTRODUCTION

One reason why so many women have accepted the idea of abortion as a woman's right is that the unborn have been "defeminized." The use of male pronouns as generic terms for any person leads many to think of every unborn child as "he." We think of baldness as a male trait; most pictures of a fetus show a little bald person; so there is a tendency to identify that individual as male. Scientifically, of course, we know that half of the unborn are female, but scientific fact often fares badly when it collides with our psychological quirks.

Do unborn women have rights, including a right to control their own bodies? How can they do that if their bodies are torn apart by suction machines, or destroyed by salt poisoning, or delivered so early by hysterotomy that their lungs cannot breathe the air? If they have rights, don't their little brothers have rights, too? These are some of the questions that many feminists have ignored in their haste to make a case for absolute reproductive freedom for those women who have been born. So relentless has been the drive for such freedom that it seems a classic case of ideology gone wild.

Not only have unborn women been left out of the equation. Many adult women who oppose abortion have also been left out. Public opinion polls generally find that more women than men are opposed to abortion.[1] Mary Segers notes that women constitute a

---

[1]George H. Gallup, *The Gallup Poll: Public Opinion 1935–1971* (New York: Random House, 1972), 3 vols., vol. 3, pp. 2225–2226; *The Gallup Poll: Public Opinion 1972–1977* (Wilmington, Del.: Scholarly Resources, 1978), 2 vols., vol. 1, pp. 54, 94, 247–249, 379, 509–519, and vol. 2, pp. 669–673; *The Gallup Poll: Public Opinion 1978* (Wilmington, Del.: Scholarly Resources, 1979), p. 29; *The Gallup Poll: Public Opinion 1979* (Wilmington, Del.: Scholarly Resources, 1980), pp. 132–135; *The Gallup Poll: Public Opinion 1980* (Wilmington, Del.: Scholarly Resources,

---

MARY MEEHAN ● Free-lance writer, 23 2nd Street, N.E., Washington, D.C. 20002.

small percentage of Congress and that "for the most part, men dominate political decision-making on the issue of public policy on abortion." Yet, the women in the 1983–1984 session of Congress included eight prolifers. In the previous session, prolifers comprised 40% of the women in Congress.[2] These facts are of special significance because women's political groups discriminate quite openly against prolife women. The National Women's Political Caucus and the Women's Campaign Fund, for example, refuse to support women candidates who favor restrictions on abortion.[3]

## PROLIFE FEMINISM

Three themes are stressed in the writing of prolife feminists. One is that we cannot advance the rights of women by denying the rights of the unborn. As Daphne de Jong said:

> Human rights are not exclusive. Any claim to a superior or exceptional right inevitably infringes on the rights of someone else. To ignore the rights of others in an effort to assert our own is to compound injustice, rather than reduce it.[4]

A second theme is that abortion is one of many ways in which men exploit women. Jo McGowan referred to the "sexist assumption . . . that a woman's body is only acceptable (to men) when it is 'perfect,' i.e., 36-24-36 on the one hand, and not pregnant on the other."[5] And de Jong said that

> today's women's movement remains rooted in 19th century thinking, blindly accepting patriarchal systems . . . processing women through abortion mills to manufacture instant imitation men who will fit into a society made by and for wombless people.[6]

---

1981), pp. 171–174; *The Gallup Poll: Public Opinion 1981* (Wilmington, Del.: Scholarly Resources, 1982), pp. 112, 114, 116. There is an even more striking difference in the attitudes toward abortion of whites and nonwhites, with the latter opposing abortion more than the former.

[2] These statements are based on checks of voting charts prepared by the National Abortion Rights Action League and the National Right to Life Committee and, in the case of new members, on reports of their positions on the abortion issue.

[3] *Women's Political Times* (April 1980), p. 3; *Campaign Practices Reports* (1 February 1982), p. 5; Mike Feinsilber, "Ranks of Women in Politics Swelling," an Associated Press story in *Missoulian* (4 October 1982), p. 15.

[4] Daphne de Jong, "The Feminist Sell-out," in *Pro-Life Feminism* (Milwaukee: Feminists for Life of America, 1980), p. 6.

[5] Jo McGowan, "The Body as Battleground," Ibid., p. 24.

[6] de Jong, "Feminist Sell-out," p. 5.

Others have noted that abortion, often called a great convenience for women, is, in fact, a much greater convenience for men. It is a cheap way for them to buy out of any responsibility or commitment to women and unborn children.

The third theme is nonviolence. Prolife feminists encourage the kind of approach that Mary Segers notes in two feminist philosophers who stress women as nonviolent. But prolife feminists insist that words like *caring* and *nurturing* be honored even when it is very difficult to do so. We cannot celebrate women as caring and nurturing and nonviolent people if, every time a hard case comes along, they decide that the best way out is to take a human life. Prolife feminists believe that support of abortion is not a logical or a necessary part of feminism. We think it is contrary to the best feminist ideals. It is a tragic mistake, but one that can be remedied without tearing down the entire philosophical structure of feminism.

With the alternative of prolife feminism in mind, I would like to turn to specific points of Mary Segers's paper.

## COMMON GOOD, INDIVIDUAL GOOD

Segers says that legal positivists view the law "simply as a system of coercive sanctions keeping the citizen from external actions harmful to the community." Yet, our laws, both common and statutory, are also designed to keep individuals (and not just citizens) from harming other individuals. This harm, rather than harm to the community, is what most criminal cases and civil lawsuits involve. Later, Segers suggests that it is objectionable to legislate against abortion "when no substantive harm would be done to the common good by removing legal compulsions." I believe that abortion does harm the common good. But even if it did not, it should be outlawed because it does irreparable harm to individual humans by taking their lives. It is the first work of law and ethics to take care of specific individuals, and only after that to worry about more general concepts of the "common good." Indeed, we cannot decide what the common good is unless we know what is good for individuals. Similarly, it is difficult to understand what harms the common good unless we first know what harms individuals. When this point is missed, discussions of abortion are too abstract and bloodless.

Such discussions tend to overlook the fate of the individual most directly affected by abortion: The unborn child. Segers says that the mother must consider the interests of the child, but she insists that the mother alone have the right to decide whether that child lives or dies. The one most affected by her decision has no say in the matter—not even through the other parent or through a guardian. The mother, who is an interested party, is supposed to make a detached, wise, moral decision. Expecting such an outcome goes against reason and history. What we should expect instead is what we have today: a terrible death toll from abortion and many women with bad consciences. New systems of ethics, feminist or otherwise, cannot solve the problem.

## CONSENSUS IS POSSIBLE

Segers says that we have no consensus on abortion now, and she is right. There has been an abortion revolution in this country, one accomplished largely by a judiciary that is not accountable to the people. The legal revolution has resulted in more public acceptance of abortion, although polls find that substantial portions of the American people still oppose it strongly. Others are ambivalent; some have genuinely open minds. I believe that it was G. K. Chesterton who observed that the point of having an open mind, as in having an open mouth, is eventually to close it on something. We have an obligation to try to find answers, to form a consensus, on issues, like abortion, that are not just theoretical in nature but also have great practical consequences for individuals and for society.

The point of political action is either to register a consensus that already exists or else to build a consensus. In working for a legal ban on abortion, prolife advocates are trying to rebuild a consensus that existed before the 1960s. In their educational and political work, they are following the example of other human-rights movements throughout our history: the antislavery movement of the nineteenth century, the women's suffrage movement of the early twentieth, and the movements to abolish the death penalty in both centuries.

I believe that rebuilding a consensus on abortion is possible, though I concede that it will be difficult and may take many years. My limited optimism is based on three factors. First, the tremendous strides in scientific knowledge about the unborn helped turn around a leading proabortionist, Dr. Bernard Nathanson.[7] It takes courage to say that one was wrong about such a crucial issue; I hope that

---

[7] Bernard N. Nathanson and Richard N. Ostling, *Aborting America* (Garden City, N.Y.: Doubleday, 1979), pp. 159–169, 195–205. Dr. Nathanson was a founder of the National Association for Repeal of Abortion Laws, which is now the National Abortion Rights Action League (NARAL).

others will find that courage. Second, there is great commitment and talent in the prolife movement. Most of its members do not have access to sources of institutional power in the media and the courts, but that situation could change. Third, both prochoice people and those who are ambivalent about abortion tend to rely on natural rights theories in dealing with other life-and-death issues. The way we deal with abortion cannot be forever compartmentalized from the way we deal with other issues.

## OVERLOOKED POINTS ABOUT ABORTION AND THE CULTURE

What does it mean for a society when the taking of human life becomes legal, routine, systematized, and profitable? When it becomes a business and part of the gross national product? Although abortion is a small industry when compared with the military-industrial complex that President Eisenhower warned us about, it *is* an industry. Dr. Bernard Nathanson has estimated that it takes in about $325 million a year.[8] Gwynn McDougal, former director of an abortion clinic in Rhode Island, wrote in 1979 that "a handful of individuals have been criss-crossing this country for several years setting up abortion clinics for various private investors." Her clinic was one of a chain. She said that another clinic in the chain, which did from 70 to 90 abortions a week, made a net profit of $35,000–$40,000 per month. She said that a doctor at that clinic could earn "upwards of $1,000 each day for performing abortions from ten in the morning until two or so in the afternoon."[9]

The abortion industry has a trade group (or "professional organization," as its members prefer to call it), the National Abortion Federation. I attended its 1980 convention and found that continental breakfasts were served in the exhibit room, buffet-style, so that conferees could chat with one another and view the commercial wares. They sipped coffee and munched rolls as they looked at literature on pregnancy tests, picked up free samples of laminaria tents, and examined curettes and other abortion instruments. I spoke with the representative of the Columbus Pathology Lab, Inc. (Columbus, Ohio), who revealed that after examining fetal remains, the lab sent them

[8]Bernard N. Nathanson in U.S. Congress, Senate, Committee on the Judiciary, Subcommittee on Separation of Powers, *The Human Life Bill: Hearings on S. 158,* 2 vols., 97th Cong., 1st sess., 18 June 1981, vol. 1, p. 1048.
[9]Gwynn McDougal, *Women's Medical Clinic of Providence: A Story of Private Enterprise in the Abortion Arena* (Providence: Scorpio Press, 1979), pp. 7, 12, 101.

to a funeral home for disposal, and that the funeral home charged by the pound for their service.[10] Neither he nor the abortion clinic workers circling through the exhibit area seemed to find anything unusual or gruesome in all of this. They seemed like nice people. Have-a-nice-day kind of people. What are we coming to?

Those whose livelihoods depend on abortion are not the only ones who have been corrupted. I find it impossible to accept Segers's statement that abortion is "unique" and her suggestion that it does not lead to other kinds of killing. The 1982 Bloomington baby case, in which a Down's syndrome baby starved to death because his parents refused to authorize an operation, was not unusual in its general outline. Many similar cases have not reached the courts.[11] What was doubly shocking about the Bloomington case was that, after it did reach the state courts, they refused to intervene and save the child's life, despite Indiana statutes forbidding child neglect and discrimination against the handicapped. But no one should have been too surprised: Discrimination against the handicapped unborn, through the amniocentesis–selective-abortion package, has become increasingly common in our society. Some people who have emotional, aesthetic or moral objections to late abortions nevertheless support their legal authorization precisely so that selective abortion of the handicapped can be accomplished.

Nor is infanticide limited to handicapped babies. In the past several years, there have been many news reports of healthy newborns who were dumped in trashcans or abandoned out-of-doors.[12]

---

[10]Mary Meehan and Elizabeth Moore, "Forced Abortion Suggested at Clinic Owners' Conference," *National Right to Life News* (2 June 1980), pp. 1, 13, 16, 17.

[11]Harold M. Schmeck, Jr., "A Film Examines Right to Life of a Mentally Retarded Infant," *New York Times*, (15 October 1971), p. 31; Anthony Shaw, "Dilemmas of 'Informed Consent' in Children," *New England Journal of Medicine* 289 (25 October 1973), pp. 885–890; Raymond S. Duff and A. G. M. Campbell, "Moral and Ethical Dilemmas in the Special-Care Nursery," *New England Journal of Medicine* 289 (25 October 1973), pp. 890–894; Diane Brozek, "Defective Newborns Are Dying by Design," *Hartford Courant*, 14 June 1981, pp. A-1, A-25.

[12]Headlines in the *Washington Post* over a 41-month period outline the problem: "District Heights Woman Guilty in Death of Her Newborn Son" (7 September 1979); "Birth of Baby in Street Sets Off a Downtown Drama" (22 January 1980); "Woman Held for Attempting to Kill Baby" (6 December 1980); "Police Seek Parents of Baby Boy 'Discarded' in Trash Bin" (11 May 1982); "Infant in Trash Can Send Mother to Jail" (3 June 1982); "Baby Left in Bag Wins the Heart of Paramedic" (16 August 1982); "Abandoned Baby Found in Md." (5 November 1982); "Baby Found in Woods" (11 November 1982); "Baby's Body is Found in College Park" (9 January 1983); "Abandoned Baby's Mother Charged in Murder Attempt" (2 February 1983); "Body of Infant Found in Trash Room in Md." (10 February 1983).

Most of them survived because, unlike the unborn, they could attract attention by crying. But what does the phenomenon of "throwaway babies" say about our society and its attitudes toward children? Widespread abortion encourages people to think of babies as expendable.

Killing and violence spill over from one area to the next, both intellectually and emotionally. Rationalizations accepted for one type of killing—abortion, for example—are transferred to others, such as infanticide, euthanasia, and suicide.[13] And once defenses are down, what is to prevent the acceptance of any type of warfare, as long as the objective is reasonably utilitarian? Many leaders of the peace movement, because they support legalized abortion, lack intellectual credibility when they speak of the sanctity of life in relation to war and peace. The same is true of people (and groups like the American Civil Liberties Union) who oppose the death penalty but support abortion. They put themselves in the strange position of defending the right to life of the guilty at the same time that they deny the right to life of the innocent.

When a high fever threatens a patient's life, a doctor does everything possible to bring the fever down quickly. So it should be with the fever of violence. There is an urgent need to reduce the level of violence everywhere, as soon as possible, before it engulfs us all.

[13]Duff and Campbell, pp. 891–894; "Doctor Wants Clinic for Painless Suicide," a United Press International report in *Philadelphia Evening Bulletin* (13 August 1977), p. 22; Ellen Goodman, "Who Lives? Who Dies? Who Chooses?", *Washington Post* (22 August 1981); p. A-23; Richard Cohen, "It Depends," *Washington Post* (20 April 1982), p. B-1; "Can America Stop Footing the Bill for Those Ready to Die?", an Associated Press report in Hagerstown, Md., *Morning Herald* (13 October 1982), p. B-8.

## CHAPTER 10

# Abortion, Autonomy, and Community

## LISA SOWLE CAHILL

### AUTOBIOGRAPHICAL STATEMENT

*Although any worthwhile moral argument must stand unsupported by authorial expressions of intention, the nature of this project on "abortion and values" creates a special context for indicating the experiences and commitments out of which particular arguments have evolved. Though my essentially conservative attitude toward the fetus is not entirely relative to my personal history, I acknowledge that familial, religious, and academic influences can augment an inclination to highlight certain features of abortion (and its relation to broader cultural values) and to downplay others.*

*In my case, it is difficult to disentangle religious from more properly "intellectual" sources of influence, as my academic discipline is theological ethics. I was raised a Roman Catholic, a communion with which I continue to affiliate, and was educated generally to think of unborn humans as "babies" who are to be cherished. Abortion, however, appears not to have loomed as large on the Catholic moral agenda of the 1950s and 1960s as it does in the post-1973 prolife movement. In the moral universe of my upbringing, it was taken for granted that abortion was wrong, but that fact was not belabored. Perhaps for that reason, I regard a single-issue focus on abortion as a distortion of what ought properly to be a Christian and human concern about the value and the quality of human life in all its forms and conditions. I understand the essence of the Catholic position on abortion (as permitted only when the life of the mother is endangered, and only then under special circumstances) to be congruent with the historically*

LISA SOWLE CAHILL • Department of Theology, Boston College, Chestnut Hill, Massachusetts 02167.

*positive valuation of prenatal life in the Christian tradition. My own view of the very limited justifiability of abortion is consistent with this traditional thrust, though I would modify the contemporary Church's teaching in the direction of more flexibility in exceptional instances.*

*As a professional ethicist I do not identify my research or teaching as "Catholic" in an exclusive sense. I graduated from one Jesuit university (the University of Santa Clara) and am now on the faculty of another. My studies for the master's and doctoral degrees were completed at the University of Chicago Divinity School, currently an interdenominational institution of Baptist origin. In graduate work and subsequently among colleagues, I have enjoyed exposure to contrasting points of view well argued, and thus, I have been privileged to pursue a critical sense of my own religious tradition. The work of my dissertation director, James M. Gustafson, represents the sort of accomplished moral analysis to which I aspire, along with many more of his students and former students. His moral evaluation of abortion differs from mine, but the ecumenicity and the circumspection of judgment with which he approaches controverted questions continues to be instructive.*

*My theoretical position on abortion (that the fetus deserves serious but not absolute consideration) has been confirmed rather than challenged by my experiences of pregnancy and parenthood, with the difference that my view of the mother–fetus relation is now "from the inside out" rather from detached observation. Motherhood has heightened my sensitivity to the vulnerability of the fetus and its concomitant need for protection, as well as to the "otherness" of the fetus and the burden that it imposes when the needs of mother and fetus are incompatible.*

Within the circle of Christian theological ethicists who converse in "the academy," as I do, it is definitely not in vogue to voice opposition to the prochoice position. This position is often believed to be entailed in a serious commitment to sexual autonomy, to feminism, and to enlightened, humanistic causes in general. To some extent, my contribution to this project is a reaction against that assumption.

In formulating my position, and in evaluating the relation of positions on abortion generally to the values affirmed and denied in contemporary North American culture, I have drawn on resources both theological and philosophical. The relevant religious resources are those biblical stories, symbols, and thematic patterns that support a willingness to sacrifice personal interests in order to protect the weakest or the "neighbor" most in need. (The latter category includes both women, who suffer the effects of injustices in the spheres of sexuality, domesticity, and reproduction, and fetuses, as dependent and unable effectively to assert claims.) Also central are the resources of the Roman Catholic tradition in social ethics, which has been considerably more "progressive" than the tradition in personal ethics, medical and sexual.[1] However, I dissent from the proposition that abortion is a narrowly religious issue. Both biblical themes and Catholic natural-law social analysis are presented here in terms congruent with many secular or humanistic perspectives on the relations of persons in community (though not all, e.g., utilitarianism). The possibility of assuming in principle an alliance between religious and rational ethics is itself a fruit of the Catholic, Thomistic, natural-law tradition of moral insight.

The principal value at stake in this essay is the existence of the fetus itself, for it must be established *who* are considered members of the "human community" before the moral relationships among these members can be addressed. The question of the status of fetal life in the human community is the most divisive and the least easy to resolve in the entire abortion debate; it is also the most fundamental. Although it is not my purpose here to defend a certain view of the fetus, of its rights, or of the rights of its mother, I have yet to be persuaded that these issues can be avoided successfully. For this reason, I feel a need to briefly indicate my own evaluation of fetal life, fully realizing that any position on the status of the fetus is vulnerable. I then proceed to my major task of broader reflections on abortion and the culture, where assumptions about the fetus also influence social attitudes and policies.

I am convinced that the fetus is from conception a member of the human species (having an identifiably human genotype, and being of human parentage), and, as such, is an entity to which at least some protection is due, even though its status may not at every phase be equivalent to that of postnatal life. (See the following section on "Dualism and Corporeality" for a further discussion of the relation between biological facts and moral value.) Further, I believe that there exists, even in our pluralist culture, a relatively broad consensus that the fetus does have some value and status in the human community, even among those who maintain that "hard choices" about sustaining its life must be left finally to the woman who bears it. My

---

[1]The twentieth-century popes have taken a persistent and sometimes prophetic interest in redressing imbalances in the social and economic orders, whether precipitated by socialism or by capitalism. Examples are Leo XIII's *Rerum Novarum* (1891), Pius XI's *Quadragesimo Anno* (1931), John XXIII's *Mater et Magistra* (1961) and *Pacem in Terris* (1963), Paul VI's *Populorum Progressio* (1967) and *Octogesima Adveniens* (1971), and John Paul II's *Laborem Exercens* (1982).

position on fetal status might be characterized as "developmentalist"[2] insofar as I view its value as incremental throughout gestation. The fact that few, if any, give absolutely equal value to the mother and the fetus is attested to by the fact that all are willing to prefer the mother in at least some "life-against-life" cases, and by the fact that virtually no one perceives the abortion of a 7-month-old fetus as the moral equivalent of the use of an abortifacient method of birth control, such as the IUD (even though both may be viewed as wrong). Nonetheless, I see the fetus as having a value at conception that is quite significant and that quickly increases; but it never overrides the right of the mother to preserve her own life. Even relatively early in pregnancy (for example, in the first trimester), I think serious considerations must be present to justify abortion. Threat to life is the classic case, although I would not exclude the possibility that other threats might justify abortion, particularly when the interest that the mother has at stake is equal to or greater than her interest in her life. (To specify such interests and to stipulate circumstances in which they might be threatened remains a perplexing task.) In summary, I endorse a strong bias in favor of the fetus and rest a heavy burden of proof on those who would choose abortion. This endorsement will in obvious ways influence my assessment of the values that form the backdrop for our culture's permissive policies regarding abortion. At the same time, I trust that much of what I have to say about such things as community, corporeality, suffering, physical or mental disabilities, and family will find agreement among many who do not share my evaluation of fetal life or my grounding in Catholic Christianity.

## LIBERALISM AND THE COMMON GOOD

A central focus of my analysis of abortion and the culture is the relations between individuals and the communities in which they associate. Often, these relations are articulated in terms of "rights" and "duties." It has been observed, however, that these terms encourage moral individualism and isolation of the moral agent(s) from the social relationships in which decision making occurs.[3]

I continue to think it legitimate to use "rights" language to

[2]Daniel Callahan, *Abortion: Law, Choice, and Morality* (New York: Macmillan, 1970), pp. 384–390.
[3]See, for example, Larry R. Churchill and José Jorge Simán, "Abortion and the Rhetoric of Individual Rights," *The Hastings Center Report* 12 (February 1982), pp. 9–12; and Sandra Harding, "Beneath the Surface of the Abortion Dispute," in this volume.

discuss abortion, but I want to remove that language from the context of moral and political liberalism. To shift attention away from the rights of the fetus or the woman understood individualistically does not mean that the value and rights of either thereby become irrelevant. It means, rather, that their respective rights must be defined in relation to one another (and, in a less immediate sense, to the rights of others, for example, family members). Where those rights can conflict, neither can be absolute. The rights of both are *limited*, but still significant.

Fundamentally, then, I want to speak of rights in the context of sociality and of community. Of particular relevance to the abortion dilemma is the fact that duties or obligations can bind humans to their fellows in ways to which they have not explicitly consented. Such obligations originate simply in the sorts of reciprocal relatedness that constitute being a human. The mother–fetus relation is characterized by obligations of this sort, as are all parent-child relations.

Abortion represents a conflict between, most directly, the rights of the mother and the rights of the fetus. In contemporary American culture, this conflict is settled in favor of the pregnant woman's right to dispose of the fetus as she deems necessary to protect her own rights or interests. A warrant often adduced in support of such an adjudication of claims is the woman's right to autonomous self-determination, particularly regarding her body and its reproductive capacities. Thus, a restriction of the right to choose abortion is perceived as an infringement of personal liberty in a most intimate and private sphere.

The present dominance of the prochoice position on abortion (that is, every woman has a right to decide for herself, and on the basis of her own religious and moral convictions, whether or not to have an abortion) represents *positively* the view that women must be taken seriously as autonomous moral agents. Societal and legal protection of the freedom to control childbearing, through abortion if necessary, represents a challenge to those dimensions of marriage, family, and employment that continue to oppress and subordinate the female sex. In addition, to leave abortion decisions to the discretion of the agent most directly involved is to acknowledge the individuality that attends every moral decision, especially decisions that are complex, filled with conflict, and even tragic.

However, I believe that our culture's general willingness to grant to women the exclusive power to terminate their pregnancies has other, too frequently unexamined, implications that can be described *negatively*. First, and perhaps most fundamentally, the single-minded affirmation of the rights of the pregnant woman (e.g., her "right to privacy" or "right to reproductive freedom") virtually circumvents the equally important but incorrigibly difficult problem of the status of fetal life. What sort of being is it that threatens the welfare of the pregnant woman? Does it in turn have rights? And if so, how do they weigh in the balance against those of the woman? Furthermore, the subordination in the legal and practical spheres of any right to life of the fetus (at least, if previable) to a whole spectrum of rights, needs, or interests of the mother manifests a widespread and often uncritical cultural acceptance of political and moral liberalism.

By *liberalism,* I mean a family of views concerning the person and the society resembling or rooted in the social contract theories of John Locke, Thomas Hobbes, and Jean Jacques Rousseau, who have influenced, at least indirectly, Western democracy and the American constitutional tradition. In such views, persons are seen essentially as free and autonomous agents who come into society to protect self-interest by a series of mutually advantageous agreements. Society or community is thus secondary to the existence of the individual; persons are not social by nature and have no natural obligations antecedent to their free consent.[4] A woman, for example, has no *prima facie* moral obligation to sustain a pregnancy that she has not undertaken voluntarily; to do so would constitute a supererogatory act (Judith Jarvis Thomson[5]).

Other competing theories—for example, some Marxist and feminist social theories, or the Thomistic notion of the "common good" as reinterpreted by the modern papal social encyclicals—begin from the contrary premise. That is, persons are by definition interrelated in a social whole whose fabric of reciprocal rights and duties constitutes the very condition of their individual and communal fulfillment. The concept of the *common good* envisions society in a way that is neither liberal nor utilitarian. The community is understood as prior to the individual; however, each individual is equally entitled to share in the benefits that inhere in the community. The common good is not identified with the interests of any particular group. Rather, it is a normative standard or ideal by which to criticize and reform any existing social order. Undeniably associated with this notion are some intransigent problems of definition shared with other attempts to elucidate "normative" or "essential" humanity or human community. Still, fidelity to the common good as the primary framework for social analysis guarantees, at least that *individual* and *community,* as well as *rights* and *duties,* will be taken as a pair of com-

---

[4]See the critiques of liberalism by Sandra G. Harding, "Beneath the Surface of the Abortion Debate"; and Jean Bethke Elshtain, "Reflections on Abortion, Values, and the Family," both in this volume.
[5]Judith Jarvis Thomson, "A Defense of Abortion," *Philosophy and Public Affairs* 1 (Fall 1972), pp. 47–66.

plementary terms. Above all, it suggests that human society is characterized by an intrinsic interdependence or cohesiveness for which paradigms that construe society as voluntary affiliations of individuals whose mutual obligations are purely contractual do not adequately account.[6]

From the viewpoint of the common good, understood in these terms, one indeed has a duty, premised on the mutual interdependence and obligations implied by common humanity, to help another person when to do so involves relatively little self-sacrifice and a proportionate gain for the other. Because gestation is a primordial, prototypical, and physically concrete form of sociality and interdependence, some obligations to the fetus may exist even when they have not been undertaken deliberately. One consequence of the individualistic liberal view of the pregnant woman as moral agent, besides the obvious one of minimizing restraints on her free power of self-determination, is that it reduces the obligations of other individuals or of the community to offer support during and after a burdensome pregnancy. Moral and social dilemmas are regarded as the business and the burden of individuals, to be resolved or borne alone.[7]

[6]The papal social encyclicals have been largely *ad hoc* in nature, addressing themselves in the name of the common good to actual abuses and imbalances of rights and duties, rather than attempting to articulate any exhaustive list of rights and duties or to formulate precisely enduring relationships among them. For instance, Leo XIII addressed in *Rerum Novarum*, against socialism, the right of the worker to own private property; Pius XI in *Quadragesimo Anno* asserted the rights of the worker against capitalistic property owners who neglected duties to others and to the community as a whole. Among the best concise definitions of *common good* in the encyclicals is that offered by John XXIII in *Pacem in Terris* (Paragraphs 55–58). I have furthered developed this analysis of common good, rights, and duties in "Toward a Christian Theory of Human Rights," *Journal of Religious Ethics* 8 (Fall 1980), pp. 277–301.

In a recent essay ("Abortion and the Pursuit of Happiness," *Logos* 3, 1982, pp. 61–77), Philip Rossi, S. J., similarly asserted the connection between human freedom and interdependence and linked it with Kant's characterization of moral agency in accord with membership in a "kingdom of ends." Rossi argued effectively that "rights-in-conflict" language is insufficient to handle the morality of abortion in the absence of a unified view of happiness or the human good.

[7]In *The Heretical Imperative* (Garden City, N.Y.: Doubleday, 1979), Peter Berger dubbed the "modern consciousness" a phenomenon akin to the liberal ethos. The modern man or woman is under the necessity of making choices rather than of acquiescing to fate. However, he or she also is confronted with a plurality of world views, rather than with a cohesive tradition that shapes social roles and gives them significance. A crisis of belief results because beliefs about reality, including religious and moral beliefs, require social confirmation, and that is widely unavailable in modern society. As a result, morality and religion become subjectivized and contingent on the sheer choice or "preference" of the individual (Chapter 1, "Modernity as the Universalization of Heresy," pp. 1–31).

## Dualism and Corporeality

Twentieth-century philosophy and theology have been accustomed to repudiating the "dualism" of ancient Greece and its remnants in Christianity or its facsimile in René Descartes. In sexual ethics, for example, we resist any attempts to define the body as "bad" and the spirit as resistant to it, and instead, we insist on attention to bodily experience in definitions of moral obligation.[8] The unity of body and spirit in human experience should also be taken into account seriously in discussions of pregnancy. The facts that a fetus is ineluctably dependent for its very existence on the body of another, and that this relation of dependence is not *prima facie* pathological or unjust, but physiologically normal and natural for a human being in its earliest stages of existence, should count as *one* factor in a moral evaluation of pregnancy and abortion. The morality of abortion is not reducible to the issue of "free consent" to pregnancy. This is not to say that abortion can never be justified (given the presence of countervailing factors), but only that we have not grasped the reality of the moral situation when we define freedom only as "freedom over" the body and not also as "freedom in" or "freedom through" the body. The body makes peculiar demands, creates peculiar relationships, and grounds peculiar obligations.

The Catholic moral theologian Louis Janssens has reformulated the notion of a normative human nature in a way that affirms the historicity, equality, sociality, and corporeality of all persons:

> That we are corporeal means in the first place that our body forms a part of the integrated subject that we are; corporeal and spiritual, nonetheless a singular being. What concerns the human body, therefore, also affects the person himself.
> That we are a subjectivity, or a conscious interiority, in corporeality . . . is the basis for a number of moral demands.[9]

Conversely, our culture as liberal denies both determinations of "freedom" by our concrete embodied nature and obligation without consent (as a contradiction in terms). The former denial is related to the latter as partial cause. Examples of the tendency to ignore, repress, or negate the demands of corporeality can be seen at many levels: in the rapid increase in medical litigation over the past two decades, which seems to represent the unrealistic demand that the physician free us from the vulnerability of the human body and the

---

[8]See, for example, James B. Nelson, *Embodiment: An Approach to Sexuality and Christian Theology* (Minneapolis: Augsburg, 1978), and Robert Baker and Frederick Elliston, eds., *Philosophy and Sex* (Buffalo, N.Y.: Prometheus Books, 1975).
[9]Louis Janssens, "Artificial Insemination: Ethical Considerations," *Louvain Studies* 8 (Spring 1980), pp. 5–6.

fallibility of the medical arts; in the denial in popular mores and in sexual ethics that there is any morally significant connection whatsoever between sex and procreation; and in the recalcitrant refusal of denizens of the developed nations to curtail their supposed right to pursue life, liberty, and happiness at the expense of the material needs of Third World citizens.

At the same time that we avoid the exaltation of autonomy to the detriment of corporeality, it is important to avoid biologism, another form of dualism, in which freedom is completely constrained by physiological functions or conditions. Examples of the latter can be found in traditional Roman Catholic analyses of sexual and medical ethics. Since the negative response of the Holy Office of the Vatican in 1869 to the inquiry whether craniotomy is licit, magisterial teaching regarding abortion has been that a fetus may be sacrificed to preserve its mother's life only when the procedure that destroys it is aimed *physically* at some other objective. Thus, the removal of the cancerous uterus of a pregnant woman would be allowed, insofar as the physically indirect method of killing the fetus (though a surgical procedure related directly to a condition other than pregnancy) "guarantees" that the intention of the agents involved is not primarily to bring about the death of the fetus, but to protect the woman. By the same token, it would be permissible to remove the entire fallopian tube in a case of ectopic pregnancy; but it would not be permissible to remove the embryo from the tube, leaving intact the tube and the woman's potential to conceive again. Much less would it be justified to remove a potentially viable fetus directly from the womb to curtail the potentially fatal strain of pregnancy on a woman suffering from renal or coronary disease. The crucial question in such dilemmas is whether the moral key ought to be the indirectness of the physical procedure of resolution or the simple fact of two lives in conflict.[10]

[10]More complete discussions of the evolution of the Catholic position on abortion are offered in John T. Noonan, Jr., "An Almost Absolute Value in History," in John T. Noonan, ed., *The Morality of Abortion* (Cambridge: Harvard University Press, 1970); and John Connery, S.J., *Abortion: The Development of the Roman Catholic Perspective* (Chicago: Loyola University Press, 1977). Critiques have been developed by Bernard Häring, "A Theological Evaluation"; James M. Gustafson, "A Protestant Ethical Approach; and Paul Ramsey, "Reference Points in Deciding About Abortion," in *The Morality of Abortion*. Charles Curran examined the problem of "physicalism" in Roman Catholic ethics generally in "Natural Law and Contemporary Moral Theology," *Contemporary Problems in Moral Theology* (Notre Dame, Ind.: Fides, 1970). Several discussions of the "principle of double effect" operative in the Catholic analysis of abortion appear in Charles E. Curran and Richard A. McCormick, S.J., eds., *Readings in Moral Theology No. 1: Moral Norms and Catholic Tradition* (New York: Paulist, 1979). Unfortunately, to cite these resources is only to skim the surface of those available.

Another nexus of dualistic arguments about abortion is the problematic relationship of the biological development of the fetus (for example, its appearance) to its status in the human community. Equally prone to oversimplification are those who claim that a recognizably human genotype or human form is of no relevance at all to the respect accorded some particular being and those who assume that a demonstration of the membership of the fetus in the species *Homo sapiens,* or its resemblance to a baby, settles the issue of full "humanity" or "personhood," and thus of abortion. Few are unfamiliar with the attempts of some prolife advocates to substitute enlarged photographs of aborted fetuses for rational argument. More subtle are the efforts of prochoice proponents to eliminate critical recognition of the matter–spirit link in abortion. Michael Tooley and Laura Purdy asked rhetorically, "If pig fetuses resembled adult humans, would it be seriously wrong to kill pig fetuses?"[11] Dualism is the premise that allows such a question to be posed at all, as it requires us to dissociate from our notion of "humanity" what it means to exist materially and corporeally in a human (or porcine) manner. The reader is induced to answer, "No," and thus to agree with the proabortion argument framing the question, because the hypothetical situation is nonsensical.

A more thoughtful treatment of the problem is presented by Joseph Donceel's revival of the Aristotelian-Thomistic notion of "hylomorphism."[12] Donceel suggested that the material aspect of any being is naturally appropriate to its "form" or spirit. Thus, the increasingly human appearance of human offspring during gestation may be relevant to their developing status within the community of persons. Donceel suggested that the possibility of the "delayed hominization" of the fetus is not inconsistent with the acceptance by some traditional Christian authors (such as Anselm, Aquinas, and Alphonsus Liguori) of the idea that "ensoulment" takes place at some point subsequent to conception, for example, at "quickening." Abortion, although always sinful, becomes the sin of homicide only after that point.

The merit of a position such as Donceel's lies in its recognition that scientific or empirical evidence (e.g., about genotype or appearance) can be relevant to moral decisions, even if it is not in itself decisive. An integral view of the person urges recognition that neither human spirit, freeom, and valuing, on the one hand, nor the

[11]Michael Tooley and Laura Purdy, "Is Abortion Murder?," in Robert Perkins, ed., *Abortion: Pro and Con* (Cambridge, Mass.: 1974), p. 134.
[12]Joseph Donceel, S.J., "Animation and Hominization," *Theological Studies* 31 (March 1970), pp. 76–105.

material conditions, realizations, and manifestations of same, on the other, ought to be taken alone as definitive of moral obligation. Normative ethics is dependent on the empirical sciences and other "descriptive" (as distinct from "normative") accounts of the human situation for two reasons at least: (1) the ethicist must have a realistic appreciation of the act or the relation that he or she proposes to evaluate; and (2) the fact that an entity or relation is "normal" or "abnormal" in, for example, a sociological, physiological, or psychological sense will count for or against the conclusion that its existence ought or ought not to be chosen or encouraged. (However, to determine the precise weight that empirical or statistical normality or abnormality ought to have in normative ethics is not a simple matter. It joins the ranks of the highly debated questions in ethics.) Donceel's point is not only that the entity to be evaluated, the fetus, has a corporeal dimension, but also that what is known about normal fetal development should be correlated with any normative account of fetal status.

## SUFFERING

The liberal ethos discourages making personal sacrifices and encourages at best a minimal appreciation of the virtue and even the necessity of constructive suffering. Our culture has a low tolerance of the burdens and failures of life and tends to deny that life has value when conducted in irremediably painful conditions. There are an expectation of ready resort to the "technological fix" and an inability to appropriate suffering in meaningful ways.[13] To these sorts of attitudes might be contrasted the Christian ideals of reconciliation or redemption of the conditions of brokenness and evil in which we consistently find ourselves.

The notion of ability and responsibility to constructively redeem tragedy under circumstances of difficulty is not incompatible with the feminist concern that women be regarded as and regard themselves as mature moral agents who do not need protection from and do not avoid the exigencies of adulthood in the human community. I do not recommend masochism, nor the martyrdom of women who sacrifice themselves out of unwillingness or inability to assert their legitimate claims; rather, I recommend a recognition that some hu-

---

[13]I perceive a concern similar to mine in David Peretz's "The Illusion of 'Rational' Suicide," *Hastings Center Report* 11 (December 1981), pp. 40–42. Peretz sees planned suicide as an attempt to gain control over feelings of pain and helplessness by idealizing the freedom and autonomy of the "self as agent."

man situations have unavoidably tragic elements and that to be human is to bear these burdens. We cannot be freed from all infringements on our self-fulfillment, and to persistently demand that is to avoid moral agency in the complete sense. The decision to continue a pregnancy might be construed as a decision by the stronger to assume burdens that would otherwise fall on the most defenseless. However, "the stronger" includes not only the woman, who is also a victim, but the larger community of which she and the fetus are a part. (This is not to deny that the tragic elements of conflictual pregnancies may justify some decisions to abort.) As a final note, an important element in constructively assimilating suffering, and also in alleviating suffering to the extent possible, is communal support, both of the difficult pregnancy and of the abnormal fetus, child, or adult. In another context, Daniel Callahan (himself a prochoice advocate) has perceptively commented on the kind of community needed to successfully weather moral conflicts for which there appears to be a dearth of satisfactory resolutions:

> Hard times require self-sacrifice and altruism—but there is nothing in an ethic of moral autonomy to sustain or nourish those values. Hard times necessitate a sense of community and the common good—but the putative virtues of autonomy are primarily directed toward the cultivation of independent selfhood. . . . Hard times need a broad sense of duty toward others, especially those out of sight—but an ethic of autonomy stresses responsibility only for one's freely chosen, consenting-adult relationships.
> Whether suffering brings out the best or the worst in people is an old question, and the historical evidence is mixed. Yet a people's capacity to endure suffering without turning on each other is closely linked to the way they have envisioned, and earlier embodied, their relationship to each other.[14]

## STANDARDS OF HUMAN EXISTENCE

Our culture tends to estimate the value of human life in direct proportion to its level of physical and intellectual perfection or achievement. This attitude leads to the inability of parents and others to envision creatively or positively the task of raising an abnormal child, and it creates widespread support of abortion for so-called fetal indications. A question that often could be pressed more critically

[14]Daniel Callahan, "Minimalist Ethics," *Hastings Center Report* 11 (October 1981), pp. 19–20. Callahan addressed the question of whether a morality that stresses the autonomy of the individual is a "good-time philosophy," able to sustain a society in times of affluence but not in times of economic and political stress.

is whether the abortion is intended primarily to serve the interests of the family (in its "freedom") or of the fetus (in a "happy" life), and in either case, what criteria of evaluation are used.[15]

The liberal individualistic theory of moral responsibility comes into play not only in the moral weight usually given to freedom, but also because society often seems to see parents as responsible for avoiding the births of defective (and hence burdensome) children; social willingness to provide structures of assistance for severely handicapped individuals and their families decreases correspondingly.[16]

One Christian ethicist, Stanley Hauerwas, has developed a critique of the further implications of liberalism for the nature of the family.[17] Hauerwas, who is noted for his emphasis on the narrative qualities of religion and theology, on the centrality of character in morality and ethics, and on the importance of community in embodying religious and moral commitment in life and action, observed that the modern nuclear family is perceived as a complex of intimate relationships whose purpose is the personal fulfillment of its members. Such an account of family life has lost both the connection of the "self-sufficient" family with the larger community and its institutions and any resources for understanding the purposes of family life, including having children, beyond the gratification of the couple. Hauerwas proposed that the family ought not to be understood as "a contractual social unit"[18] and that "marriage is not sustained by

[15]A provocative example of a criterion of the life worth preserving has been offered by Richard McCormick in a discussion of whether and when to treat infants suffering from serious congenital anomalies. McCormick suggested that physical life can be a worthwhile good for the person living it if it offers at least "relational potential," that is, the capacity to give and receive love, and even if it does not offer "normal" intelligence or physical competence ("To Save or Let Die," *Journal of American Medical Association* 229, July 1974, pp. 172–176).

[16]Those who have counseled or interviewed parents of abnormal infants have commented that the availability of aminiocentesis and abortion in cases of genetic defect has altered the nature of the parent–child relationship after such a birth occurs. John Fletcher commented, "If an infant is born with a severe genetic defect which might have been diagnosed pre-natally, will it not occur to the physicians and parents, that this infant might have been tested and aborted? Such thoughts will, presumably, intensify the rejection of the infant" ("Moral and Ethical Problems of Pre-natal Diagnosis," *Clinical Genetics* 9 October 1975, p. 25). See also John Fletcher, "The Brink: The Parent-Child Bond in the Genetic Revolution," *Theological Studies* 33 (September 1972), pp. 457–485; and Raymond S. Duff and A. G. M. Campbell, "Moral and Ethical Dilemmas in the Special-Care Nursery," *New England Journal of Medicine* 289 (October 1973), pp. 890–894.

[17]This is accomplished most extensively in Stanley Hauerwas, *A Community of Character* (Notre Dame, Ind,: University of Notre Dame Press, 1981), especially Part 3, "The Church and Social Policy: The Family, Sex, and Abortion."

[18]Hauerwas, p. 171.

being a fulfilling experience for all involved, but by embodying moral and social purposes that give it a basis in the wider community."[19]

The language of rights is criticized by Hauerwas because it seems to represent the liberal commitment to the autonomy of the individual and his or her freedom to enter into moral obligations electively via contracts.[20] He also seems to detect a liberal agenda hidden behind attempts to hinge the abortion discussion on whether the fetus has or has not a "right to life." Hauerwas suggested that the precise status of the fetus as a "human being" may not be crucial as long as it is agreed that it is a "child." (These terms are not clarified precisely, but by *human being* I take Hauerwas to mean a member of the human community with full status and by *child* to mean human offspring.)

> Thus the preliminary question must be inverted: "What kind of people should we be to welcome children into the world?" Note that the question is *not* "Is the fetus a human being with a right to life?" but "How should a Christian regard and care for the fetus as a child?"[21]

I concur with Hauerwas that our evaluations of the morality of abortion, and particularly a commitment to its avoidance, cannot be understood apart from communal values and commitments. My discussion, too, concerns essentially the kinds of community (the kinds of values, attitudes, and virtues that community encourages) that will support or not support nascent life in difficult circumstances. However, I am not convinced of the wisdom or even the possibility of setting aside the question of the status of the unborn offspring, because the presupposition that we *should* support it (even as a sign of hope in the future) seems to involve a certain understanding of its value. Our protectiveness and hope do not include in the same way other forms of sentient and nonsentient life. The point is well taken, however, that the virtue of hope embodied in inauspicious situations enables the perception of at least a *prima facie* obligation to sustain fetal life, even if that life is not clearly of equal value to postnatal human life. Indeed, this takes us far from the position that it must be demonstrated beyond a reasonable doubt that the fetus is a "person" in the full sense of the word as a precondition for according it protection. If relatedness to and concern for others and for the sort of community in which we all associate is more important to us than "defending our own territory" (by defining the precise limits of our minimal obligations not to prevent other equal beings

[19]Ibid., p. 191.
[20]Ibid., pp. 198–199.
[21]Ibid., p. 198.

from promoting their own self-interested welfare), then it becomes less important to show whether or not the fetus is a human with exactly the same right to consideration as our own. If we are able to foster a sense of duty to others and to our common society, a duty that precedes and grounds our own rights as individuals, then it also becomes possible to envision a moral obligation to support the cohesion in the human community of even its weakest members, those with the least forceful claim to consideration, whether they be the unborn, the sick, the poor, or the socially powerless.[22]

## CONCLUSIONS

The precise value and rights of human fetal life remain questions awaiting resolution, perhaps indefinitely. However, without at least a provisional answer, the abortion discussion cannot proceed coherently, for the participants will not avoid hidden presuppositions about the consideration due the fetus as such. My own conviction that the fetus deserves considerable respect from conception may not represent a common denominator in the abortion debate. Nevertheless, I believe that there is now more of a consensus in our culture than is usually recognized that a policy on abortion attributing to the fetus no value that can ever outweigh its mother's choice to terminate pregnancy is not consonant with its membership in the human community, disputed though the exact nature of that membership may be. Failing agreement on the precise status of the fetus, we may hope still for concurrence in a generally protective attitude toward the fetus, a bias in its favor, and an expectation that those seeking to kill it will be able to claim reasonably that its continued existence imposes on others unjust and intolerable burdens. For such an attitude to be genuinely life-enhancing, rather than simply restrictive and destructive of the lives of pregnant women and their families, will require a move beyond the liberal ethos. It will require nourishment by a renewed and even redirected sense of community, one in which not only the fetus is protected, but also all who suffer disadvantage at the hands of fellow humans, nature, or chance. "Human 'flourishing'"

---

[22]In an essay entitled "The Christian, Society, and the Weak: A Meditation on the Care of the Retarded," *Vision and Virtue* [Notre Dame, Ind.: Fides, 1974] pp. 187–194, Hauerwas argued that the Christian's task of caring for the weak exemplifies the obligation to live the love revealed in the Cross, rather than either to try to eradicate all suffering or to attribute the existence of suffering to God's hidden purposes.

is a phrase invented by G. E. M. Anscombe to describe what grounds, defines, and constitutes the virtues that human beings ought to cultivate.[23] A community in which the "right to abort" could be overshadowed by rather than entailed in the "duty to encourage human well-being" would be one in which human interdependence in the spheres not only of personal freedoms and civil liberties, but also of physical prosperity and amelioration of suffering, corporal and spiritual, is recognized as the very condition of human flourishing, and so as bounty, not burden.

[23]G. E. M. Anscombe, "Modern Moral Philosophy," *Philosophy* 33 (January 1958), p. 18.

# Commentary to Chapter 10

VIRGINIA ABERNETHY

## A Personal Statement

Lisa Cahill begins with her views on the value of the fetus. Although she does not say so explicitly, the reader is to understand that these value judgments are supported by the subsequent philosophical and theological discussion. My discussion addresses Cahill's initial propositions, and then the main body of her paper.

To begin, two early statements that have a potentially *factual* status can be distinguished from all others that are, by their nature, beliefs or attitudes. Cahill writes first, "I am convinced that the fetus is from conception a member of the human species (having an identifiable human genotype, and being of human parentage)." In my own paper, the human fetus is also identified as an instance of human life as opposed (for example) to dog life or cat life; I propose that there are no scientific or other rational grounds on which one could challenge the logic or the accuracy of this one idea.

Cahill continues with a second proposition, in which fact is again determinable in principle: "I believe that there exists . . . a relatively broad consensus that the fetus does have some value and status in the human community." This statement is verifiable, in theory, if one first specifies what proportion of what political or geographic entity would have to agree in order to satisfy the standard of a "relatively broad consensus." However, given that the decisive data are unavailable, I am constrained to state my contrary opinion: I think that this second statement is factually dubious, especially when the term *fetus* is loosely applied to include the undifferentiated blastocyte, as is clearly Cahill's intention.

Thereafter, her position develops beyond the reach of empiricism and into assertions of belief: "I see the fetus as having a value

VIRGINIA ABERNETHY ● Department of Psychiatry and Director of Program on Human Behavior, Vanderbilt Medical School, Nashville, Tennessee 37203.

at conception that is quite significant and that quickly increases."
This belief becomes the premise for decisions in which fetal rights
(are there fetal duties?) lie in the balance with correlative maternal
rights and duties. It is a value statement that deserves close scrutiny
because, as with other beliefs, it seems likely to subsume points with
which reasonable persons might reasonably disagree.

There is, first, the questionable notion that the conceptus has
any value at all, or (if it has some value) that the value is "quite
significant." Reasonable people might also disagree with Cahill's "developmental" idea that the fetus gains value continuously. Why not
a discontinuous model, in which there is a time before which the
fetus has no value, and after which it has a qualitatively different
status, *some* value? There are traditions in which this discontinuity is
expressed around the event of quickening. Again, reasonable people
differ widely on how much value a fetus has even after negotiating
the threshhold of acquiring *some* value.

These reservations are disarmed by Cahill's personalization of
each statement. She does not claim universality, but rather the contrary. Thus, this part of the analysis finds its purpose in a second
issue: illumination of the qualitative contrasts among the premises.
Cahill's first two statements are potentially verifiable, and of these,
the first is probably factual. This approach relaxes our critical posture
so that we are not prepared for, nor is there a stylistic marker to
alert us to, the shift from an empirical to a value orientation. We are
smoothly led from what is clearly fact to what is possibly factual to
what can be revealed, with equal clarity, as belief.


## PHILOSOPHY

From personal statement, Cahill turns to the central thesis of
her paper, a challenge to the philosophical tradition of moral and
political liberalism that is "rooted in the social contract theories of
John Locke, Thomas Hobbes, and Jean Jacques Rousseau." She views
this tradition as the wellspring of the prochoice position on abortion
because it entails the use of "rights" language and "encourages moral
individualism and isolation of the moral agents from the social relationships in which decision making occurs." Cahill offers a contrary
premise: "That is, persons are by definition interrelated in a social
whole whose fabric of reciprocal rights and duties constitutes the
very condition of their individual and communal fulfillment."

I could use the present platform to defend social contract theory.
It would be appealing to strip away the pejorative connotations placed
on "moral individualism" by noting that the reciprocal and comple-

mentary play of rights and duties creates interdependence, mutuality, and a lively sense of community. These qualities do not need to be posited as preexisting elements of the human condition; they are continuously and dynamically re-created in human relationships. Moreover, the centrality of accountability, or the capacity for moral agency, as the distinguishing feature of personhood[1] challenges the view that self-centered hedonism is exalted by moral individualism. On the contrary, moral individualism demands maturity, self-discipline, responsibility to fellow persons, and the capacity to postpone gratification.

But no. I will not defend social contract theory because a poor anthropologist is not needed at these battlements; they are better manned by philosophers. I prefer a more playful enterprise.

## SOCIOBIOLOGY

I proposed to accept Cahill's premise that "persons are by definition interrelated in the social whole," assuming that her phrase, "by definition," is congruent with a notion of some inherent characteristic entailed by species membership. I think Cahill would also agree that the phrase "interrelated in the social whole" has its biological counterpart in the proposition that the totality of humanness includes a long evolutionary history of group living. That is, through a necessity imposed by our genetic inheritance, we do not live individually, but socially.[2]

The biogram that encodes our sociality seems likely to contain associated behavioral predispositions (or call them *traits*) that have evolved as adaptations to group living. A successful adaptation is, by definition, one that increases survivorship for those who exhibit that trait. Through the mechanism of the differential survivorship of those who bear the gene(s) that control a trait, there is selection over time for the gene(s) and the corresponding expression of the gene in behavior.[3]

Relatives are most likely to have genes in common, and the closer the relationship, the greater the proportion probably shared.

[1]H. T. Engelhardt, Jr., "Viability and the Use of the Fetus," W. B. Bondeson, H. T. Engelhardt, Jr., S. F. Spicker, and Daniel Winship, eds., *Abortions and the Status of the Fetus,* (Dordrecht, Holland: Riedel, 1984).
[2]L. R. Churchill and J. J. Simon, "Abortion and the Rhetoric of Individual Rights," *The Hastings Center Report* 12, no. 1 (1982), pp. 9–12.
[3]S. B. Hrdy, *The Woman Who Never Evolved* (Cambridge: Harvard University Press, 1981).

Genes spread through communities when the behavior that they control increases the probability of individual survivorship, with the constraint that the trait must not have an effect so antisocial as to destroy the community of which the individual is a part.[4,5]

Within this theoretical framework, I shall show that abortion as an optional response to pregnancy is most probably part of the human biogram. That is, abortion is a choice inherent in human nature. The mechanisms of evolutionary selection that I will discuss pertain first to the community, and second to the individual.

## COMMUNITY AS A UNIT OF SELECTION

A trait that (on the face of it) enhances the probability that a gene will spread, but that may ultimately destroy the community and thus all individual bearers of the gene, is the tendency to reproduce up to one's biological maximum. Human and many nonhuman communities that experiment with this reproductive strategy are decimated when their numbers outrun the environment's carrying capacity, which is a way of saying that, in the long run, there is selection *against* unrestrained fertility. Conversely, there is selection *for* reproductive restraint in the context of resource scarcity. It is both logical and empirically demonstrable that a community growing beyond the carrying capacity of its total environment is eventually ravaged by famine and disease.[6]

Through the action of natural selection processes, individuals in *surviving* communities are likely to have, as part of their genetically coded behavioral repertoire, a sensitivity to the environmental cues that signal the state of the resource base. Evidence of the existence of such sensitivity can often be observed in the various behaviors that reduce population when resources are scarce. In seed-eating birds, for example, a sparse seed crop correlates with laying claim to larger territories, so that fewer birds than usual can obtain a territory and fewer, consequently, mate. Similarly, there are numerous examples of human societies where unusual, even grotesque, patterns of behavior are most economically explained by their population-limiting function. In primitive societies, cultural patterns often include some combination of infanticide, widow murder or suicide,

[4]Stephen Jay Gould, "Darwinism and the Expansion of Evolutional Theory," *Science* 216 (April 1982), pp. 380–387.
[5]Edward O. Wilson, "Group Selection and Altruism," in *Sociobiology—The New Synthesis* (Cambridge: Harvard University Press, 1975).
[6]Virginia Abernethy, *Population Pressure and Cultural Adjustment* (New York: Human Sciences Press, 1979).

abortion, coitus interruptus, penile subincision, postpartum sex taboos, delayed marriage or sexual intercourse, celibate lifestyles, ritual abstinence, and a belief in the finite quantity and interchangeability of a man's blood and semen, which also appears to encourage abstinence.[7]

These assorted behaviors are easily understood when the community is taken as the unit of evolutionary selection. The only alternatives in a closed social system are to restrict population density to some critical level consistent with the long-term carrying capacity of the environment, or to suffer (near) extinction of the breeding community because the ecosystem on which it depends will ultimately be severely damaged.

## INDIVIDUALS AS THE UNITS OF SELECTION

Under certain circumstances, an individual can also increase his or her genetic success through the fertility-limiting behaviors listed above. This paradoxical idea, known as *inclusive fitness,* refers to the sharing of one's own genes with relatives. Inclusive fitness may be enhanced by restricting one's fertility if the fitness of those bearing genes in common is thereby increased by the mathematically appropriate multiple. For example, one may attain greater inclusive fitness by having two offspring rather than many if the ensuing better opportunities for the small family lead to greater reproductive success in the grandchildren's generation. A more mathematically explicit example is the increase in inclusive fitness from forgoing an extra child (who shares 50% of one's genes) when this altruism *more than doubles* the fitness of one's niece (who shares 25% of one's genes, on average): Consider that a loss of 50% and the doubling of 25% represent a balanced transaction from a genetic point of view.

I will not give extensive examples. But I do ask the reader to note the familiarity of the reproduction calculus: upper-class parents delay and restrict their childbearing in order to increase each child's opportunities; they then acquire a lively interest in becoming grandparents because each generation is expected to reproduce (although not so mightily as to plunge the family into poverty). In another scenario, an estate claimed by many children would be split into insignificant shares; here, the parents may urge one or more children into celibate lifestyles (for example, a religious vocation), so that their share of the estate and even their lifelong efforts can benefit their nieces or nephews (the parent's grandchildren). Among the

[7]Ibid.

poor, births are so devalued that three out of five pregnancies to black women ended in abortion during the early years of legal abortion in New York.[8]

I do not deny that numerous rational and conscious incentives and values may underlie these fertility-limiting patterns. But such explanations depend on postulating a multiplicity of factors. The power of the inclusive fitness concept is that it alone can account for an enormous number of patterned behaviors. It is an economical and elegant hypothesis; and it is strongly supported by an accumulating research base.

So far, I have described two mechanisms of natural selection that probably maintain facultative abortion within the human biogram. These mechanisms are selection through the *extinction* of whole communities that fail to exercise reproductive restraint, and selection through *inclusive fitness* for reproductive behavior that is maximally beneficial to an individual and her or his close kin. As a counter intuitive corollary of inclusive fitness, an individual can sometimes maximize genetic success through a strategy of reproductive restraint.

But why abortion? Consider alternate means for restricting fertility in human evolutionary history. Contraception hardly appears as a blip in recent time. Other than contraception, what?

*Infanticide* is widely used and has the obvious advantage of delaying a reproductive choice until very late, so that estimates about what resources will be available for child rearing are based on the most current data. On the other hand, the woman wastes high energy in maintaining a whole pregnancy, but perhaps the waste is not greater than that for the repeated pregnancies and abortions that might otherwise occur within a nine-month gestational period.

*Abstinence,* especially episodic rather than lifetime abstinence, is widespread; but a disadvantage stems from its conflict with the continuous human sex drive. This continuousness (and concealment of female estrus) was itself possibly selected because it promotes male investment in a given pregnancy as a function of the probability of being the genitor; this, in turn, increases the probability that a male will tolerate or even help to rear a female's offspring, thus improving the latter's chances of survival.[9]

*Widow murder* has a very limited distribution (traditional only in Brahmin Indian and some New Guinea societies, to my knowledge), and it probably depends on a very special concatenation of circumstances. For example, the victim's acquiescence certainly de-

[8]Ibid.
[9]Hrdy.

pends on an unusually strong religious or social rationalization, which would develop only when the threat to the community from over-population was extreme *and* when the coefficient of relationship within the community was high so that the widow's very close kin would benefit from her altruism. Moreover, to have a significant population effect, widow murder must occur when the woman is still young, so associated cultural patterns have to be either large age disparities between spouses or practices such as militarism and dangerous hunting that regularly kill off men at a young age.

In short, very little works well in primitive societies today—or could have worked well for our progenitors—except infanticide and abortion. Abortion requires rather more skill and sophistication, but it is the rare society that does not know and practice it.

## CONCLUSION

In conclusion, the very facts that the human adaptation is a group adaptation and that sociality is intrinsic to humanity predispose persons to choose abortion in certain exigencies. Protection of the community as well as benefit to kin sometimes demands individual reproductive restraint, and the means to this end are limited.

It follows that a philosophical perspective on the human community as factually and morally prior to the individual in no way precludes abortion as a moral choice. This conclusion challenges what I take to be Cahill's central assumption, namely, that a philosophical argument based on community is more likely than an individual orientation to support an antiabortion position.

## CHAPTER 11

# Value Choices in Abortion

### SIDNEY CALLAHAN

## AUTOBIOGRAPHICAL STATEMENT

*I come from an Alabama family, which migrated north to Washington, D.C., but never abandoned the curious mix of conservatism and populism often found in the rural South. My father and his brothers were U.S. Navy and Army officers, so moving around was standard operating procedure. Although we had to become adaptable and socially sophisticated to cope with changing people and places, there remained an inner narrowness of view. My parents had left behind the strict Baptist, Methodist, Presbyterian Calvinism of their forebears, but they were definitely superiorly Protestant and southern, prejudiced against Catholics, Jews, Italians, Irish, Slavs, blacks, and so on, and all Yankees.*

*The values I received were that it was important to be smart; to work hard; to be successful, honorable, and athletic; and to have great personal charm and style. Even more virtue and goodness was expected of all southern ladies, including, of course, modesty and chastity. My father, as a believer in science, medicine, and progress, made sure that I was instructed early about all the sexual facts, including contraception, but the ideal was also imparted that, as a good woman, I should not kiss anyone until I was engaged. I don't remember ever hearing abortion discussed, but then sex, like religion, death, and money, was reserved for rare, very private discussions.*

*In my subsequent rebellions against my background, I determined to be more intellectual, feminist, and religious than was acceptable. I went north to Bryn Mawr College on a scholarship, became a Quaker-like liberal in politics, and embraced Roman Catholicism. Marrying an Irish, Roman*

SIDNEY CALLAHAN • Department of Psychology, Mercy College, Dobbs Ferry, New York 10522.

*Catholic philosopher and having many babies in a row, while living in poverty, was a bracing vigorous personal statement. As a follower of Dorothy Day's Catholic Worker movement and as a Commonweal Catholic, I was dedicated to an intense intellectual life combined with intense familial and social commitment. Professionally, this all gradually took the form of writing and lecturing, followed by work toward a Ph.D. in psychology. Now I have a desirable mix of teaching, research, and writing, with all of my six children in and out of college and graduate school. I mainly look forward to more time to do research and write.*

*During all of this growth and change, I have always remained un-waveringly prolife in my views. One serious moral problem that I faced was whether contraception was morally acceptable. I finally decided that it was, wrote a book about it, and tried to influence others. But although I accept contraception, I cannot accept abortion, despite my intense sympathy for, empathy with, and understanding of women's present situation. I remain feminist, pacifist, and prolife. Unfortunately, I usually do not fit into any group, and I rarely find much social support—not even at home. With the times as they are, I am constantly challenged on my views by my spouse, my children, my friends, and my students.*

*But the fruit of a long struggle to go one's own way against the grain is stubbornness and self-sufficiency. I have always lived between worlds, constantly moving back and forth. I have to carve out my own territory in my own way and stand by it. And so I come back to my heritage. Robert E. Lee, a distant progenitor, was the hero and idol held up to us at home. These days, I often think of his wily, superb campaigns against superior forces. But we loved and admired him for more than his skills as a strategist: He was the quintessential man of honor and integrity, who followed his conscience but always did so with graciousness, tact, and magnanimity. It's really the only way to fight.*

Abortion is a public and private problem that does not fade away. Private moral decisions, public policy conflicts, and theological and philosophical debates over abortion keep attention focused on the question. Prolife and prochoice activists continue to struggle for their opposing points of view. Americans remain divided, and there seems little hope of a quick consensus or a rapid resolution of the abortion controversy. Why does this conflict remain so intractable?

Abortion persists as a troubling issue because it is closely linked to our personal world views and our central life commitments. Certainly, economic factors, education, and ethnic and class member-ships affect attitudes toward abortion, but no deterministic expla-nation invoking only sociological variables seems to account fully for individual attitudes and convictions. Even religious affiliation, which does seem to relate to a person's attitudes toward abortion,[1] may do so because religious memberships and allegiances often, if not invariably, express life commitments and personal views of the world.

Although many have asserted that abortion is invested with implicit symbolic meanings and value commitments, few have focused attention directly on these symbolic linkages. My goal in this paper is to try to understand the constellations of values and world views that undergird the different positions in the abortion debate. I seek an answer to a basic and troubling question: How can it be that so many wise and good people can know all the same facts, be familiar with all the same arguments, and yet reach different conclusions? What are the prior assumptions, ideologies, or value linkages that produce such different outcomes from the same evidence?

When considering which basic assumptions lead to opposing abortion positions, I think that critical issues are found in attitudes toward sexuality, meaning, suffering, and emotion. On these issues, different beliefs and values discriminate between a prolife and a prochoice position. I write from my experience as a participant-observer in these debates, and as an advocate of a prolife position. In a sense this paper, along with others in this collection, is trying to tap the personal knowledge informing those taking different sides in the abortion controversy.

## SEXUALITY, PROCREATION, AND THE HUMAN SPECIES

How one interprets and defines sexuality is critical to abortion discussions and debate. Answers to certain questions about sexuality may produce predispositions to either a prochoice or a prolife point of view. Is sexuality intrinsically procreative in nature, as well as being an expression of love, desire, and unity? Is sexuality a central, necessary dimension of human personality that must be fully and frequently expressed if one is to have a good life? The prior assumptions and constructions of sex and human nature involved in these questions implicitly inform much of the abortion debate's outcome.

Today, in American culture, a certain ideology of sexuality has triumphed, or almost triumphed, as the commonly received wisdom.[2]

---

[1]Donald Granberg, "The Abortion Activists," *Family Planning Perspectives* 13, no. 4 (July–August 1981), pp. 157–163.
[2]Paul Robinson, *The Modernization of Sex* (New York: Harper and Row, 1977).

Sexual identity and sexual functioning have been appraised as being at the core of human personality. Healthy sex equals a healthy human being. Sexual health is judged by the frequency and the adequacy of one's sexual functioning and by subjective individual feelings of satisfaction.[3] Although many experts, like Masters and Johnson, emphasize the "pleasure bond" as psychological in origin, and as best experienced in exclusive pair bondings, others have a more straightforward recreational view of sexuality.[4] In either model, a great deal of sexual experience and experimentation is necessary for the proper development of mature sexuality. The idea of suppression, sublimation, or the confinement of sexual expression to procreative contexts has become almost unthinkable. Given fallible human nature, interacting with imperfect contraception, unplanned pregnancies are all but inevitable, and so they are excused as the unfortunate side effects of sexual function and development. When the subjective expression of sexuality is given priority and is seen as a basic human need not to be denied, the procreative dimension of sexuality becomes less important, and more or less an additive option.

If procreation is seen as additive rather than intrinsic to sexuality, a different time focus is set up in regard to pregnancy and childbirth. In the additive model, conception is a discrete event that begins at a special point in time. Pregnancy is a state building up bit by bit, and birth is one more moment in time. Because each moment is additive and isolated in character, there seems to be a greater predisposition to take a prochoice position and to view the moments as discretionary and stoppable. As procreation is separated from sexual intercourse, so conception is separated from pregnancy, and pregnancy from birth. In the additive model, each additional step may be intended, consented to, or refused, day by day, in discrete acts of consent or nonintervention. Thus, to refuse to allow intervention at any discrete point is to impose "compulsory pregnancy" or forced childbirth.

Another view of sexuality that I and most prolife advocates share sees procreation as equal to the values of love, desire, and unity. The link between sex and procreation cannot and should not be broken. Sexual expression should be confined to those committed pair bondings that can serve procreation if need be. Persons taking

---

[3]Helen Singer Kaplan, *Disorders of Sexual Desire* (New York: Simon and Schuster, 1979).

[4]See William H. Masters and Virginia Johnson, *The Pleasure Bond* (Boston: Little Brown, 1979), versus Albert Ellis's discussion of "Love Slobbism" in "Sex and Love Problems in Women," in Albert Ellis and Russell Grieger, eds., *Handbook of Rational-Emotive Therapy* (New York: Springer, 1977), p. 155.

this view of sex differ on whether each sexual act must be open to procreative potential or whether the whole ongoing sexual relationship can be seen as procreative. Many, like myself, accept contraception and even voluntary sterilization as acceptable means to further the nurturing potential of a committed procreative pair.[5] And once procreative potential has gone with age, there is surely no problem, for in the synthesis proposed, sexual expression as an erotic manifestation of love and unity is equal in value to sexuality as procreative. Neither dimension can be denied or discarded or can displace the other in importance. Manufacturing test-tube babies without love is as unacceptable as recreational promiscuity without personal commitment.

Keeping a hold on both the erotic and the procreative dimensions does full justice to the reality of sexuality. Human sexuality fuses the biological and the psychological; we have evolved as one animal species among many, but we are more than biological organisms. If we retain an emphasis on procreation, we can grant the claims made by sociobiologists who see sexuality as existing for the service of selective reproduction and evolutionary processes. Erotic pleasure is viewed as nature's ingenious way of ensuring genetic selection. Courtship, love, and sexual preference are means of selecting the best genes for the next generation and ensuring reproductive success. The pleasure of sex ensures the bond between participants; it evolved to further successful human parenting. Whatever strategies further genetic fitness are incorporated in the gene pool.

But this is not the whole picture of human sexuality by any means. Human sexuality is also malleable and can become an intensely subjective personal experience for the participants. Individual subjective motivations for sexual activity have long been recognized as other than reproductive. Sexual activity has been motivated by erotic desires, as well as by almost every other known motivation. The desire to experience pleasure and the desire to express love have often coexisted or have been supplanted by desires to control, dominate, profit, placate, aggress, rebel, explore, and so on. Social learning and cultural conditioning influence subjective experiences of sexuality.[6]

A recognition of sexuality as procreative and a channeling of sexual functioning within committed relationships can be strengthened by cultural approval and teaching. I think human sexuality can be shaped, conditioned, sublimated, and suppressed because it is *not*

[5]Sidney Callahan, *Beyond Birth Control* (New York: Sheed and Ward, 1968).
[6]Ann Oakley, *Sex, Gender and Society* (New York: Harper and Row, 1972).

necessarily the core of psychological identity or the most vital ingredient of human personality. Healthy human beings can exist without frequent, satisfying sexual functioning. The prolife call for disciplined procreative sexual functioning rests on a view of human personality in which sexuality does not have to play an overriding, all-important role. A balanced view of sex as good, but not compulsory is difficult to express. Rebecca West, in an early feminist essay, succeeded when she said:

> Because sexual love is the most useful and common type of excitement we are apt to think it necessary to life, when the truth is that it is excitement itself that is life's essential.[7]

Excitement, love, and emotional fulfillment may be necessary for the good life, constant sexual expression is not. When human beings can have access to many other emotional joys and pleasures equal to sex, then it is possible to preserve the procreative dimension inherent in human sexuality by reserving sexual expression for procreative contexts of commitment and love.

If sexuality is seen as procreative, then conception, pregnancy, and birth are inevitably and tightly linked to sexual functioning. Acts of sexuality "naturally" serve reproductive ends and may have reproductive consequences. To totally separate sexual activity from reproduction becomes the exceptional case. Procreative purposes are validated by taking an objective, long-range view of the species as evolving over eons.

And a different time sense emerges in regard to any individual pregnancy. When procreation is intrinsic to sexuality, then the ongoing process of conception-pregnancy-birth is seen as whole. There is little comprehension of how one can look at pregnancy as discrete stage following on discrete stage, without considering the future outcome of the whole process. In my view the words *compulsory pregnancy* are as meaningless as the use of the term *compulsory aging* to describe being alive. Ongoing human life processes continue of their own accord, following dynamic, lawful sequences of development that are goal-directed. Intention and intervention may be appropriate in initiating or engaging in sexual activity, or even in efforts to control fertility. But once conception has taken place, a dynamic, goal-oriented, holistic process begins whose end is in its beginning. With this time focus, it is appropriate to see potential "babies" rather than embryos. Indeed, most abortions are chosen to avoid the coming "baby," not to avoid the dangers of a pregnancy. Potentiality and

---

[7]Rebecca West, "The Schoolmistress," *The New Republic* (January 22, 1916); (reprinted April 11, 1983).

developing processes through time are recognized implicitly by all. The difference is that abortion for some is late contraception, and for others, early infanticide. In the holistic time focus, the burden of proof rests on those who would intervene to pull apart a process that is intrinsically whole. Stopping a pregnancy is in the same category of act as stopping any dynamic, ongoing human life.

Emphasis on the procreative dimension of sexuality has a further corollary. It is possible to take the individual as the basis of a primary perspective, or one can look first to the group and the human species as a whole. The procreative perspective on sexuality keeps the focus on the ongoing collective life of the species. The individual is seen not as an isolated, subjectively motivated unit, occasionally coming together with other units to form social contracts. Rather, the group or the human species exists first and primarily, and individuals are separated from the collective whole in a secondary process of differentiation. Moreover, the differentiated unit can have value as a member of the collective human species apart from its developed qualities of intelligence, achievement, competency, or whatever. With this view of the primacy and the value of the collective human species, a prolife bias can emerge that views as superfluous discussions of whether the fetus is a person with rights. To be a member of the human family is enough of a criterion for value.

In a thoroughgoing collectivist view, the famous analogy used in abortion discussions, of the woman who wakes up and finds herself connected to the life support system of a violinist,[8] is most inapt. No one could ever wake up and find that such a new connection exists, because each human being is already connected to all others —genetically, ecologically, and socially. The fundamental unity and interdependence of humanity are weighted far more than individual differences, and many images express this unity: "solidarity," "family of man," "brotherhood of man," "one body," "members of one another," "humankind."

Emphasizing the collective unity of human beings correlates, I think, with a view of human beings as equal in worth. All who share membership share resources and claims to equally good treatment. Once a developing human life has been granted species membership, there is the assumption of its equality with its fellow members. Taking the larger, long-term view of the species as a whole, individuals as members in the species are of equal worth. This view undercuts claims arising from passing differences in age, sex, family relation-

---

[8]Judith Jarvis Thompson, "A Defense of Abortion," *Philosophy and Public Affairs* 1, no. 1 (1971), pp. 47–66.

ships, competency, power, health, or other qualities. In particular, worth is not assigned or granted in relationship to the claim of the individual family or its members, be they mother, father, grandparent, or siblings. Although the nuclear and the extended family are important in nurturing and socialization, that function does not necessarily give the family a claim to primary privileges or power over individuals, if one puts the human community's rights first.

Arguments over the role of the family are particularly instructive of the way in which various alignments can be made across prolife and prochoice positions in abortion debates. Prochoice positions often cite the welfare of the existing nuclear family as a legitimate justification for elective abortions. The welfare of mother, father, and siblings is seen as reason enough not to add another child, especially if a fetus is damaged in some way and may become a burden. Young, unmarried girls and women are thought to be justified in choosing abortions because their future family life may be handicapped, or because their own parents will be overburdened with the addition of a grandchild to the household. In fact, one could guess that more abortions are performed for the family's sake than for any other reason.

Prolife proponents have often been the advocates of more family involvement in abortion decisions. Such proposals seem to be based on the assumption that potential fathers, grandparents, and other family members will be in favor of sustaining a pregnancy or will be willing to rear a child. Although in some cases this assumption may be correct, it is doubtful how generally true it would be. Many women who choose abortion report that their pregnancies were not supported by boyfriends, spouses, or parents. In many cases, it is the family that exerts the most pressure for an abortion. Moreover, a particularly painful paradox arises when the family is invoked in prolife efforts to get pregnant women to consider the alternative of adoption rather than abortion.

In order to persuade a woman to continue a pregnancy, appeals are often made to "give your baby a chance to be born." Or in efforts to allow a girl's parents to become involved in the decision, the grandparent–grandchild relationship is invoked: "Shouldn't you have some say in your grandchild's fate?" If the father is being considered, the paternal relationship is stressed: "It is your baby, too." Such appeals emphasize the familial possessive relationship in order to induce feelings of duty and obligation to protect and nurture offspring. But ironically, this appeal to the possessive feeling of familial ownership and obligation can work against giving away one's child for adoption. The child will be illegitimate, and it will be stigmatized as rejected by its family. How can one know it will be reared well? The sorrow of seeing one's own flesh and blood, a family member, given away to outsiders and an unknown fate becomes too hard to face. If possessive familial ties are stressed, the thought of giving up one's own baby becomes one more pressure for aborting a child that one cannot rear. The decision tends to become an all-or-nothing decision, with all of the pressures working toward abortion.

An alternative prolife strategy that might encourage more completed pregnancies and adoption decisions would deemphasize the possessive familial relationship. Each developing fetus can be pictured as a unique, individual new life, sharing membership in the human species or the larger human family. A nonfamilial, nonpossessive appeal to continue a pregnancy can be made in order to give a new innocent life its chance to join the human family and to be reared by those ready and able to enjoy the privilege. A shift can be made from viewing this as *my* baby, which I shouldn't have and then give away, to giving this small, unique fellow human being its equal chance.

## CHANCE, PLANNING, AND MEANING

Attitudes toward chance occurrences may also be crucial in discriminating between a prolife and a prochoice weighting of facts and arguments in the abortion debate. An involuntary pregnancy is, by definition, something that occurs by chance, sometimes despite efforts at contraception. How one responds to a surprise pregnancy may be shaped by more general attitudes toward unplanned, involuntary happenings.

It may be that people respond to the unplanned, involuntary chance events of life on a continuum. At one end of the spectrum, there might be a totally fatalistic acceptance, and at the other, a total dedication to planning, personal control, and the rejection of unplanned chance occurrences.[9] In any case, an expectancy of being able to control reproduction and attitudes toward uncontrolled chance pregnancies may be related. If one can prevent conception, or if one can abort a fetus, then the attitude toward the pregnancy and the birth may change. Is there some subtle pressure to move from "one-can-do-it" assessments to "one-ought-to-do-it" judgments? Many people today worry over the imperialism of technological advances

---

[9]Lawrence S. Wrightsman and Kay Deaux, *Social Psychology in the 80s*, 3rd ed. (Monterey, Calif.: Brooks/Cole, 1981), pp. 392–401.

in many fields. Abortion can be seen as just one more instance of the technologically possible becoming first acceptable and then mandated.

But in the face of an unplanned chance event a basic question becomes inevitable. If an event, specifically a conception, is an unplanned or a chance event from the woman's perspective, is it a chance event from all perspectives? Is there an order in the universe in which nothing is unplanned or bereft of meaning? Answers to this perennial philosophical question have had great import. I think beliefs, or cognitive constructs, or images of the universe do make a difference in the expectancies brought to abortion decisions.[10] This influence seems to be mediated through presuppositions about order, purpose, meaning, and goodness. My own set of assumptions is shared by many in the prolife movement.

Perhaps the most relevant ultimate presupposition is the affirmation of existing benevolence and order in the universe. The idea is rejected that some evil creator deceives or tortures humankind, as in the despairing cry in Shakespeare's *King Lear:* "We are to the Gods as flies to wanton boys, they kill us for their sport." Nor are explanations invoking absurd coincidence or random chance events accepted as plausible. When the question arises as to why there is something rather than nothing, believers in benevolence and order affirm that a good universe has emerged out of ultimate goodness. This belief undergirds a basic affirmation of life; those making this affirmation not only "accept the universe" with Margaret Fuller, they gratefully celebrate all that is seen and unseen as basically good. The particulars may be dim and perhaps unknowable, and arguments rage over questions of processes or origins, but basic benevolence is assumed to be at the core of reality.

The prolife belief in benevolence and the response of gratitude contribute to the view that life is good. Life is a precious gift and is better, far better, than the absence of life. There is an ultimate bias in favor of life, fruitfulness, abundance, and procreation that influences where a person begins any discussion of issues such as abortion. Moreover, human life is considered the most special form of life we can know, and if this be "speciesism" from an animal liberationist point of view, so be it. Humankind, with its special powers, has special responsibilities for responsible stewardship of the earth. Thus, in any debate over bringing life into the world, a believer in ultimate goodness will probably cast the question as one of "Why not?" rather than "Why?"

[10]George A. Kelly, *The Psychology of Personal Constructs* (New York: Morton, 1955).

Another important cognitive construct is the affirmation of purpose and meaning in the universe. All of this amazing process is going somewhere; there is a meaning to the flow of events. Instead of meaningless absurdity or the despair of hopelessness, some story is being enacted that is going to have an outcome. There is meaning in life, and we can discover it. Viktor Frankl has been the psychologist most concerned with the importance of meaning.[11] Meaning is not simply some placebo that people invent to make themselves feel better, but a real discernment of the purposes of reality and the unique individual's course through life. We discover meaning, we do not make it up; in another way, meaning is revealed to us through unexpected opportunities to respond to unforeseen events. Human beings should be asking what life demands of them in way of response rather than constantly focusing on what they demand of life. Whatever the origin of chance events, the believer in meaning affirms that what occurs is ultimately meaningful. Therefore, there can be little justification for judging all involuntary things as negative occurrences. Individuals are expected to respond properly when events occur and not simply to exert control on behalf of personal agendas. No matter how hard one works to control and bring order into existence, surprises and untoward events, such as unplanned pregnancies, will occur, and they should be accepted as part of the challenge of life.

This affirmation of purpose, meaning, benevolence, and an emphasis on responding, which I share with other prolife advocates, could be described as a position of basic trust toward life.[12] Trust engenders hope in a future that will work; therefore, taking risks and accepting unplanned events is valued. A trust in larger purposes and meaning also implies a move toward two-dimensional values. What is here and now apparent may not represent ultimate reality. What you see is not what you get. In this perspective, the "real world" is dense with unseen transcendent values and meanings that may not accord with the accepted view of those determining the *status quo*. In fact, the powers-that-be may be least in tune with ultimate purposes, as they have invested so heavily in things as they are. In a real way, a basic trust in an order beyond what we see engenders distrust of "worldly wisdom" or "realpolitik."

When one accepts values other than those guiding the "realism" of the day, there arises an impetus to defend, champion, and succor those who will be ignored in most cost–benefit calculations based

---

[11]Viktor Frankl, *Man's Search for Meaning* (New York: Simon and Schuster, 1963).
[12]Erik H. Erikson, *Childhood and Society*, 2nd ed. (New York: Norton, 1963).

on efficiency or productivity. The poor, the handicapped, the imprisoned, the sick and dying—all those who are without power are seen as having special claims. For many in the prolife movement, advocacy for the unborn is only an extension of a concern for the helpless, the hidden, the powerless ones of the earth. If the unseen is as real as the seen, and reality is not simply what humans decide to construe as real, the fact that one cannot see the embryo does not alter the conviction that empathy and concern should be extended. In psychological terms, one could say that we should be constantly exhorted *not* to let our attention be captured by the presently visible and to remember that things still exist when we are not looking at them.[13]

Furthermore, an emphasis on human equality despite appearances to the contrary results in discounting physical differences between developing fetal life and mature forms of adult life. So, too, the mutilated leper or the aged, ravaged, sick person differs from us but may be no less valued in the ultimate scheme of things. Different races, from time to time, have also been denied human equality, and women as a sex have been seen as less than fully human. Those who hold a different view of ultimate reality must fight the world's "realism."

The argument that the fetus is treated as women once were motivates the many feminists who are prolife; they work with groups such as Feminists for Life, or Pro-Lifers for Survival, an antinuclear, antiabortion group that carries the argument further. My own prolife convictions stem from a feminist, Quaker-influenced, pacifist tradition. From this feminist, prolife, pacifist viewpoint, all the arguments asserting the value of women's development in the face of male power and hostility to feminine equality can be made on behalf of the fetus. Immediate affirmative legal action is needed to protect women, the unborn, and all life on earth from violence.[14] Consciousness must be raised on behalf of all the powerless. Women, of all people, should not identify with the traditional male aggressor and extinguish fetal life, reasoning that it is insufficiently developed. After all, women were once though to be so undeveloped that their rights and their participation in the larger world were denied. Prolife feminists insist that pregnancy is not a disease that disqualifies women from participating in the male world. The nonpregnant male body is not the human norm. Faced with a choice between men and women, prolife feminists choose women, and faced with a conflict between women

---

[13]For Piaget, the development of intelligence depended on freeing oneself from the egocentric stance and the power of the immediate perception.

[14]Mary Meehan, "The Other Pro-Lifers," *Commonweal* (January 18, 1980), pp. 13–16.

and the fetus, the choice is made for the fetus, by analogous reasoning. In tragic conflicts and choices, one must give the benefit of the doubt to the more powerless and renounce solutions that do harm to human life. Thus, most feminist prolife advocates are, like myself, not only for the ERA, but also against capital punishment, against nuclear arms, against the draft, and for redistribution of income. Perhaps the most important feminist prolife demand is for family allowances, health care, day care, and the end of society's virtual abandonment of women and children, which increases pressures for abortion as the quick, less expensive solution. To be consistently prolife, we must challenge the status quo and all the expedient utilitarian values so embedded in a world indifferent to suffering.

## SUFFERING AND EMOTION

The question of suffering is, of course, the crux of the matter. In all prolife positions, the problem remains that one is also going to inflict suffering by supporting the claims of the fetus to be protected by a change in the law. As prochoice advocates correctly point out, women most often choose abortion in order to avoid suffering: their own, their family's and sometimes (in the case of birth defects) the potential child's. How can those who believe in a benevolent universe, or who claim to care for the powerless, how can they be willing to inflict so much suffering in the defense of fetal life? Those who believe that the fetus may suffer pain in the process of abortion, especially in late abortions using saline solutions, can answer that in a sheer calculus of suffering, fetal pain will outweigh the social and psychological suffering that drives women to choose abortion.[15] Others espouse the argument that psychological and social suffering, even the suffering of economic deprivation, is relative, in that it is a human construct. As a socially constructed reality, such suffering is capable of being adjusted and changed by social interventions. In this argument, sociopsychological pain is not equal to the definitive ending of a human life, which destroys both physiological life and potential psychological life. Besides, say some, women still suffer psychologically and physically when they do have readily available access to elective legal abortion.[16] Women decide in anguish and

---

[15]John T. Noonan, Jr., "The Experience of Pain by the Unborn," *The Human Life Review* 7, no. 4 (1981), pp. 7–19.

[16]Magna Denes, *In Necessity and Sorrow: Life and Death in an Abortion Hospital* (New York: Basic Books, 1976).

ambivalence; their health can be harmed from repeated abortions; and they suffer the loss of the potential child, which they may mourn.

But it is still the case that many, many women regularly choose abortion as the way of lesser suffering, so the problem of suffering cannot be bypassed. Dealing with the question of why there is suffering is central for all thinking beings, but especially so for believers in a benevolent reality. Approaches to suffering must be complex. Some suffering seems to be justly related to the free and evil choices made by individuals who receive immediate and commensurate punishment. Other suffering seems totally disproportionate to a person's wrong action or the moral lapse that precipitates it. Much more suffering is endured by completely innocent persons in absolutely unjust and unfair measure. On the other hand, the evil prosper or at least escape unscathed, living happily ever after. Our world as we know it is grotesque in the overwhelming suffering regularly visited on innocent people. One response to all this unbearable injustice has been to say that on some final judgment day, a just reckoning will be made. The good will be rewarded and comforted, every tear will be wiped away, and the evil will be denounced and punished.

In the interim, where our daily life takes place, the example of the great and good encourages us to liberate, heal, reconcile, and relieve the suffering of everyone, whenever possible. However, when suffering cannot be relieved, or when it is freely taken on for the sake of others, the suffering will not be meaningless for those who live in basic trust. The hope is that pain and suffering can be used in the ongoing transforming work of the world and individual lives. Even human suffering can be given meaning by being joined to some larger order of reality. Human beings are to relieve the suffering of others, to avoid suffering, but when *necessary,* to bear suffering patiently in the belief and hope that their suffering can have meaning.

But how to tell the difference between necessary and unnecessary suffering? When suffering is imposed from without and cannot be avoided, it is obviously necessary. However, suffering may also be necessary in order to avoid doing evil, or letting wrongs be done to others, especially to those who cannot protect themselves and are the least members of the human community. How are such altruistic decisions made or avoided?

Emotions have to be taken into account in determining how people make difficult decisions on matters in which there are strong opposing arguments. In all rational arguments and decisions, there are also emotional styles, configurations, and forces at work. Human emotions are now seen to be more than physiological arousal or the result of drive or deficit needs. The rise of sophisticated evolutionary theories descended from Darwin's initial investigations has convinced many investigators that qualitative, built-in species-specific emotions are found in every culture.[17] Primary human emotions, such as anger, joy, shame, fear, disgust, and sorrow (there are different versions of the exact list and the possible blends), are more powerful and far more complex and complicated than those of other species.

One reason that human beings differ in their emotions is that their ability to reason interacts with their feelings. Although certain feelings and emotions may be pretty much preprogrammed and universal in certain situations, other emotions depend on complex cognitive operations of appraisal and interpretation of events before the particular emotion is felt.[18] The cognitive operation may not be totally conscious or may not operate in full awareness, so some emotions may be decided at preconscious levels. Advertisers, seducers, preachers, politicians, and artists made use of this fact, long before psychologists ever researched the phenomenon.

Certainly, each side in the prolife–prochoice abortion debate, consciously or unconsciously, appeals to emotional responses to further its cause. Emotional responses that already exist are invoked; disapproved emotions are discouraged; and emotions that are presumed to be latent and undeveloped are encouraged. Such strategies cannot help but be effective if they do not provoke reactions and backfire. A whole range of emotions can be appealed to, from the personal and self-serving all the way to the most subtle altruistic and social emotions. Should such appeals be made?

On the whole, I think appeals to emotion are both inevitable and acceptable. If attitudes and behavior are shaped by complex cognitive and emotional interactions, then it makes sense to strive to capture emotional allegiance as well as rational agreement. Emotions can be viewed as warmly held beliefs, which also seem to produce action. Moving a cause or a concern from the cold, intellectual periphery of a person's belief system to the warm, emotional center is a form of conversion that produces activists for a cause.

But the vast majority of Americans are still ambivalent, pulled in two directions in their emotional reactions to the different appeals of the opposing abortion arguments. In one sense, the abortion debate revolves around which emotional reactions are more appropriate and should be culturally dominant.[19] Primary emotions are displayed

[17]Carroll E. Izard, *Human Emotions* (New York: Plenum Press, 1977).
[18]Richard S. Lazarus, "Thoughts on the Relations between Emotion and Cognition," *American Psychologist* 37, no. 9 (September 1982), pp. 1019–1024.
[19]Arlie Russell Hochschild, "Emotion Work, Feeling Rules, and Social Structure," *American Journal of Sociology* 85, no. 3 (1979), pp. 551–575.

and invoked on each side of the debate, but different emotions are evoked, encouraged, or suppressed by the two sides. What do these different emotional configurations look like to an observer?

The prochoice side encourages individual self-esteem and self-realization through a courageous assumption of responsibility for hard choices. Deep empathy and sympathy for the physical and psychological suffering of women is invoked. Desires to relieve suffering and to help women, children, and overburdened families are present. At the same time, ambition and the desire for success in work and careers through planning, education, and energetic striving are endorsed. Self-realization through work and sexual activity is admired, along with individualism, autonomy, and independence. There also appears to be a commitment to temperate emotions: A person should not be too emotional about life but should take a cautious, careful, prudent assessment of costs and benefits in every situation. The emotions to be avoided and repressed are guilt, romantic self-sacrifice, sentimental overidentification with a fetus, and a passive acceptance of events. Judgmental criticisms or indignant censure of others' abortions is discouraged. In general the emotions encouraged are those of the Enlightenment model of a rational, pragmatic human being.

The emotions encouraged in the prolife movement are quite different and could be described as romantic. Feelings of sacrificial love and gifts of self to others are called for. Empathy and nurturing feelings are focused on the fetus, which is fiercely identified with, either as a family member or as a powerless, helpless being in need of protection. Communal memberships and the giving and receiving of love are seen as the highest emotional fulfillments, and attractions to achievement and independent autonomy are secondary. Life is with people, and being a good person is the all-important goal. Creative receptivity to unplanned events is admired as a display of basic trust in the goodness of life and the universe. One has a duty to meet new personal demands with love and sacrificial work, even if they entail suffering, for relief of suffering is not the most important human goal. To suffer is preferable to doing harm or choosing evil because trust in the order of the universe delivers the individual from the lonely exercise of control and from a final autonomous responsibility for the future.

But trust in the universe is not matched with complete trust in human nature in the prolife configuration of emotions. Everyone must suppress and be on guard against selfishness, exploitation, and expediency at the expense of others. Standing up against pressure from the world's materialism or reductionist utilitarian ethic is seen as the proper use of autonomy. Expanding the heart and curbing the power drive are seen as difficult; therefore, society's laws and structures must be shaped to support right actions. Educating and disciplining the emotions are seen as necessary to character development, for emotional growth is possible. A woman, for instance, who may not want a child can change her emotional reactions through reflection, self-mastery, and the power of love. Self-mastery and self-control are valued more than mastery and achievement in the world of work. The desired goal is to feel more deeply for others than for oneself. Danger comes from selfish emotions, or from deadening the emotions so that one becomes callous or habituated to evil.

I contend that many choose or find themselves on one side or the other of the abortion debate because they are more attracted to or repelled by the different emotional configurations of one position or the other. Once attracted, they attend to and give more weight to certain arguments and facts than others. The arguments convince because they are rational, and because they connect with our other beliefs and our deepest emotions and aspirations. I take the prolife position because I judge it to be closer to the truth of reality, and also because it appeals to me emotionally as the more compelling embodiment of human life and feeling. I think human beings feel now—and can be educated to feel more deeply—the emotions I admire in the prolife position. Emotional change or progress is possible in our collective human history as well as in individual lives. Every great humanitarian social reform has involved a change in emotional response—empathy extended or indignation newly aroused. My commitment to the prolife position involves a commitment to the configuration of emotions that I believe does humanity more honor.

# Commentary to Chapter 11

DANIEL CALLAHAN

I find it difficult to respond to my wife, Sidney, in the formal manner of a paper destined to be published in a book. For one thing, it is considered a fallacy in lofty quarters to engage in *ad hominem* arguments. But of course marital disputes luxuriate in such arguments. For another, it is by no means easy to focus entirely on the written word, putting out of mind all the oral versions of the same ideas that we have wrestled with in private.

Yet the most difficult part of attempting a response is that I must put myself in an awkward position. Whether it is also a compromising position is best judged by others. The problem is that those prolife values of Sidney's that I want in part to reject are values that, lived out in one's house and daily company, are decent, warming, and constructive. Prudence, truth, and goodness, however, do not necessarily always follow parallel tracks. The values that may make some people admirable as individuals are not always those that can or ought to wholly govern our common life together in society.

My sense of awkwardness stems, then, from a profound ambivalence. I would not want to persuade Sidney to give up the constellation of values that have shaped her stand on abortion; they are neither base nor self-serving. Yet I also think that they represent a kind of moral reverie, one neither sufficiently true to the world or human nature nor internally coherent and consistent. If they are values that fail, as I think they must in some essential respects, they fail at a high level. They suffer not from a deficiency in ideals, but from an excess. One cannot readily, therefore, reject them in the name of some higher good. Instead, they must be rejected in the name of a lesser morality, but one perhaps better suited to the lesser beings that we as humans are.

---

DANIEL CALLAHAN ● Director, The Hastings Center, Hastings-on-Hudson, New York 10706.

There are three parts to Sidney's paper, and I will respond to each in turn. In the first part, a holistic sexuality is espoused, one that would fuse the unitive and procreative functions of sexuality in the individual with the individualistic and social functions in the species. That desire for wholeness, and specifically for a sexuality always understood within a "procreative context," expresses an admirable ideal. But is it a meaningful ideal? In the first place, it is evident biologically that sexuality is possible (and morally unexceptionable) in contexts that are not procreative, that is, during a woman's infertile time of month prior to menopause, and altogether after menopause. Whatever nature may have been up to with that bifurcation, it surely indicates a biological distinction between sexuality and procreation. The result is that sexual activity can have a procreative significance but is evidently not limited to it.

Sidney says that "to totally separate sexual activity from reproduction becomes an exceptional case." Exactly the opposite seems true: It is reproductive sexuality that is the exceptional case. Why, then, hold out as an ideal that which is simply not consistent with ordinary biology? One rationale might be that one will thereby encourage a higher or purer form of sexuality. But I see no reason to suppose that would be the case; one might expect, on the contrary, a lower, more functional view—women as "breeders." Another rationale might be that, lacking such a standard, there are no natural norms by which to judge, limit, or set sanctions on sexual activity. But why assume that conclusion? Biology does not necessarily provide a better guide to developing moral standards than reason and sober human reflection on experience. As a moral alternative, it is possible to invoke not a "procreative context" as the *only* possibility for a moral foundation, but what might be called a *commitment context.* By that, I mean a context in which a couple commits themselves to an enduring monogamous relationship. Procreation as a potential is possible within such a relationship, but the relationship itself would transcend that particular potential, encompassing a broader conception of the sexual relationships. Why could not that concept prove as morally helpful as a "procreative context"—and do much the same work that Sidney seems to look for in procreation as a standard?

I propose that solution because it seems the only way that a contradiction (or at least the appearance of one) can be avoided. On the one hand, Sidney objects to what she calls an "additive model" of sexuality, in which sexuality is understood as divisible into "discrete acts of consent or nonintervention." On the other hand, she also says that "many, like myself, accept contraception and even voluntary sterilization as acceptable means to further the nurturing potential of a committed procreative pair." But the *conceptual* possibility of contraception and sterilization suggests that the "additive model" is fully compatible with the biological reality. Moreover, I fail to see how that model can in general be rejected whereas contraception and sterilization—both decisive interventions—can in particular be accepted. As far as I can make out, the only "additive" possibility that is actually rejected is abortion. But perhaps the crucial phrase in the passage (and argument) is "nurturing potential." If so, I am still baffled. I see no reason why people cannot be nurturing even if they are not or cannot be procreative. It is a common occurrence.

I take it to be a mark of human progress that many, including myself, have come to reject the view that sexuality and procreation are " a process that is intrinsically whole." On the contrary, the process is divisible, and our common moral problem is to decide how to make the proper distinctions and divisions. If abortion is to be morally rejected, that can be done far more plausibly by rejecting *that* intervention into *that* part of the procreative process than by rejecting the principle of intervention altogether—something that, in any case, Sidney does not, in fact, do, and that most others cannot do either.

In the second part of her paper, Sidney notes that she shares a belief held by many in the prolife movement, an "affirmation of existing benevolence and order in the universe." The view expressed is that of a scarcely veiled religious perspective, one that affirms that even chance events, or harmful occurrences, can have meaning. I'm afraid I simply don't share those assumptions, however attractive they are in theory and however beneficial many of their consequences are in practice. I wish they were true, but I can't bring myself to believe that they are. Nor does Sidney offer an argument for that position. It is called a "belief"—and it sounds like one. A rejection of such a belief does not, however, entail that everything involuntary is necessarily negative. It would be literally crazy for any person to assume that anything and everything beyond human control, or in a state of disorder, is of necessity harmful or somehow an offense to human dignity and rationality. The issue is to decide what ought to be accepted and what should be rejected. Cancer, broken legs, and auto accidents are "unplanned events," but we work hard to avoid them, and we do not take a desire to avoid them as a failure of virtue. Since Sidney, as noted above, accepts contraception—thus sharply dissociating herself from many of the prolife activists whom Kristin Luker describes—it cannot be said that she wholly values "unplanned events."

I think Sidney serves her own cause better when she moves

from a high, truly abstract principle of trust in the universe to the lower but firmer realm of accepting unexpected fetuses and unplanned pregnancies. But the argument is very different here. We are not asked simply to have benevolent biases about chance and mischance in general, but more specifically to beware of self-interested acts of violence carried out by those with power, whether they be women with power over fetuses, men with power over women, or political leaders who have power over the fate of nations. It is reasons of that kind, rather than assumptions about the sweet disposition of reality, that are powerful arguments against abortion. Neither the hard-nosed "realism" (which I reject along with Sidney) nor the too-tender trust that Sidney would like us to embrace seems to me right. There is, I hope, a mean between those extremes.

Sidney's third section rests on a moral premise that is as attractive as it is problematical: "To suffer is preferable to doing harm or choosing evil." The emotional correlate of that proposition is warmth, empathy, giving, and trusting. The moral premise is attractive because, if it were lived out, ours would be a better world, and our communities, large and small, would be more civilized and humane. But it is problematical because, for many, to kill a fetus is not, morally speaking, to do great harm; and many would also argue that, say, an abortion to avert having a child born with a crippling genetic defect would be an act of good, not harm, to the fetus. To say that is not to embrace moral relativism. It is only to note that what one counts as an evil action is, in part, a function of a moral judgment. Statements about suffering of the kind that Sidney makes do not, therefore, take us very far. They seem to assume that sheer passivity must necessarily be the best response to suffering; that no evil can be done if one does nothing (about, for instance, a pregnancy). Yet, that is part of what the moral argument is all about, and Sidney's position begs the question. The emotions that she espouses create similar problems. As she seems to recognize, lavishing the same emotions on women with troubled and unwanted pregnancies, rather than on their fetuses, gives one a very different moral outcome. In its own way, the pro-choice position argues for a kind of loving passivity as well; that is, let women be their own judges, and stand aside from impeding their decisions.

The standards that Sidney would have us admire, although laudable enough, are essentially loose and indiscriminate. It is hard to see how anyone could live by them without eventually running into serious problems. If they were applied at every turn, contradictions would result. Yet if they are not always to be applied, and other principles or biases are more appropriate on occasion, then we need some criteria for making such distinctions.

The most significant problem that I see in Sidney's position is that it is far from sufficient to form the legitimate basis of a prolife legal or public policy stance. Her position, I take it, is that abortions should be banned, or at least severely curtailed in their availability. Yet the moral standards that seem implicit in Sidney's stance toward reality seem to be marked by aspiration and hope—what we should strive for in our personal lives rather than what, strictly taken, we are obliged to do as part of our life in society. At any rate, I find the distinction between an ideal and a duty highly unclear; and that ambiguity, in turn, leaves opaque the difference between what we may hope for in others and what we can legitimately demand of them. We might, in short, hope that others would believe that the universe is ultimately benevolent; that all events (including unwanted pregnancies) have a redeeming meaning; and that out of those convictions they would deny themselves abortions. But are we to make it a matter of law that people feel that way about the universe? If that can't be done, how could it be legitimate to force them to abstain from abortions, a position that requires certain convictions about the universe and its foundations?

As these remarks suggest, I do not think that the threefold set of values that Sidney presents are sufficient either as a personal moral foundation for opposition to abortion or as a basis for a public policy that would restrict the availability of abortion. Both the analytical style of my objections and their skeptical content suggest, to use Sidney's term, that the "emotional configurations" that attract me are different from those that grip her. Yet the values that she would advance exert a powerful attraction. It is far easier to imagine the creation of a morally healthy community with those values dominant than with those that I find more congenial. Moreover, I would hope that in my personal life I could display many of the virtues that are part of her cluster of values. They are surely more attractive virtues than most of those inherent in the prochoice position, one that is not notable for a transcending of the calculating self. Yet, in the end, I cannot take the extra steps of belief and hope required to bring me over to her side. I cannot soar but can only muddle through at a more pedestrian level. I am still available around the house to be worked on, however.

CHAPTER 12

# The Abortion Debate
## Is Progress Possible?

DANIEL CALLAHAN

## AUTOBIOGRAPHICAL STATEMENT

*Sociologically, I suppose, the combination of values that I hold on abortion is utterly predictable. My Roman Catholic background predisposes me toward a moral condemnation of abortion, and a good part of me is inclined in that direction. But I am also by background upper middle class, highly educated, and an inhabitant for most of my adult life of what might loosely be described as "liberal" circles. That combination, of course, inclines me toward a permissive view of abortion, and it would hardly surprise pollsters that I count myself among the "prochoice" supporters. The likelihood of that outcome is all the more enhanced by the fact that I am, at best, only a cultural—as distinguished from an active—practicing Catholic these days. Yet, even as a Catholic, I was influenced by that powerful movement in the American church during the 1950s and 1960s that sharply distinguished between the requirements of personal morality and those of public policy.*

*The late and distinguished theologian John Courtney Murray was one of my early teachers and heroes. His pioneering work on Catholicism and pluralism set the stage in my own thought for differentiating between the morality of abortion and what might constitute sensible policy on the subject. Father Murray died before the advent of the abortion dispute, and it is hard to guess how he would have come out on that issue. But he did provide me (and many others) with a rough map for making our moral way in a pluralistic society. In sum, my own intellectual and moral formation, in*

DANIEL CALLAHAN • Director, The Hastings Center, Hastings-on-Hudson, New York 10706.

*both religious and secular terms, was of a kind likely to produce a prochoice advocate.*

*I confess to that sense of social determinism with no great cheer. It would do my spirit much good if I could believe that my own thinking effortlessly rose above the determinations of class and time. To be sure, I see in myself only free will, pure reason, and* ex nihilo *originality. But I am ruefully able to appreciate that I may appear less so from the outside. The only interesting question, I think, is whether anyone might be able to predict whether and to what extent my views might be different 20 or 30 years from now (assuming my views could be distinguished from my senility). For anyone who would care to make such a prediction, here is the data with which to work.*

*I was born of Catholic parents and raised in Washington, D.C. My father was an executive in the early years of radio, and a few of my childhood years were spent in New Orleans and Boston. After World War II, my father started a business publishing newsletters in Washington, and I spent my high-school years at a Catholic military school in the city. My mother, a sophisticated woman who was once called by a newspaper in the 1920s "the most beautiful woman in Washington," was a somewhat stronger Catholic than my father, but for both of them, religious life and secular life existed comfortably together. I cannot recall ever hearing the subject of abortion discussed, and about the only thing my mother ever said came in my adult years, when she once remarked that she had known a number of women during her younger years (she was born in 1895) who had had illegal abortions. She was not shocked by the social reality of abortion.*

*I initially stumbled across the subject of abortion during the mid-1960s, when the abortion reform movement first came to significant public attention. At that time, I was an editor of the liberal Catholic magazine,* Commonweal, *and gingerly wrote a few editorials on the subject. By 1967, I had become interested enough to decide to write a book on it all. When I began the book, I was firmly in the prolife camp (though the term was not used then), but as my research and thinking proceeded, I gradually changed to a prochoice position: My principal reason for writing the book, however, was not to promote that particular point of view. Instead, I wanted to examine the question of how a subject like abortion ought to be morally understood and analyzed (a reflection of my philosophical training), and how our country could devise a wise public policy (a reflection of my long-standing interest in the relationship between law and morality).*

*I think it is important to note that my interest in abortion has always been principally an intellectual one. It is an issue that serves wrenchingly yet beautifully to touch on a wide range of moral considerations and their social implications. Though my wife and I have raised six children—not all of them "planned"—I cannot say that abortion ever arose as a debatable option in my own case. To this day, I find it hard to imagine any circumstances whatever that would impel me toward abortion—though I can imagine many reasons that might impel others, without condemnation from me. In that respect, then, I have always felt an emotional repugnance toward abortion that I do not feel is shared by some of my prochoice allies. My reason, not my feelings, has led me to my prochoice position. At least, I hope it has been my reason, and not just some confluence of social determinants that has deceived me into thinking that I am not deceiving myself.*

Abortion, I once thought with the confidence in rationality of a young philosopher, was a moral issue much like any other. Given enough careful thought and ethical sensitivity, it could find an adequate resolution. As a political issue, I believed, it was no less subject to a solution. If the opposing parties would pay due attention to the convictions of their opponents, giving a bit here and there, then a decent compromise could be worked out, in the great tradition of American brokerage politics.

I was wrong. Sophisticated moral arguments now exist on both sides, whether on the question of when life, or personhood, begins; or on the rights of women or fetuses; or on the beneficial (or harmful) effects of abortion. No one moral position, on any of those points, has triumphed. The U.S. Supreme Court decision in *Roe* v. *Wade,* which might have signaled an end to the political struggle, only exacerbated it. It served primarily to galvanize and generate a more organized opposition to abortion; and it led those favorable to the option of abortion to dig in their heels, to defend the notion of free choice all the more tenaciously. Far from the emergence of a satisfactory political and legal compromise, the past decade has seen an intensification of the battle. In great part, the reason is that abortion touches on many other fundamental matters. It carries a symbolic weight beyond abortion itself and encapsulates a wide range of competing general moral, political, and cultural perspectives.

With that discouraging recent history in mind, I want to pose the question of whether progress is possible in the abortion debate, and if so, what it might require. "Progress" can be understood in at least three senses. One sense would be that of a clear-cut victory for one side or another in the debate. For the prolife forces, I assume that progress would be defined as the outlawing of legal abortion, give or take a few nuances here and there. For the prochoice group, progress would be not only a continuation of *Roe* v. *Wade* as the law of the land, but also an extension of the economic availability of abortion to those not yet fully served.

Another sense of progress could be that of more finely tuned, carefully honed moral and political arguments. Although mutual hostility and orchestrated passion have been a mark of the public debate, a more muted struggle has been waged in legal, philosophical, theological, and social science writings. In the latter, though ideology and moral conviction have been present, the emphasis has been on precision of analysis, solid scholarship, and a careful weighing of opposed arguments and positions. Even better scholarly work could then be counted as another form of progress.

Still another sense of progress could be that of a different kind of public debate, one that somehow found a way of combining the self-restraint of the scholarly arguments with a different vision of what was required in the public and political arena. That is the sense of progress that I want to concentrate on here. Is it possible, at least as an ideal, to imagine a public debate on abortion marked by civility, by empathy for the values of those who hold different positions, and, most important, by a conviction that our society ought to understand abortion as a problem requiring a shared communal effort to work out a solution?

I am a bit embarrassed by the possible naiveté of even imagining such a possibility. There are at least three obvious obstacles. The first is that for those who represent the most intransigent prolife and prochoice views, too much seems to be at stake to risk the danger of defeat. They apparently believe that they cannot afford the luxury of empathy for their opponents, of civility toward those whom they judge dangerous, or of entertaining a solution that might require them to sacrifice any portion of their moral beliefs. The second obstacle is the nature of our political process. It rewards strong stands persistently pursued, legitimates a struggle among contending interest groups, and strongly resonates to the language of rights and entitlement (whether of fetuses or of women). If the political process as a whole is often praised for its capacity to achieve compromise, individuals who compromise are more commonly scorned than praised. A third obstacle is a widespread uneasiness with the idea of a common good or a public interest. Alexis de Tocqueville's notion of civic republicanism—of a free people using their individual liberty to seek their common human end and destiny—seems merely quaint in a society that appears to believe that only individuals, not the community as a whole, can find or judge truth and goodness. A society prone to say that the right and the good must be private, not public, discoveries is ill prepared to engage in common quests.

Nonetheless, despite those three obstacles, I want to persist in exploring the ideal that I suggested. A minimal reason for doing so is that the present debate is simply going nowhere. For the most part, much of the important scholarly work has had little impact at the political level. There, the most vocal activist groups have held sway, with little apparent interest in, or any more than partisan use of, serious probings. Self-examination and self-criticism have not been notable characteristics of those who carry the battle to courts and legislatures. At the same time, however, the available public-opinion polls suggest that the majority of Americans do not whole-heartedly identify with either of the polarized positions. They are, as Mary Anne Lamanna shows, preponderantly in favor of the pro-choice position but are troubled by those aspects of it that would support a choice in favor of abortion for any and all reasons. They would welcome a solution that would do away with the nastier aspects of the public argument and that could find a middle ground between the demands of both the prochoice and the prolife zealots.

There are other important reasons for seeking the ideal. The abortion debate has served as a general political pollutant, affecting, usually for the worse, the way in which a number of other health and welfare issues are approached. It has been a major ingredient in fostering single-issue politics and interest groups. It has set neighbor against neighbor, friend against friend, and family against family. The debate has done little, if any, good for our national self-understanding; even worse, it has brought out much that is mean-spirited, hostile, and destructive in our always uneasy life together.

Even the most spirited partisans might, if pressed, be willing to recognize that the divided state of public opinion—remarkably persistent for at least a decade now—makes it wholly improbable that either side can achieve the full-blown triumph it desires. Should the prolife side win a decisive legal victory—say, an overturning of *Roe* v. *Wade* or a constitutional amendment—widespread civil disobedience and a flouting of the law would be inevitable. Should the prochoice side hang onto its present power and succeed in its ideal of making abortion even more widely and readily available, it could count on continuing harassment, erratically available services, and a never-ending struggle to maintain its power. Any important victory that either side wins will be, to a significant extent, a victory achieved at a high price. It is possible to wish for some better future.

Now it should be clear enough, from the way that I pose the issue—as a quest for civil accord—that I am inclined toward a public policy far more favorable to a prochoice than to a prolife position. I will not rehearse in detail the various moral and legal arguments that have led me in that direction. Suffice it to say that I believe abortion can be justified morally in some circumstances and that an outlawing of abortion would not and could not command sufficient support to make it a viable public policy. When a moral issue is doubtful and ambiguous, considerable discretion ought to be left to the individual (not because in this particular case she is a woman, but only because she is a human being); and a public policy that would not command strong political support would not be good policy.

Yet there are a number of elements of the most common prochoice arguments that I find insensitive and sometimes offensive. Among them are (1) the view that moral issues labeled *private* are subject to no moral standards, and that one moral choice on abortion is as good as another; (2) that morally to oppose abortion is *ipso facto* to be antiwomen, or that only women can understand and pass judgment on abortion, or that women are the only significant moral actors; and (3) that to oppose a right to abortion is inevitably to serve the forces of regressive conservatism, injustice, and repression. I have been morally repelled by the reasons that I have heard some women give for having an abortion, reasons they would never employ, say, to kill a pet animal. I know too many feminists, including my wife, who are antiabortion to see any necessary or inevitable identity at all between the abortion issue and the more general rights of women. And the very existence of a group in our society (though not large in numbers yet) that is politically liberal and yet strongly antiabortion undercuts the fiction that such a combination of values is impossible.

The more strident prolife forces have ill served our national life, and our moral reflection, by their easy use of the words *murder, selfishness,* and *expediency,* and by their readiness to see prochoice advocates as incipient infanticides, killers of the elderly and the defective, and stokers of genocidal furnaces. But my own group, for better or worse the prochoice phalanx, has done almost as great a disservice by fostering religious bigotry (especially against Catholics), by labeling its opponents as hostile to women or the poor, and by making it appear that its position is the only one compatible with morality, freedom, and justice. The kindest thing that one can say about the more monomaniacal supporters of either the prolife or the prochoice position is that they deserve each other. The rest of us, I suspect, would like to find some other company.

Yet that is not always easy to do, particularly if one would hope also to have some political impact. A number of aspects of abortion as both a moral and a political issue make it resistant to compromise, middle-ground solutions. The most obvious moral feature is that a pregnant woman can either have or not have an abortion; there is no third option. Like pregnancy itself, there is no such thing as "just a little" abortion. Politically and legally, the options are almost as limited, and each has significant drawbacks. Abortion can be banned altogether, an action guaranteeing a high illegal abortion rate, with its attendant high morbidity and mortality. Or it can be made legal under some circumstances, but not under others. "Indications," medical or social, can be specified. Systems of that kind were tried in many countries in the 1960s and the early 1970s, and in some states prior to *Roe* v. *Wade*. That kind of a solution pleased very few, led to a hypocritical application of the "indications," and often broke down in practice.

Finally, abortion can be made wholly legal, requiring nothing more than the desire of a woman for an abortion and a physician prepared to carry it out. Although *Roe* v. *Wade* did establish restrictions after the twenty-fourth week of gestation, that is the present system in the United States. Its principal drawback is that it leads to a large number of abortions and a significant proportion of repeat abortions, undercuts to some extent a motivation to use effective means of contraception—and of course, enrages that not insignificant part of the citizenry that considers abortion the immoral taking of life. Moreover, if the government supports abortion services for the poor—which is imperative if it is to be equally available to all—then that same portion of people who believe abortion immoral will be forced to pay for something that they believe is fundamentally wrong. A move from a woman's right to be free from state interference in her choice (leaving it wholly a matter of personal liberty) to a right to an abortion at public expense (making it a matter of subsidized public policy) has the additional effect of a not-so-subtle moral legitimation of abortion on the part of the government. It puts abortion in the same category as the provision of free food, housing, and medical care, all morally approved basic goods.

Given these limitations on the available moral and legal choices, it is not difficult to see why a satisfactory resolution of the debate is elusive. Even if one is willing to compromise, the viable ways of doing so are exceedingly limited.

I stress the various traps that the available choices offer not only because it is important to keep them in mind in trying to find a decent solution, but also because they help to explain the mutual frustration, indignation, and anger that mark so much of the debate. We are forced into never-ending arguments with ourselves and others, as if subject to a chronic illness for which all of the various possible cures are as painful as the disease itself. I am tempted to say that those whose apparent stance is a serene embracing of simple prolife or prochoice are not afflicted with that kind of illness. They can appear impregnably sure of their own convictions and no less certain of the bad faith of their opponents. They cannot resist the *ad hominem* argument because, by their lights, only a bad or distorted moral character could possibly explain their opponents' actions and convictions.

Yet my own experience in talking off the record and in private to many who so conduct themselves publicly is that they have more doubts than they are willing to admit in the public arena. They know, if pushed to candor and self-revelation, that these issues are inherently hard, that doubts now and then assail them, and that the victory they seek will have at least some bad consequences. They have continually to convince themselves, as well as others, of the rightness of their cause, a noxious combination that invites overstatement, public rigidity, and a deadly fear of compromise. The response of putatively true, but secretly troubled, believers when faced with an objection or a criticism is not to ask, "Is that right?" or "Is there some truth in that?"—but to seek out their allies to ask, "What's our answer to that?" or "What's a good counterargument"? The purpose of fellow believers then becomes that of keeping one's spirits up, of supplying answers to objections that one can't discover oneself, and, most of all, of continually reinforcing a desperate hope that one is right. Anger—with oneself for harboring hidden doubts that cannot be allowed to come out, and with others of a different persuasion because their probings and counterconvictions trigger one's own doubts—is a hardly surprising corollary.

No less important in the abortion debate has been the effort, on all sides, to make abortion fit into some overall coherent scheme of values, one that can combine personal convictions and consistency with more generally held social values. Abortion poses a supreme test in trying to achieve that coherence. It stands at the juncture of a number of value systems, all of which continually joust with each other for dominance, but none of which by itself can do full justice to all the values that, with varying degrees of insistence and historical rootedness, clamor for attention and respect.

The values that sustain and give theoretical legitimacy to the prolife movement are numerous. They are respect for an individual's right to life, even if that right is uncertain or in doubt in borderline cases (or even if there is doubt about whether it is "life"); protection of the weak and powerless, at the least in order to preserve them from the harm that can be done by the more powerful, and at the most to provide them with an opportunity to develop their full potential; the legitimacy of writing moral convictions and principles into law, particularly when that seems necessary to protect the rights of others (as in the civil rights movement, which denied a "prochoice" option to southern segregationists); the value, not of fatalism, but of accepting accidents and mischance as a part of life, and a denial of violent solutions as a way out of such vicissitudes; an obligation on the part of the community, whether through mediating institutions or the state, to provide support for those whose troubles (for example, an unwanted pregnancy) might lead them to forced, destructive choices; and, finally, the conviction that moral values and ideals should be upheld even at the cost of individual difficulties and travail.

The values that I have identified as integral to the prolife position are a mixture of those ordinarily labeled *liberal* and *conservative*. As many of the papers in this volume indicate, the prolife movement cannot, in its essence, be reduced to a simple conservative nostalgia or backlash. In the formulations of some, it can just as well go in a recognizably liberal direction. What probably most distinguishes it in that rendering is its willingness to live with—and accept—externally imposed tragedy as a part of life. That has not been a traditional part of secular liberalism, which has always been far more inclined toward instrumental rationality than the version that has surfaced in the prolife movement. The liberal community itself, however, has engaged in some sharp criticism of the part of its tradition that has stressed "rationalization" (a rational, socially engineered solution to personal and political problems) and "emancipation" (freedom from the restraints of society and a rejection of moral traditions). Hence, not only can the prolife movement make a strong claim to upholding traditional liberal values, it can also (in some important formulations) lay claim to reflecting some recent developments internal to liberalism's self-definition.

The prochoice movement can lay an equally strong claim to an important piece of the American and Western tradition. By stressing freedom of choice, it gives centrality to the sovereignty of the individual conscience, especially in cases of moral doubt. It also recognizes a closely related principle: that those who must personally bear the burden of their moral choices ought to have the right to make those choices. By its emphasis on the unique burden of women in pregnancy and child rearing, it has fostered the enfranchisment of women in controlling their own destinies. In its polity, the prochoice movement is at one with that recently emergent tradition that would free procreational choices from the control of the state and, more generally, give the benefit of uncertainty in matters of conscience to the individual rather than the government. Its recognition of the injustice inherent in the known pattern of illegal abortion— that of *de facto* discrimination in favor of the affluent and the powerful—makes an important contribution to a more just society. Through its concern for choice and control in procreation, it has focused attention on parental responsibility, helping to remove childbearing from the realm of biological chance and sexual inevitability. By sundering a once necessary relationship between sexual activity and procreation, it helps provide an adaptation to a world that no longer needs, nor can afford, unlimited childbearing.

Just as the prolife movement can be said to have its conservative and liberal wings, the same is true of the prochoice movement. In its libertarian formulation, it is heavily weighted toward the maximization of individual choice and the privatization of moral judgment. The basic concern is not so much with the social and economic conditions under which choices are made, nor with the ethical criteria by which they ought to be made, but solely with preserving a right to make a choice. But that is not the only prochoice formulation. In a different rendering—what might be called liberal communitarianism—the prochoice movement recognizes that a socially forced choice in favor of abortion is not a fully free choice; that a lack of communal, economic, and social support often coerces an abortion that would not be necessary in a more just society; that private moral choices are subject to moral judgments and standards; and that what ought to be an inherently difficult, tragic choice can easily be trivialized and routinized—tacitly sanctioned and advanced by a society that promotes narcissism, prefers technological fixes to structural change, and is all too happy to see abortion put to the service of reducing welfare burdens.

If my attempt to characterize the prolife and the prochoice movements have any validity, then we are confronted with two different debates taking place at two levels. At one level, that which most meets the public eye (and is well illustrated by Kristin Luker's findings on prolife and prochoice activists), a fairly primitive, monochromatic struggle is taking place. There is a prolife movement dedicated to the preservation of the nuclear family, the centrality of childbearing in the life of women, a denial of choice in the name of an acceptance of life's burdens, and a religious rather than a secular view of life. As a mirror image of that movement, there is a prochoice ideology dedicated to female emancipation from the body and a repressive nuclear family, a subordination of childbearing to other personal goals, a celebration of rational control of self in place of the acceptance of fate, and a secular rather than a religious view of life.

At that level, the debate admits of no accommodation. It is a living out, in bold relief, of the struggle between modernity and

traditionalism that has been waged since at least the age of the Enlightenment. For both the prochoice modernizers and the prolife
traditionalists, abortion serves as a pefect symbol for such pervasive
issues as the roles and rights of the sexes, the family, the relationship
between law and morality, the nature and malleability of social reality,
and the place of reason and choice in human life. But by choosing
to cast the issues in those fundamental terms, and by making abortion
carry the weight of a Manichaean-like struggle between the good
(evil) past and the good (evil) present, each side has doomed itself
to an utter inability to talk with the other side, the certainty that
neither side can wholly triumph in the future, and the disheartening
prospect of never-ending, never-decided civil strife for everyone
else.

For all of those reasons, it is the debate at the other level that
bears attention, cultivation, and development. The collection of papers in this book, and the spirit of the meetings behind them, is a
manifestation and an explication of that discussion. Four features of
that discussion are worth noting. The first, already alluded to, is that
participants from each side combine both liberal and conservative,
modernizing and traditionalist, ingredients in their respective positions. Each side is uncomfortable with the more stark options and
tight combinations of values pursued at the extremes of the debate.
They have thus felt free—and indeed, in many ways, compelled—
to appropriate and adapt from both poles to fashion a different kind
of synthesis. Both, strikingly, borrow from the various civil-rights
struggles of the recent past. The prolife groups point out that a
fundamental aim of the civil rights efforts was to protect and give
voice to those without power—to give them an equal moral standing
in the community. For them, the task is to extend to the fetus the
rights won by women and racial minority groups. The prochoice
group, sensitive to the deprivations of women who are given no
options in their reproductive lives want to provide women with a
choice about something central to their lives. Yet, though they may
differ about the meaning of the various civil-rights struggles, those
battle serve as a common reference point for both. Most critically,
neither side finds the understanding and interpretation of the other
outlandish or implausible.

Second, both sides share a distrust of that form of libertarianism
that would wholly sunder the individual from the community, setting
up the private self as an isolated agent bound by no moral standards
other than those perceived or devised by the agent. In this, they not
only share some of the conservative and neoconservative critiques
of liberalism, but share as well a similar questioning that has become

part of the liberal tradition itself, whether from Marxist or other sources. They are, however, hardly less distrustful of that form of traditionalism that believes the past must be preserved in all of its purity. They want to be able to use the past selectively, preserving what remains valuable, rejecting what has been either harmful or wholly overtaken by time, and in general seeing the past as a resource requiring constant adjustment and adaptation for life in the present.

Third, they are uncomfortable with the labels *prolife* and *prochoice*. Those terms, they are well aware, were devised for polemical and political purposes, not for carefully nuanced distinctions. *Prolife* is misleading because it begs the question of what actually serves human life and welfare; *prochoice* is no less misleading because it begs the question of whether freedom of choice ought to be made an ultimate moral value, regardless of the nature of the choice to be exercised. Put another way, *prolife* begs the question of moral ends, and *prochoice* begs the question of moral means. The labels are also disliked because of a suggestion that one must be wholly one or the other. But the more complex reality is that many in the prolife group will not condemn out of hand all women who have abortions, whereas many in the prochoice group are repelled by the banal moral arguments used to justify many abortions. Neither group, in short, is happy when *prolife* or *prochoice* seems to require a *reductio ad absurdum,* or inflexible, insensitive moral rules, to be pursued regardless of consequence.

Fourth, both sides are concerned about the conditions that lead or drive women to abortions, and about the social, economic, and cultural contexts of abortion decisions. They reject, on the one hand, that rendering of the prolife position that construes all choices in favor of abortion as merely personal convenience or crass expediency; and, on the other, that version of the prochoice position that is interested only in the easy availability of abortion, regardless of cause or motivation. They are willing to pursue together an understanding of ways to limit a forced choice of abortion because of poverty or the oppression of women, or lack of social support for childbearing; and they are no less willing to pursue together those social reforms that would be more supportive of troubled pregnancies.

Why, then, sharing so much in their beliefs about how the abortion problem should be understood, and sharing some mutual criticisms of the assumptions and premises of those who fight at what I have called the first level, do they still differ? In part, they can differ because of the relative weight they give to various considerations; ever so faintly tilting one way or another can be decisive when the political and legal choices are so narrow. In my own case, I am what might be called a 51% prochoice advocate; that is, the intellectual margin I give to that position is very slight, I am voting no overwhelming mandate to the prochoice bloc, and a good part of my mind accepts many prolife arguments. But, for public, voting purposes, that 51% is decisive, as much as I wish that I could avoid such a stark choice in the first place. I am certain that I am not alone in this kind of a balance, whether in a prolife or a prochoice direction.

Yet there is one element of the debate, I suspect, that might account for my own 2% bias in favor of abortion, and the 2% bias of others against it. It comes down to what is perhaps one of the most profound and subtle value differences of all. That is the matter of one's general hopes and beliefs about the world, human nature, and reality. Put simply, for many of us who are prochoice, abortion is a necessary evil, one that must be tolerated and supported until such time as better sex education, more effective contraception, and a more just social order make possible fewer troubled pregnancies. And even then, there will still be some justifiable reasons for abortion; it will never disappear. For the prolife group, a ban on abortion is a necessary evil, one that must be advanced as a long-term step in devising a social order that is more supportive of women and childbearing and more dedicated to an eradication of violence as a solution to personal or social threats.

Both sides, then, are prepared to agree that abortion is undesirable, a crude solution to problems that would better be solved by other means. The crucial difference, however, is that those on the prochoice side believe that the world as it is must be acknowledged, and not just as it might or ought to be. Here and now, in our present social reality, there are women who need or desire abortions. Future solutions to the general problem of abortion, at some unspecified date, will do them no good. They have to live with the reality they encounter. They cannot be asked to bear personally the burden of helping to create a better future, which, even if possible, is not within their individual power to bring about. By contrast, the prolife group believes that a better future cannot be achieved unless we begin now to live the ideals that we want to achieve, unless we are prepared to make present sacrifices toward future goals, and unless aggression is denied, however high the individual cost of denying it. The acceptance of reality as it is implicitly legitimates the *status quo*, undercuts efforts to bring about social change, and sanctions violence as an acceptable method of coping with problems.

Differences of that kind run deeply, pitting fundamentally discrepant attitudes and predispositions against each other. The dichotomies are expressed in our ordinary language when "idealists" are contrasted with "realists," when the "hard-nosed" are pitted against the "starry-eyed," and when the "tough-minded" dispute with the "tender-minded" (to use William James's phrase). The prolife group, it sometimes seems, favors an equivalent of unilateral disarmament on abortion and is willing to bear the hazards of a stance that will put many women at risk of disaster. They are willing to make a moral bet that the violence inherent in abortion will, in the long run, be repudiated; the public, they think, will eventually respond to the principled witness of those who reject it. The prochoice group, for its part, is hesitant to indulge hopes of that kind. They are unwilling to ask women to give up a viable solution to their present problems in the name of a yet-to-be future, one that might never come. If the prochoice group can accuse its opponents of ingenuousness about the world and its possibilities, so also it can charge them with evading a straight look at the consequences in real life of their lofty principles. Unrealistically high, rigid principles can wreak havoc. If the prolife group can accuse its opponents of capitulation to the world, so also it can charge them with a failure to confront the consequences of the lack of a moral principle more rigorous and demanding than that of free choice, which makes no substantive demands at all.

Can progress be made in the abortion debate? That is the question with which I began, and which I must now answer. I believe that it can, but if and only if those on the opposing sides are willing to undertake the following steps in the future:

1. There must be a more extensive discussion among those who represent the middle range of the spectrum on abortion. Although they can have some profound differences, they are normally more sympathetic toward the positions of their opposites than those who argue at the extremes. That sympathy enables them to serve as helpful rather than as hostile critics.

2. Each side should argue against the best and strongest positions of the other side, and each should also help the other to formulate the best way of putting its case. A standard tactic in many abortion polemics is to seize on the worst manifestations of behavior and logic of the opposed position and then to treat those examples as representative of the whole. Yet the most gross offenses are committed by fringe representatives, for whom the more moderate adherents in the center bear no responsibility. At the same time, it is important that those who behave badly be resolutely disavowed. It is not sufficient to condemn them and yet kindly

to "understand" them on the grounds of their sincere convictions and strong feelings.

3. Each side should reject a quest for total victory. Some degree of compromise will be necessary, not only because neither side is likely ever to command sufficient public opinion to win, but also because a due respect for the beliefs of others (even if considered wrong) is a necessary part of life in a pluralistic society.

4. Instead of beginning with those points of conviction that are the most different, discussion would best begin with those points where there is the most agreement. It is all too easy for the public, primarily exposed to black-and-white differences through the media and legislative struggles, to fail to note those areas where some degree of consensus does exist. They need to be stressed and, where possible, made the point of departure. The hardest, most divisive issues should come last, not first.

5. Each side should recognize that at least some elements of the position of the other side represent long-standing American values. Neither side has a monopoly either on old tradition or on the most recent new values. A synthesis of the old and the new is needed for the future, one yet to be discovered. A prolife position does not necessarily entail a defense of the patriarchal family, a suppression of women, or a higher defense budget. Nor does a prochoice position on abortion necessarily entail an acceptance of infanticide, a socialist society, or a nihilistic morality. Many different combinations of values are possible and require further exploration. Nothing is more important for the quality of the debate than a rejection of the mutual stereotypes that the two sides have held about each other. The fact that they accurately reflect important regiments of the opposing sides ought not to be allowed to overshadow the larger truth that a more complex and subtle debate is emerging, one that has the possibility of breaking a now rigid and sterile mold.

I cannot pretend to promise that, if those guidelines were accepted, a solution to the problem of abortion could be found in the near future. It is a subject that has divided individuals and society for as long as there has been a human history. The profundity of the questions that it raises goes to the heart of personal morality and the nature of political society. There is no reason to expect easy answers, nor any reason to expect a smooth process in trying to achieve any answers. What can be hoped for, however, is a debate that illuminates the broader issues that it raises, one where the means and the spirit of the debate foster greater self- and societal understanding. I continue to believe that such understanding will incline our society toward a prochoice position, and I have yet to be persuaded to abandon that position. But I would be failing in my own moral duties and ideals if I did not continue to allow my prolife friends to continue working on me. If they will not dismiss me, I will not dismiss them. Or—even more strongly—even if they dismiss me, I will not dismiss them.

# Commentary to Chapter 12

SIDNEY CALLAHAN

I find much to praise in Daniel Callahan's paper. He gives a fair, perceptive analysis of the abortion debate, displaying subtle understanding of the values involved. I agree with many of his points, but I also, unfortunately, fundamentally disagree with much of what he has to say.

To start on a positive note of agreement, let me say how accurate I think the paper is in describing what is going on. I also think that the debate is being carried on at different levels with varying degrees of commitment. There *are* muted scholarly struggles going on at the same time that extremists battle fiercely to control the political process. But I am not so sure that it is right to dismiss the extremist on either side too quickly.

After all, as Daniel Callahan's paper puts it so well, taking either a prolife or a prochoice position is, in a sense, a choice of lesser evils, or a forced choice that is going to scant important values. One of the ways in which one may be influenced in a hard either/or dilemma is to look at the dreadful extremes that each side can exhibit and decide which set of extremists is less appalling or dangerous. With an inevitable shudder of repugnance, I still ought to be able to see my crazies as less horrible than yours. I think I can do that with the prolife movement, and I do not mind being labeled prolife.

Perhaps one thing can be said for the abortion debate (and here again I disagree with Daniel Callahan's paper, which claims that the abortion debate is a "general political pollutant"): It does force clarification of certain issues. Neighbor has been set against neighbor, and friend against friend, because real principles are at stake. I, for one, think some principles are important enough to justify single-issue politics. At times, it may be appropriate to make a stand on one issue. A position on nuclear disarmament may be a single political

SIDNEY CALLAHAN • Department of Psychology, Mercy College, Dobbs Ferry, New York 10522.

issue that is worthwhile, and peace issues also create a great deal of social conflict between people.

Perhaps the most important insight clarified in the abortion debate is the shocking lack of support available to American women in childbearing and child rearing. The strongest argument of the prochoice position is that because a woman must bear and rear a child alone, with no guaranteed support, she alone has the right to make the decision to continue a pregnancy. This bald statement of a truth points out that Americans do not really value children very much, as there are no family allowances, guaranteed day-care programs, free medical care, or the other social aids that other countries provide. What little help exists is too little, too late, and mostly reserved for the destitute. Churches, unions, neighborhood communities, the extended family, and the other "mediating institutions" can hardly be said to do much better by women and children. Single women raising children alone are the fastest growing poverty group in America.

Daniel Callahan makes a good case for the possibility of a prolife–prochoice consensus on the needs of women and children. Prochoice advocates wish women to have reproductive freedom, which means being able to say yes as well as no. But who can easily say yes to reproduction when economic forces are all against a decent life. Prolife groups want to support women and children in order to encourage completed pregnancies and births and to avoid abortion. Together, they may do something about changing the patterns and policies of employment, which make it so difficult for women (and men) to nurture and care for their children. Already, some changes in adoption practices are making this option more flexible and available. Concerted practical work on behalf of women and children is ready and waiting.

A more subtle issue that has not been much explored is how prolife and prochoice forces could work together to increase women's sense of self-esteem and strength. Some feminists have tried to identify feminism with a prochoice position, and some prolife forces are reactionary; but some consensus is possible. The key issue here is how sexuality relates to identity. Women need to respect their own sexuality and to stop measuring themselves by male models, or seeing feminine sexuality as valuable only in relationship to male demands. Some feminists have begun to explore what it means for women to heal the body–mind dualism rife in Western thought. Is a feminine body different from a male body, and if so, how? Taking female reproductive power and sex-specific concerns more into account may be one way to move society toward meeting women's needs. Feminists and prolife forces both agree that women have to be more powerful and responsible. They differ in that prochoice advocates see women growing stronger through free, responsible decisions to abort or not, and prolife advocates see women becoming more mature and responsible by accepting and fulfilling their reproductive potency. Surely, some common thinking about women and sex might result in a creative approach to the future sex education of young women.

In the meantime, the number of adolescent pregnancies increases, and more and more abortions are performed. As Daniel Callahan says so well, "Like pregnancy itself, there is no such thing as 'just a little' abortion." One can have an abortion or not. At this point, there is no alternative way out of the dilemma. We may hope that human inventiveness may develop an artificial placenta and/or a fail-safe contraception. Then basic decisions might be faced in a new context, but present arguments have to be based on present options—all less than satisfying.

Considering these options, I advocate the prolife demand that prenatal fetal life be considered as valuable as other human life and be protected under the law. In medical emergencies, some abortions may rightly be sanctioned in order to protect a woman from life-threatening pregnancies. But when elective abortions are performed to avoid the resulting child, it seems to me that we are solving a psychosocial problem with a medicalized solution and immorally using technology to destroy life. Any political solution that can protect innocent and powerless human life from arbitrary destruction would be better. And for me, an ideal solution should also include measures to follow through and support women and children in both childbearing and child rearing.

But if the ideal solution cannot be obtained now, I think compromise is in order. Daniel Callahan's paper too quickly dismisses the old, messy "indications" approach that applied in other countries and in some states prior to *Roe* v. *Wade.* If, as polls repeatedly show, most Americans take an in-between "indications" approach to the morality of abortion, why not explore the possibilities of a return to the middle of the road? If a return to some form of committee approval in hospitals or facilities can be envisioned, perhaps women and others besides male physicians should be in on the decision. It is ironic that, because of advances in bioethics, a physician cannot perform medical experiments on a fetus without the consent of his or her institution's ethical review board, but the same physician can privately kill the fetus at the mother's behest. In the prochoice position, a woman becomes judge and jury. Women now have over the fetus the same unlimited power that men used to have over "their" women and children. Some more equal redistribution of power seems only just. Indeed, it has always been a principle of justice that those who are involved in a conflict of interest do not decide their own case. Yes, a woman will bear the burden of the pregnancy and so does have the greatest interest in the decision, but this very interest can also prejudice her in the making of a fair decision. This is why the researchers desiring to do experimental research on human (and animal) subjects is not allowed to make the final decision on the ethics of the case. The common good of all necessarily involves a curtailment of individual liberty.

I also think that the prolife forces are correct in their assessment of how one does *not* get to the utopian society in which abortions are no longer needed or seen as necessary. Liberalizing abortion laws and making abortion a readily available, acceptable procedure can only strengthen the practice. The increase in the number of "trivial" and repeated abortions has given pause to some prochoice advocates. Abortion is now a quick, relatively easy, individual, private solution to a common problem. As more and more women elect abortion as the best solution, it becomes more difficult not to do so. Peer pressure makes any practice more prevalent once it is permitted. Psychologists and moralists know that behavior influences judgment, so that having had an abortion, one is more likely to justify her behavior than to judge it as wrong. Habituation to what was once seen as unacceptable is otherwise known as callousness.

At the same time, all the alternatives to abortion take effort, money, time, and commitment. To use contraception properly, or to carry through a pregnancy, or to raise a child is far more difficult than eliminating the fetus in the course of a morning. As far as society goes, it is far, far easier to give individual women permissive access to abortion than it is to collectively support child care, health care, or even preventive programs of sex education. Something in human nature is powerfully attracted to the easy way out. How tempting it is to suppress moral qualms rather than make efforts to change things. Easy abortion works against everything needed to promote sexual responsibility.

I also think abortion corrupts the parent–child bond by emphasizing the "wanted child" and the idea that parental obligations to children are intentional contracts. Following this line of thought, fathers will soon refuse claims to support children whom they did not want, or children who were unplanned. The idea that the parental contract can be reversed up until birth is insidious. Although abortion may not lead to euthanasia and other life-threatening practices aimed at fellow adults, I think it does lead to an acceptance of infanticide for those babies who do not meet parental criteria of acceptability. Infanticide has been so much a part of so many cultures (including our own) that the voices now being raised on its behalf are as disturbing as the forced abortions reported in Communist China.

The prolife stand and resistance to permissive abortion here and now reflect a shrewd appraisal of psychological truth. Present inertia about quick immoral solutions leads to a future that is even less attractive. How can one reverse a trend except by reversing the means by which the trend is maintained and strengthened? Similar problems, I should add, face the peace movement. How can one move toward disarmament and peace if nations increase armaments and do nothing either to reverse this trend or to seek alternatives? The more our economy is entrenched in arms manufacture and defense spending, the harder it is to reverse our society's direction. For many in the prolife movement, institutionalizing abortion can *never* lead to a better state of things. Why should it? If the social factors that produce "problem" pregnancies can be "cured" or "disposed of" by permissive abortion, why look for other solutions? Take away the irritant, and the body politic refuses to stir.

It takes a committed minority with a moral sense of outrage on behalf of others to change the world. As we have seen in the civil rights movement and the women's liberation movement, you don't get change by waiting for the whole country to support the claims of justice. I do not agree with Daniel Callahan when he says that a policy that does "not command strong political support would not be a good policy." Social policy and the law must lead, educate, and at times coerce in order to stand up for the powerless. Compromise and brokerage politics can help any cause, but not everything is open to negotiation. To me, the prolife movement seems more tough-minded and realistic than the prochoice group. The realism of the prolife movement lies in its understanding that the tendency of human nature is to take the easy way out and in its insight that change in law coerces both behavior and changes moral attitudes.

The prolife movement is also courageous in committing the offense of moral judgment. In relativistic, pluralistic, permissive America, it is damned hard to say something is a damnable practice. Perhaps right-wing fundamentalist groups collect followers because they are still willing to say that certain things are wrong and immoral. But the new fundamentalists seem to have forgotten the old message about hating the sin and loving the sinner. As wrong as I believe almost every abortion to be, I thoroughly and completely understand why women have them. My dearest friends and most beloved relations have had abortions, so I am never tempted to think that it is wickedness or evil character that sends women to the abortionists. Many are too desperate to think, or to reflect; others truly believe that abortions are like appendectomies; still others feel that abortion is the lesser of two evils and has to be. In my view, these women are the equivalents of men in the trenches or foxholes or strategic air commands, or the loving fathers and husbands employed in the napalm factories. They all inhabit a world full of pressures that drive them on, and for the most part they are doing what seems necessary to them. My idea of progress is to change the world so that it is easier for us all to do good and avoid evil. I respect many of those who disagree with me, especially Daniel Callahan, and in his case, my effort to persuade and to win my case begins at home.

# Index